INTERVENTIONAL CARDIOLOGY CLINICS

www.interventional.theclinics.com

Editor-in-Chief

MATTHEW J. PRICE

Complex Coronary Intervention

April 2016 • Volume 5 • Number 2

Editor

MICHAEL S. LEE

ELSEVIER

1600 John F. Kennedy Boulevard • Suite 1800 • Philadelphia, Pennsylvania, 19103-2899

http://www.theclinics.com

INTERVENTIONAL CARDIOLOGY CLINICS Volume 5, Number 2
April 2016 ISSN 2211-7458, ISBN-13: 978-0-323-41759-4

Editor: Lauren Boyle
Developmental Editor: Susan Showalter

Interventional Cardiology Clinics (ISSN 2211-7458) is published quarterly by Elsevier Inc., 360 Park Avenue South, New York, NY 10010-1710. Months of issue are January, April, July, and October. Subscription prices are USD 195 per year for US individuals, USD 436 for US institutions, USD 100 per year for US students, USD 195 per year for Canadian individuals, USD 520 for Canadian institutions, USD 150 per year for Canadian students, USD 295 per year for international individuals, USD 520 for international institutions, and USD 150 per year for international students. To receive student/resident rate, orders must be accompanied by name of affiliated institution, date of term, and the signature of program/residency coordinator on institution letterhead. Orders will be billed at individual rate until proof of status is received. Foreign air speed delivery is included in all Clinics subscription prices. All prices are subject to change without notice. POSTMASTER: Send address changes to Interventional Cardiology Clinics, Elsevier Health Sciences Division, Subscription Customer Service, 3251 Riverport Lane, Maryland Heights, MO 63043. Customer Service: Telephone: 1-800-654-2452 (U.S. and Canada); 1-314-447-8871 (outside U.S. and Canada). Fax: 1-314-447-8029. E-mail: journalscustomerservice-usa@elsevier.com (for print support); journalsonlinesupport-usa@elsevier.com (for online support).

Reprints. For copies of 100 or more of articles in this publication, please contact the Commercial Reprints Department, Elsevier Inc., 360 Park Avenue South, New York, NY 10010-1710. Tel.: 212-633-3874; Fax: 212-633-3820; E-mail: reprints@elsevier.com.

CONTRIBUTORS

EDITOR-IN-CHIEF

MATTHEW J. PRICE, MD
Assistant Professor, Scripps Translational
Science Institute; Director of the Cardiac
Catheterization Laboratory, Scripps Green
Hospital, La Jolla, California

EDITOR

MICHAEL S. LEE, MD, FACC, FSCAI
Interventional Cardiologist, Cardiology
Division; Associate Professor, Department of
Medicine, UCLA Medical Center, Los Angeles,
California

AUTHORS

KHALDOON ALASWAD, MD
Department of Cardiovascular Diseases,
Henry Ford Hospital, Detroit, Michigan

BASIL ALKHATIB, MD
Division of Cardiology, Winthrop University
Hospital, Mineola, New York

SUBHASH BANERJEE, MD
Department of Cardiovascular Diseases, VA
North Texas Healthcare System, University of
Texas Southwestern Medical Center at Dallas,
Dallas, Texas

GAURAV BANKA, MD
Cardiology Division, Department of Medicine,
UCLA Medical Center, Los Angeles, California

ANN N. BEHRENS, BS
Science and Research Department,
Cardiovascular Systems, Inc, St Paul,
Minnesota

MAROUANE BOUKHRIS, MD
Department of Clinical and Experimental
Medicine, University of Catania, Italy; Faculty
of Medicine of Tunis, University of Tunis El
Manar, Tunis, Tunisia

EMMANOUIL S. BRILAKIS, MD, PhD
Department of Cardiovascular Diseases, VA
North Texas Healthcare System, University of
Texas Southwestern Medical Center at Dallas,
Dallas, Texas

LESZEK BRYNIARSKI, MD
Department of Cardiology and
Hypertension, Jagiellonian University
Medical College, Krakow, Poland

DAVIDE CAPODANNO, MD, PhD
Dipartimento Cardio-Toraco-Vasculare,
Ferrarotto Hospital, University of Catania,
Catania, Italy

MAURO CARLINO, MD
Department of Cardiovascular Diseases,
San Raffaele Scientific Institute, Milan, Italy

JEFFREY W. CHAMBERS, MD
Metropolitan Heart and Vascular Institute,
The Heart Center, Mercy Hospital,
Minneapolis, Minnesota

ALAIDE CHIEFFO, MD
Department of Cardiology, San Raffaele
Scientific Institute, Milan, Italy

ALEXANDER C. FANAROFF, MD
Duke Clinical Research Institute, Durham,
North Carolina

PHILIPPE GÉNÉREUX, MD
Cardiovascular Research Foundation, New
York, New York; Department of Cardiology,
Hôpital du Sacré-Coeur de Montréal,
Université de Montréal, Montréal, Canada

ALFREDO R. GALASSI, MD
Department of Clinical and Experimental
Medicine, University of Catania, Catania,
Italy; University of Zurich, Zurich, Switzerland

JOANNA GHOBRIAL, MD
Cardiology Fellow, Division of Cardiovascular
Medicine, Department of Medicine, Beth
Israel Deaconess Medical Center, Harvard
Medical School, Boston, Massachusetts

DIMITRI KARMPALIOTIS, MD
Department of Cardiovascular Diseases, NYP
Columbia University, New York, New York

MICHAEL S. LEE, MD, FACC, FSCAI
Interventional Cardiologist, Cardiology
Division; Associate Professor, Department of
Medicine, UCLA Medical Center, Los Angeles,
California

WILLIAM L. LOMBARDI, MD
Department of Cardiovascular Diseases,
University of Washington, Seattle, Washington

GOPI MANTHRIPRAGADA, MD
Division of Cardiology, UCLA Health,
Los Angeles, California

BRAD J. MARTINSEN, PhD
Science and Research Department,
Cardiovascular Systems, Inc, St Paul,
Minnesota

PETER P. MONTELEONE, MD, MS
Division of Cardiology, Department of
Medicine, Massachusetts General Hospital,
Harvard Medical School, Boston,
Massachusetts

**SRIHARI S. NAIDU, MD, FACC, FAHA,
FSCAI**
Associate Professor of Medicine; Director,
Cardiac Catheterization Laboratory, Division
of Cardiology, Winthrop University Hospital,
Mineola, New York

MANISH A. PARIKH, MD
Director, Physician Education, Associate
Professor of Clinical Medicine, Center for

Interventional Vascular Therapy,
Columbia-Presbyterian Hospital, New York,
New York

DUANE S. PINTO, MD, MPH, FACC
Associate Professor, Division of
Cardiovascular Medicine, Department of
Medicine, Beth Israel Deaconess Medical
Center, Harvard Medical School, Boston,
Massachusetts

SUNIL V. RAO, MD
Duke Clinical Research Institute, Durham,
North Carolina

BJÖRN REDFORS, MD, PhD
Cardiovascular Research Foundation,
New York, New York; Department of
Cardiology, Sahlgrenska University Hospital,
Gothenburg, Sweden

NEIL RUPARELIA, DPhil, MRCP
Department of Interventional Cardiology,
San Raffaele Scientific Institute, Milan, Italy;
Imperial College, London, United Kingdom

JONATHAN SOVEROW, MD, MPH
Endovascular Fellow, Center for Interventional
Vascular Therapy, Columbia-Presbyterian
Hospital, New York, New York

MINH N. VO, MD
St Boniface Hospital Cardiac Science Program,
University of Manitoba, Winnipeg, Canada

LAURA WOLFE, DO
Division of Cardiology, Winthrop University
Hospital, Mineola, New York

XIAOYU YANG, MD
Cardiology Fellow, Division of Cardiovascular
Medicine, Department of Medicine, Beth
Israel Deaconess Medical Center, Harvard
Medical School, Boston, Massachusetts

ROBERT W. YEH, MD, MSc, MBA
Division of Cardiology, Smith Center for
Outcomes Research in Cardiology, Beth Israel
Deaconess Medical Center, Harvard Medical
School, Boston, Massachusetts

CONTENTS

Significant unprotected left main stem (ULMS) disease is in approximately 5% to 7% of patients undergoing coronary angiography. Historically, coronary artery bypass grafting has been the gold standard treatment of these patients. With recent advances in stent technology, adjunctive pharmacotherapy, and operator experience, percutaneous coronary intervention (PCI) is increasingly regarded as a viable alternative treatment option, especially in patients with favorable coronary anatomy (low and intermediate SYNTAX (Synergy Between Percutaneous Coronary Intervention with TAXUS and Cardiac Surgery) scores). This article aims to discuss the evidence supporting PCI for ULMS disease, current guidelines, and technical aspects.

Saphenous vein graft interventions compose a small but important subset of percutaneous coronary revascularization. Because of their unique biology, percutaneous angioplasty and stenting require tailored patient and lesion selection and modification of intervention technique to optimize outcomes. The use of embolic protection and appropriate adjunctive pharmacology can help minimize periprocedural complications, such as the no-reflow phenomenon. Recommendations for best practice in saphenous vein graft interventions continue to evolve with emerging research and therapy.

The presence of moderate and severe coronary artery calcification (CAC) is associated with higher rates of angiographic complications during percutaneous coronary intervention (PCI), as well as higher major adverse cardiac events compared with noncalcified lesions. Diabetes mellitus, a risk factor for CAC, is increasing in the United States. Vessel preparation before PCI with atherectomy can facilitate successful stent delivery and expansion that may otherwise not be possible. We review here CAC prevalence, risk factors, and impact on PCI, as well as the currently available coronary atherectomy devices including rotational atherectomy, orbital atherectomy, and laser atherectomy.

In-stent restenosis (ISR) is the narrowing of a stented coronary artery lesion. The mean time from percutaneous coronary intervention (PCI) to ISR was 12 months with drug-eluting stents (DES) and 6 months with bare metal stents (BMS). ISR typically presents as recurrent angina. The use of DES has significantly reduced the rate of ISR compared with BMS. Predictors of ISR include patient, lesion, and procedural characteristics. Intravascular ultrasound, optical coherence tomography, and fractional flow reserve are important tools for the anatomic and hemodynamic assessment of ISR. Treatment options for ISR include percutaneous coronary intervention with DES.

Platelets play a key role in mediating stent thrombosis, which is the major cause of ischemic events immediately after percutaneous coronary intervention (PCI). Antiplatelet therapy is therefore the cornerstone of antithrombotic therapy after PCI. However, the use of antiplatelet agents increases bleeding risk, with more potent antiplatelet agents further increasing bleeding risk. In the past 5 years, potent and fast-acting $^{P2Y}12$ inhibitors have augmented the antiplatelet armamentarium available to interventional cardiologists. This article reviews the preclinical and clinical data surrounding these new agents, and discusses the significant questions and controversies that still exist regarding the optimal antiplatelet strategy.

Numerous agents are available for anticoagulation during percutaneous coronary intervention (PCI). These agents have been evaluated in a variety of clinical settings, including elective, urgent, and emergent PCI. Although unfractionated heparin remains a frequent choice, accumulating data support the use of newer agents to mitigate bleeding risk, especially in the setting of femoral access and concomitant use of glycoprotein IIb/IIa receptor inhibition. With several antithrombotic agents available, an assessment must be made regarding the ischemic and bleeding risks. This article summarizes existing data examining the benefits and limitations of the various anticoagulants and guidelines for their use.

The Synergy Between Percutaneous Coronary Intervention with Taxus and Cardiac Surgery (SYNTAX) score is a semiquantitative angiographic score developed to prospectively characterize the disease complexity of the coronary vasculature. With more than 50 validation studies, the SYNTAX score is the most-studied risk model in the setting of percutaneous coronary intervention. In this article, the evolutionary journey of the SYNTAX score is reviewed, with emphasis on its sequential modifications and adaptations, now culminating in the development and validation of the SYNTAX score II.

This article focuses on specialized techniques and devices used in the most challenging cases of acute myocardial infarction. Areas where high-quality evidence is either clear or absent are avoided. Controversies in the use of support or thrombectomy devices, the addition of adjunct pharmacology, and the decision to treat nonculprit lesions are discussed. Recent years have seen a shift in guidelines to downgrading the use of assist devices in cardiogenic shock and aspiration thrombectomy, whereas consideration of nonculprit coronary intervention has been revived. These changes come in the wake of a series of large, practice-changing clinical trials.

COMPLEX CORONARY INTERVENTION

ISSUE OF RELATED INTEREST

Cardiology Clinics, November 2015 (Vol. 33, No. 4)
Adult Congenital Heart Disease
Karen K. Stout, *Editor*
Available at: http://www.cardiology.theclinics.com/

THE CLINICS ARE NOW AVAILABLE ONLINE!

Access your subscription at:
www.theclinics.com

PREFACE

The New Era of Interventional Cardiology: Tackling Complex Coronary Intervention

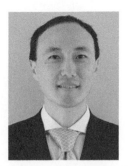

Michael S. Lee, MD, FACC, FSCAI
Editor

Since I first started my career in interventional cardiology in 2004 until now, I have seen the field dramatically change with the introduction of new technology, refinement in technique, and data from clinical trials demonstrating the safety and efficacy of percutaneous coronary intervention. In particular, drug-eluting stents have redefined how we treat patients with coronary disease. This revolutionary technology dramatically reduces the rate of restenosis and need for repeat revascularization, allowing for more effective revascularization.

Since then, improvements in pharmacotherapy, including antiplatelet and antithrombotic therapies, reduce the risk of ischemic events. Data continue to grow on the outcomes of complex coronary intervention, including unprotected left main disease, severe coronary artery calcification, and chronic total occlusion. Patients with severe left ventricular dysfunction can more safely be revascularized with hemodynamic support devices. The treatment of niche cases, including in-stent restenosis, saphenous vein graft intervention, bifurcation disease, and acute myocardial infarction, continues to be refined as data from randomized clinical trials continue to emerge. Risk stratification to identify which patients will benefit from percutaneous revascularization as compared with surgical revascularization can help the clinician provide the optimal treatment strategy for patients with left main and multivessel coronary artery disease.

In this issue of *Interventional Cardiology Clinics*, it is my pleasure and honor to provide a state-of-the-art update on the most relevant topics of complex coronary intervention written by a group of internationally recognized interventional cardiologists.

I am indebted to the authors, who dedicated time out of their busy practice to make this possible.

I thank my colleagues and the members of the Cardiac Catheterization Laboratory, who make it a joy to practice Interventional Cardiology at the UCLA Medical Center, one of the premier medical institutions in the United States, where we pursue unparalleled patient care, science, innovation, and education on a daily basis.

Michael S. Lee, MD, FACC, FSCAI
UCLA Medical Center
100 Medical Plaza, Suite 630
Los Angeles, CA 90095, USA
E-mail address:
mslee@mednet.ucla.edu

http://dx.doi.org/10.1016/j.iccl.2016.01.001
2211-7458/16/$ – see front matter © 2016 Published by Elsevier Inc.

Left Main Percutaneous Coronary Intervention

Neil Ruparelia, DPhil, MRCP[a,b], Alaide Chieffo, MD[a,*]

KEYWORDS

- Left main stem • Percutaneous coronary intervention • Coronary artery bypass grafting
- Drug-eluting stents • Guidelines • Heart team • Intravascular imaging

---

KEY POINTS

- Each patient presenting with significant unprotected left main stem disease should be thoroughly evaluated by the heart team on an individual basis before deciding on the optimal revascularization strategy: percutaneous coronary intervention or coronary artery bypass grafting.
- Percutaneous coronary intervention is a viable treatment option, particularly in patients with favorable coronary anatomy (low or intermediate SYNTAX (Synergy Between Percutaneous Coronary Intervention with TAXUS and Cardiac Surgery) scores).
- The stenting strategy should be determined by coronary anatomy.
- The use of adjunctive tools, including intravascular imaging and fractional flow reserve, is essential to confirming diagnosis and optimizing clinical outcomes.

INTRODUCTION

A finding of significant (>50%) disease in an unprotected left main stem (ULMS) is observed in approximately 5% to 7% of patients undergoing coronary angiography.[1] In view of the large distribution of myocardium that it supplies, ULMS disease is of prognostic importance. Medical treatment is associated with a 3-year mortality rate of 50%.[2,3] The disease may present in asymptomatic patients as stable angina, an acute coronary syndrome, in the presence of heart failure, or sudden cardiac death.

The diagnosis of ULMS disease using invasive coronary angiography can be surprisingly challenging; the role of adjunctive tools, including intravascular imaging and coronary physiology, play important roles. Treatment of ULMS is similarly nuanced. Coronary artery bypass grafting (CABG) has been regarded as the gold standard treatment of this group of patients with a significant mortality benefit in comparison with medical therapy alone.[4,5] With the introduction of drug-eluting stents (DES) (which are associated with lower rates of restenosis and target lesion revascularization [TLR] when compared with bare-metal stents[6–8]), in addition to improvements in operator experience and adjunctive pharmacotherapy, percutaneous coronary intervention (PCI) has been shown to be feasible, safe, and efficacious in this patient group.[9,10] This finding has resulted in a revision of the both the European Society of Cardiology (ESC)[11] and the American College of Cardiology (ACC)/American Heart Association (AHA)[12] guidelines on myocardial revascularization that now regard PCI as an alternative to CABG in patients without complex anatomy.

There are many factors that need to be taken account when considering ULMS PCI. During the course of this article, the authors review the evidence, current guidelines, and technical aspects of ULMS PCI.

CURRENT EVIDENCE

Data from several observational retrospective registries (Table 1) initially demonstrated that

---

Disclosures: The authors have no disclosures to declare.
[a] Department of Interventional Cardiology San Raffaele Scientific Institute, Via Olgettina 60, Milan 20132, Italy;
[b] Department of Cardiology Imperial College, Du Cane Road, London W12 0HS, UK
* Corresponding author. San Raffaele Scientific Institute, Via Olgettina, 60, Milan 20132, Italy.
E-mail address: alaide.chieffo@hsr.it

http://dx.doi.org/10.1016/j.iccl.2015.12.001
2211-7458/16/$ – see front matter

Table 1
Summary of retrospective studies

Study, Year	Patients (n)	Follow-up, (mo)	Cardiac Death (%)	MACE (%)
Palmerini et al,[13] 2006	311	12	NA	NA
Lee et al,[14] 2006	173	12	1.6 vs 2.0	25.0 vs 17.0
Sanmartin et al,[15] 2007	335	12	NA	11.4 vs 10.4
Chieffo et al,[16] 2010	249	60	11.9 vs 7.5	38.3 vs 32.4
Park et al,[17] 2010	2240	60	9.9	NA

Abbreviations: MACE, major adverse cardiovascular event; NA, not available.
Data from Refs.[13–17]

there were no differences between CABG and PCI for the treatment of ULMS disease with regard to major adverse cardiovascular events (MACEs).[9,13–19] Subsequently, several prospective randomized trials have been conducted (or are ongoing) to further explore the efficacy of PCI in this patient group (Table 2).

The landmark Synergy Between Percutaneous Coronary Intervention with TAXUS and Cardiac Surgery (SYNTAX) trial was the first major randomized trial comparing CABG versus PCI with DES.[10] The study included a prespecified subgroup of patients with ULMS (PCI n = 357; CABG n = 348). At 12 months, there was noninferiority in MACE (PCI 15.8% vs CABG 13.7%; $P = .44$), although the rate of repeat revascularization among those undergoing PCI was higher (PCI 11.8% vs CABG 6.5%; $P = .02$). Conversely, the rates of cerebrovascular events were higher in the CABG group (2.7% vs 0.3%; $P = .01$). At the 5-year follow-up, there continued to be no

significant difference in overall MACE rates (PCI 36.9% vs CABG 31.0%; $P = .12$).[23] However, subgroup analysis revealed that patients with low (0–22) and intermediate[24–33] SYNTAX scores had similar outcomes regardless of treatment strategy (30.4% vs 31.5%; $P = .74$; 32.7% vs 32.3%; $P = .88$, respectively). However, patients with high SYNTAX scores (>33) had lower MACE rates with CABG (29.7% vs 46.5%; $P = .003$).[34] The Premier of Randomized Comparison of Bypass Surgery versus Angioplasty Using Sirolimus-Eluting Stent in Patients with Left Main Coronary Artery Disease (PRECOMBAT), similarly published 5-year follow-up data of 600 patients randomized to PCI (n = 300) with sirolimus-eluting stents or CABG (n = 300). At 5 years, MACE was not statistically different with PCI and CABG (17.5% vs 14.3%; $P = .26$).[35] It is important to note that both of these studies used first-generation DES. Their use has now been superseded by second- and

Table 2
Summary of randomized controlled trials

Study, Year	Patients (n)	Age (y)	SYNTAX Score	Death (%)	MACE (%)
Buszman et al,[19] 2008	105 PCI: 52 CABG: 53	61	25	7.5 vs 1.9, $P = .37$	24.5 vs 28.8, $P = .29$
SYNTAX left main,[20] 2009	705 PCI: 357 CABG: 348	65	30	4.4 vs 4.2, $P = .88$	13.7 vs 15.8, $P = .44$
Boudriot et al,[21] 2010	201 PCI: 100 CABG: 101	68	24	5.0 vs 2.0, $P<.01$	13.9 vs 19.0, $P = .19$
PRECOMBAT,[22] 2011	600 PCI: 300 CABG: 300	62	25	2.7 vs 2.0, $P = .45$	6.7 vs 8.7, $P = .12$

Abbreviations: Le Mans, Study of Unprotected Left Main Stenting Versus Bypass Surgery; PRECOMBAT, Premier of Randomized Comparison of Bypass Surgery versus Angioplasty Using Sirolimus-Eluting Stent in Patients with Left Main Coronary Artery Disease; SYNTAX, Synergy between Percutaneous Coronary Intervention with TAXUS and Cardiac Surgery.
Data from Refs.[19–22]

third-generation DES, which are superior with regard to restenosis and late stent thrombosis rates.

With regard to the role of newer-generation DES, the PRECOMBAT 2 trial reported 18-month follow-up data in 334 consecutive patients treated with everolimus-eluting stents for ULMS disease.[24] In comparison with a historical cohort of patients treated with first-generation sirolimus-stents or CABG, there was no significant difference between the 2 groups. Longer-term follow-up data are pending. The results of the landmark trial Evaluation of Xience Prime versus Coronary Artery Bypass Surgery for Effectiveness of Left Main Revascularization (EXCEL) trial are also expected. In this study, 2634 patients with ULMS and a SYNTAX score of 32 or less have been randomized to either CABG or second-generation everolimus-eluting stents (Xience Prime, Abbott Vascular, Redwood City, CA). The primary end point is the composite incidence of death, myocardial infarction (MI), or cerebrovascular events at a median follow-up duration of 3 years.

CURRENT GUIDELINES

The current ESC[11] and ACC/AHA[12] guidelines both consider PCI for ULMS disease a treatment option in patients without complex left main stem (LMS) anatomy and in the setting of acute coronary syndromes (Table 3).

DIAGNOSIS AND ASSESSMENT

Diagnosis of significant ULMS disease is surprisingly challenging. Although invasive coronary angiography has been the gold standard test to assess LMS severity, it is also associated with the greatest interobserver variability.[25] Uncertainty is increased in the presence of a short ULMS, eccentric calcification, overlapping vessels, and in the setting of ostial lesions that may not be adequately visualized. In recent years, adjunctive tools, including intravascular imaging and fractional flow reserve (FFR), have been increasingly used to aid in the diagnosis of significant ULMS disease.

Intravascular Imaging

Intravascular imaging has a variety of roles in guiding ULMS PCI both with regard to diagnosis and post-PCI optimization. Intravascular ultrasound (IVUS) has been used and investigated the most extensively in the setting of ULMS disease (Fig. 1). A minimal luminal area (MLA) of less than 6 mm^2 has been widely accepted as significant and seems to be correlated with a significant FFR of 0.80 or less,[26] although more recently a cutoff value of 4.8 mm^2 correlated with an FFR of 0.80 in a study limited by a small number of patients and a lack of outcome data using this value.[27] In an IVUS study of intermediate LMS lesions as assessed by angiography, 33% of LMS lesions with less than 30% stenosis had an MLA by IVUS of less than 6 mm^2 and 43% of LMS lesions with greater than 50% stenosis had an MLA of greater than 6 mm^2[28] demonstrating the value of IVUS in this setting. The use of IVUS for ULMS PCI may also be associated with a mortality benefit. In the IVUS substudy of the Revascularization for Unprotected Left MAIN Coronary Artery Stenosis: Comparison of

Table 3 Current guidelines		PCI		CABG	
	Recommendation	Class	Level	Class	Level
ESC guidelines[11]	Left main disease with an SYNTAX score <22	I	B	I	B
	Left main disease with an SYNTAX score 23–32	IIa	B	I	B
	Left main disease with an SYNTAX score >32	III	B	I	B
AHA/ACC guidelines[12]	Left main disease with an SYNTAX score of <22	IIa	B	I	B
	Left main disease with an SYNTAX score of <33	IIb	B	I	B
	Left main disease with an SYNTAX of >33	III	B	I	B

Data from Authors/Task Force Members, Windecker S, Kolh P, et al. 2014 ESC/EACTS guidelines on myocardial revascularization: the task force on myocardial revascularization of the European Society of Cardiology (ESC) and the European Association for Cardio-Thoracic Surgery (EACTS) developed with the special contribution of the European Association of Percutaneous Cardiovascular Interventions (EAPCI). Eur Heart J 2014;35(37):2541–619; and Fihn SD, Blankenship JC, Alexander KP, et al. 2014 ACC/AHA/AATS/PCNA/SCAI/STS focused update of the guideline for the diagnosis and management of patients with stable ischemic heart disease: a report of the American College of Cardiology/American Heart Association task force on practice guidelines, and the American Association for Thoracic Surgery, Preventive Cardiovascular Nurses Association, Society for Cardiovascular Angiography and Interventions, and Society of Thoracic Surgeons. Circulation 2014;130(19):1749–67.

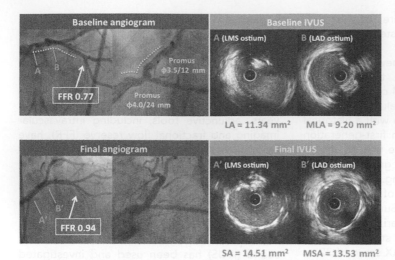

Fig. 1. Diagnosis and optimization of LMS disease. Angiography demonstrated an intermediate distal LMS stenosis (*upper left panel*), with IVUS demonstrating an acceptable minimal luminal area (MLA) (*A* and *B*). FFR was positive (0.77). Patient was treated with a single DES implanted from the LMS to the left anterior descending artery (LAD), with an excellent angiographic result (*lower left panel*), normalization of FFR, acceptable MLA, and appearance of stent on IVUS (*A'* and *B'*) (*bottom right panel*). LA, lumen area; MSA, minimal stent area; SA, stent area.

Percutaneous Coronary Angioplasty vs Surgical Revascularization (MAIN-COMPARE) study, the 3-year incidence of mortality was lower with IVUS guidance as compared with angiographic guidance (4.7% vs 16.0%, log-rank $P = .048$, hazard ratio, 0.39; 95% confidence interval, 0.15–1.02; Cox model $P = .055$).[29]

Optical coherence tomography (OCT) has also been shown to be comparable with IVUS findings (**Fig. 2**)[30] and is advantageous because of its higher resolution. However, because of the poor depth penetration, vessel diameters are often too large to be adequately imaged by OCT and often do not allow for adequate interrogation of ostial disease. For these reasons, OCT has limited value in the pre-PCI assessment of LMS disease.

Fractional Flow Reserve

The utilization of FFR in determining the functional significance of a lesion in the LMS has been shown to be useful in managing revascularization strategies.[31] Because only a minority of patients demonstrate isolated LMS disease (9%),[32] it is important to acknowledge the impact of downstream stenoses on the LMS FFR measurement, which may artificially increase the FFR reading leading to a false-negative result.[33] However, if the pressure wire is placed in a nonstenosed downstream vessel and the other vessel does not have a critical proximal stenosis,[36] then the results can be interpretable. It is important to note, however, that currently there are no large randomized studies investigating the role of FFR

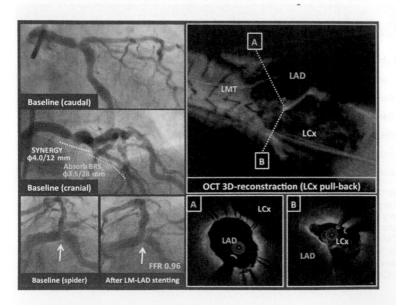

Fig. 2. OCT assessment following provisional stenting of LMS. Provisional stenting of LMS to left anterior descending artery (LAD) (*top right panel*). Excellent final angiographic result of the main branch, but angiography demonstrates compromise of the side branch ostium (*lower left panel*). FFR was unremarkable, and OCT from the side branch to the LMS demonstrated a patent ostium, with a well-opposed implanted stent (*right panels*) (*A*) OCT appearance of proximal LAD, (*B*) OCT appearance of ostial left circumflex artery (LCx)). No further intervention was carried out on the left circumflex artery. 3D, 3 dimensional; BRS, bioresorbable scaffold; LMT, left main trunk.

and long-term outcomes on the management of LMS disease.

PATIENT SELECTION

Following diagnosis of significant ULMS disease, there are broadly 3 treatment options: medical therapy, PCI, or CABG. It is important that all patients are evaluated by a heart team on an individual basis taking into account patient-specific factors before deciding on the best management strategy.

A variety of scoring systems have been devised to help with risk stratification before undergoing PCI. The traditional scores used by cardiothoracic surgeons are the Society of Thoracic Surgeons score and the Logistic European System for Cardiac Operative Risk Evaluation (EuroSCORE). However, as with all risk scores, these are associated with several limitations; more specific scores taking into account coronary anatomy based on the results of trial data have been developed.

The SYNTAX score facilitates quantification of coronary anatomy complexity, and the newer SYNTAX II score also encompasses patient risk factors. Other risk scores include the Global Risk Classification, which combines the SYNTAX score with the EuroSCORE[37] and the New Risk Stratification Score.[38]

Regardless of which tool is used, it is imperative that each patient is evaluated individually with a multidisciplinary approach to enable appropriate risk stratification and guide optimal management strategy.

TECHNICAL APPROACH

Several technical aspects need to be considered when contemplating ULMS PCI.

Guiding Catheter
The correct choice of guiding catheter is critical to increasing the chances of procedural success. Most stenting strategies, including the double-kiss (DK) and reverse crush stenting, can be performed using a 6F catheter. However, a 7F catheter is required if V-stenting or traditional crush stenting whereby the simultaneous positioning of 2 stents is required. Furthermore, larger catheters provide better support and visualization of the anatomy and also enable all burr sizes if rotational atherectomy is required.

Hemodynamic Support
Because the LMS subtends a large volume of myocardium, the use of hemodynamic support, although not mandatory, should be considered

in selected patients. In a retrospective analysis, the risk of hemodynamic instability occurred in approximately 8% of patients with high-risk features, including impaired left ventricular function or complex anatomy, or in patients with persistent ischemia.[39] The placement of an intra-aortic balloon pump may be beneficial.[39] Patients who require a higher degree of hemodynamic support may be candidates for Impella (Abiomed, Danvers, MA) or TandemHeart (CardiacAssist Inc Pittsburgh, PA).

Lesion Preparation
Appropriate lesion preparation, possibly with the aid of intravascular imaging, is imperative to maximizing procedural and long-term success, especially with ULMS PCI, as complications (eg, stent thrombosis) can be fatal or lead to large MI with hemodynamic and electrical instability.

Choice of Stent
The preferred choice of stent in ULMS PCI is DES as it is associated with lower rates of mortality, MI, and revascularization compared with bare-metal stents.[40,41] There are currently no data to support the use of bioresorbable scaffolds in ULMS PCI.

There does not seem to be a difference between various stent designs or type of drug/polymer. The Intracoronary Stenting and Angiographic Results: Drug-Eluting Stents for Unprotected Coronary Left Main Lesions (ISAR-LEFT MAIN) trial, which randomized patients to either a paclitaxel-eluting stent or a sirolimus-eluting stent, did not demonstrate a difference with regard to death, MI, or TLR at 1 year.[41] Similarly, the ISAR-LEFT MAIN 2 trial did not demonstrate any difference at 1 year with the use of a zotarolimus-eluting stent or everolimus-eluting stent, which has also been supported by findings from other registries.[42–46]

Stenting Strategy
Before embarking on ULMS PCI, it is important to plan the stenting strategy, which is predominantly determined by the location of disease. Although the overall rate of restenosis is low after stenting for LMS, PCI of the distal LMS is associated with higher rates of restenosis, with the ostium of the circumflex being particularly vulnerable to restenosis if bifurcation stenting with a 2-stent approach is performed.[47] The distal LMS is involved in most cases (approximately 70%), and the results of PCI are worse than for those patients with lesions located at

the ostium or midshaft likely representing the more complex nature of this disease.[48,49]

The treatment of ostial and midshaft LMS disease is relatively uncomplicated and can usually be treated with the implantation of a single stent. The stent should be allowed to protrude 1 to 2 mm into the aorta while attempting to avoid the distal bifurcation. Short stents (<10 mm) are at risk of dislodgement, especially during postdilatation and ongoing catheter manipulation. When selecting a stent to be implanted at the ostium, devices with minimal longitudinal deformation should be selected.

Distal bifurcation disease can be treated either by a 1-stent (provisional strategy) or a 2-stent technique. Data from observational non-randomized studies suggest that the provisional strategy, when feasible, is superior to a 2-stent technique with regard to the rate of TLR.[48–50]

However, the use of 2 stents may simply reflect more complex disease and, therefore, be associated with worse outcomes. However, a provisional strategy is not always appropriate, for example, in the setting of severe and diffuse disease in the ostium of the left circumflex artery that is 2.5 mm or greater in diameter. In these cases, a 2-stent strategy should be used.

The provisional strategy is a single-stent strategy that allows for the placement of a second stent if required. This strategy is most appropriate if plaque is limited to the LMS and main branch (MB) (which is almost always the left anterior descending artery [LAD]) alone. A stent is placed from the LMS into the LAD and postdilated as required. Depending on the appearances (or following interrogation by FFR), the side branch (SB) may be left untouched (Fig. 3) or treated with a kissing balloon inflation. In

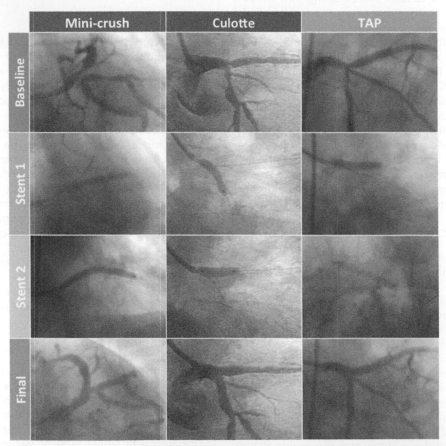

Fig. 3. Two-stent strategies. Two-stent strategies for distal LMS disease. Mini-crush (*left column*) requires stenting of the SB with protrusion into the MB. The proximal end of the stent is then crushed, and a stent is then placed in the MB followed by final kissing balloon inflation. Culotte stenting (*middle column*) is performed by stenting of the SB, followed by rewiring the first stent and implantation of the second stent into MB. The SB is then rewired, and the final kissing balloon inflation is performed. The T and protrusion (TAP) technique (*right column*) is useful to cross over to a 2-stent strategy following an initial provisional (single-stent strategy). Following placement of stent into MB, if the SB branch requires treatment, a stent is placed into the SB, followed by final kissing balloon inflation.

the case of a suboptimal result, such as SB dissection or significant residual stenosis (>50% or FFR ≤0.80), a second stent may be deployed into the SB with a kissing balloon inflation to complete the procedure.

In instances whereby disease extends into both the MB and into the ostium of the SB, then elective double stenting should be considered. The most important determining factor with regard to which bifurcation strategy to use is the internal angle between the MB and the SB. Y-shaped bifurcations demonstrate an angle of less than 70°, whereas T-shaped bifurcations have an angle of greater than 70°. Most distal bifurcation lesions are T shaped. Although it is currently unclear as to which technique is superior, outcome success is determined in part by anatomic considerations and operator experience.[51]

There are several different 2-stent strategies (see **Fig. 3**) that can be used for distal bifurcation disease.

V or Y Stenting

The V-stent or Y-stent technique (depending on how much the stents are brought back into the LMS) involves the simultaneous deployment of stents in both the MB and the SB. This technique, also known as the "simultaneous kissing stent" technique, is particularly applicable for Medina 0.1.1 (V-stent) lesions that can be treated with the creation of a minimal and very short neo-carina or Medina 1.1.1 lesions, which will create a longer neo-carina.

T Stenting

This technique is most useful when the angle between the MB and the SB is close to 90°. The SB is stented first with the careful deployment of the stent to ensure that the ostium of the SB is covered with only minimal protrusion into the MB. The LMS-LAD is then stented followed by final kissing balloon inflation.

The T and Protrusion Technique

This technique is applicable to most LMS bifurcation lesions, and it is the preferred technique when switching from a 1- to a 2-stent strategy. Following stent implantation in the LMS-LAD, a stent is placed in the SB ensuring that the proximal edge of the stent protrudes 1 to 2 mm into the MB. The stent is then deployed while keeping the deflated balloon in the MB. The final kissing balloon inflation is then performed.

Culotte Stenting

This technique is useful if the angle between the MB and SB is shallow (<60°) and the 2 vessels are of similar diameter. After stenting the SB first, the MB is rewired and a second stent is placed through the stent struts, leaving an overlap of both stents in the LMS. Following deployment of the second stent, the SB is then rewired and the final kissing balloon inflation is performed to reshape the carina.[52]

Crush Stenting Techniques

This strategy can be used when there is a size mismatch between the MB (usually larger) and the SB (usually smaller) and the angle between the branches is less than 60° (to facilitate rewiring of the SB). In the crush stenting technique, 2 stents are advanced into both the MB and the SB. After stenting the SB and then removing both the wire and balloon, the MB is then stented. The SB is then rewired through the crushed stent, and the final kissing balloon inflation is performed.[53] A modified version of this technique can be performed through a 6F guiding catheter by placing a balloon in the MB rather than a stent while the SB stent is deployed. After the SB stent is deployed, the balloon in the MB can be inflated to crush the stent followed by deployment of the MB stent. An evolution of crush technique is the mini-crush technique whereby the SB stent minimally protrudes into the MB so that the overlap of the 2 stents in the MB is minimal and final kissing balloon inflation is performed.[54] A further variation of this technique is the DK crush whereby 2 kissing balloon inflations are carried out both after stenting of the SB before MB stenting and at the end of the procedure.[55]

Post–Percutaneous Coronary Intervention Optimization

Intravascular imaging plays a central role in stent optimization following implantation by identifying suboptimal stent expansion and malposition as well as dissection. The importance of optimization in ULMS is particularly magnified because of the likely catastrophic sequelae of complications. OCT has also been used in the evaluation of LMS following PCI.[56]

FOLLOWING PERCUTANEOUS CORONARY INTERVENTION

Following ULMS PCI, a period of dual antiplatelet therapy (DAPT) is mandatory. Current guidelines suggest a minimum of 1 year of DAPT following PCI with DES,[11] although there may be additional benefit of prolonged DAPT beyond this at the risk of increased bleeding.[57]

In patients with who develop in-stent restenosis after ULMS PCI, the appropriate treatment is debated; but options include repeat DES implantation, plain old balloon angioplasty, angioplasty with drug-eluting balloon, or CABG. Repeat PCI seems to be safe and effective with favorable 2-year outcomes.[58]

SUMMARY

Approximately 5% to 7% of patients undergoing coronary angiography are found to have significant ULMS disease. Although CABG has been regarded the old standard treatment of these patients, PCI is increasingly regarded an efficacious alternative treatment strategy particularly in patients with low or intermediate SYNTAX scores. The results of large randomized clinical trials using contemporary DES and adjunctive tools (eg, intravascular imaging) are eagerly awaited, which may lead to further changes in the current guidance with regard to the optimal revascularization strategy in patients presenting with significant ULMS disease.

REFERENCES

1. DeMots H, Rosch J, McAnulty JH, et al. Left main coronary artery disease. Cardiovasc Clin 1977;8(2): 201–11.
2. Taylor HA, Deumite NJ, Chaitman BR, et al. Asymptomatic left main coronary artery disease in the coronary artery surgery study (CASS) registry. Circulation 1989;79(6):1171–9.
3. Cohen MV, Gorlin R. Main left coronary artery disease. Clinical experience from 1964-1974. Circulation 1975;52(2):275–85.
4. Yusuf S, Zucker D, Peduzzi P, et al. Effect of coronary artery bypass graft surgery on survival: overview of 10-year results from randomised trials by the coronary artery bypass graft surgery trialists collaboration. Lancet 1994;344(8922):563–70.
5. Caracciolo EA, Davis KB, Sopko G, et al. Comparison of surgical and medical group survival in patients with left main equivalent coronary artery disease. Long-term CASS experience. Circulation 1995;91(9):2335–44.
6. Chieffo A, Stankovic G, Bonizzoni E, et al. Early and mid-term results of drug-eluting stent implantation in unprotected left main. Circulation 2005;111(6): 791–5.
7. Park SJ, Kim YH, Lee BK, et al. Sirolimus-eluting stent implantation for unprotected left main coronary artery stenosis: comparison with bare metal stent implantation. J Am Coll Cardiol 2005;45(3):351–6.
8. Chieffo A, Park SJ, Meliga E, et al. Late and very late stent thrombosis following drug-eluting stent

implantation in unprotected left main coronary artery: a multicentre registry. Eur Heart J 2008; 29(17):2108–15.
9. Seung KB, Park DW, Kim YH, et al. Stents versus coronary-artery bypass grafting for left main coronary artery disease. N Engl J Med 2008;358(17): 1781–92.
10. Serruys PW, Morice MC, Kappetein AP, et al. Percutaneous coronary intervention versus coronary-artery bypass grafting for severe coronary artery disease. N Engl J Med 2009;360(10):961–72.
11. Authors/Task Force members, Windecker S, Kolh P, et al. 2014 ESC/EACTS guidelines on myocardial revascularization: the task force on myocardial revascularization of the European Society of Cardiology (ESC) and the European Association for Cardio-Thoracic Surgery (EACTS) developed with the special contribution of the European Association of Percutaneous Cardiovascular Interventions (EAPCI). Eur Heart J 2014;35(37):2541–619.
12. Fihn SD, Blankenship JC, Alexander KP, et al. 2014 ACC/AHA/AATS/PCNA/SCAI/STS focused update of the guideline for the diagnosis and management of patients with stable ischemic heart disease: a report of the American College of Cardiology/ American Heart Association Task Force on practice guidelines, and the American Association for Thoracic Surgery, Preventive Cardiovascular Nurses Association, Society for Cardiovascular Angiography and Interventions, and Society of Thoracic Surgeons. Circulation 2014;130(19):1749–67.
13. Palmerini T, Marzocchi A, Marrozzini C, et al. Comparison between coronary angioplasty and coronary artery bypass surgery for the treatment of unprotected left main coronary artery stenosis (the Bologna Registry). Am J Cardiol 2006;98(1): 54–9.
14. Lee MS, Kapoor N, Jamal F, et al. Comparison of coronary artery bypass surgery with percutaneous coronary intervention with drug-eluting stents for unprotected left main coronary artery disease. J Am Coll Cardiol 2006;47(4):864–70.
15. Sanmartin M, Baz JA, Claro R, et al. Comparison of drug-eluting stents versus surgery for unprotected left main coronary artery disease. Am J Cardiol 2007;100(6):970–3.
16. Chieffo A, Magni V, Latib A, et al. 5-year outcomes following percutaneous coronary intervention with drug-eluting stent implantation versus coronary artery bypass graft for unprotected left main coronary artery lesions the Milan experience. JACC Cardiovasc Interv 2010;3(6):595–601.
17. Park DW, Seung KB, Kim YH, et al. Long-term safety and efficacy of stenting versus coronary artery bypass grafting for unprotected left main coronary artery disease: 5-year results from the MAIN-COMPARE (Revascularization for Unprotected Left

Main Coronary Artery Stenosis: Comparison of Percutaneous Coronary Angioplasty Versus Surgical Revascularization) registry. J Am Coll Cardiol 2010; 56(2):117–24.

18. Chieffo A, Morici N, Maisano F, et al. Percutaneous treatment with drug-eluting stent implantation versus bypass surgery for unprotected left main stenosis: a single-center experience. Circulation 2006;113(21):2542–7.

19. Buszman PE, Kiesz SR, Bochenek A, et al. Acute and late outcomes of unprotected left main stenting in comparison with surgical revascularization. J Am Coll Cardiol 2008;51(5):538–45.

20. Morice MC, Serruys PW, Kappetein AP, et al. Outcomes in patients with de novo left main disease treated with either percutaneous coronary intervention using paclitaxel-eluting stents or coronary artery bypass graft treatment in the Synergy Between Percutaneous Coronary Intervention with TAXUS and Cardiac Surgery (SYNTAX) trial. Circulation 2010;121(24):2645–53.

21. Boudriot E, Thiele H, Walther T, et al. Randomized comparison of percutaneous coronary intervention with sirolimus-eluting stents versus coronary artery bypass grafting in unprotected left main stem stenosis. J Am Coll Cardiol 2011;57(5):538–45.

22. Park SJ, Kim YH, Park DW, et al. Randomized trial of stents versus bypass surgery for left main coronary artery disease. N Engl J Med 2011;364(18):1718–27.

23. Morice MC, Serruys PW, Kappetein AP, et al. Five-year outcomes in patients with left main disease treated with either percutaneous coronary intervention or coronary artery bypass grafting in the Synergy Between Percutaneous Coronary Intervention with Taxus and Cardiac Surgery trial. Circulation 2014;129(23):2388–94.

24. Kim YH, Park DW, Ahn JM, et al. Everolimus-eluting stent implantation for unprotected left main coronary artery stenosis. The PRECOMBAT-2 (Premier of Randomized Comparison of Bypass Surgery versus Angioplasty Using Sirolimus-Eluting Stent in Patients with Left Main Coronary Artery Disease) study. JACC Cardiovasc Interv 2012;5(7):708–17.

25. Lindstaedt M, Spiecker M, Perings C, et al. How good are experienced interventional cardiologists at predicting the functional significance of intermediate or equivocal left main coronary artery stenoses? Int J Cardiol 2007;120(2):254–61.

26. Jasti V, Ivan E, Yalamanchili V, et al. Correlations between fractional flow reserve and intravascular ultrasound in patients with an ambiguous left main coronary artery stenosis. Circulation 2004; 110(18):2831–6.

27. Kang SJ, Lee JY, Ahn JM, et al. Intravascular ultrasound-derived predictors for fractional flow reserve in intermediate left main disease. JACC Cardiovasc Interv 2011;4(11):1168–74.

28. de la Torre Hernandez JM, Hernandez Hernandez F, Alfonso F, et al. Prospective application of pre-defined intravascular ultrasound criteria for assessment of intermediate left main coronary artery lesions results from the multicenter LITRO study. J Am Coll Cardiol 2011;58(4):351–8.

29. Park SJ, Kim YH, Park DW, et al. Impact of intravascular ultrasound guidance on long-term mortality in stenting for unprotected left main coronary artery stenosis. Circ Cardiovasc Interv 2009;2(3):167–77.

30. Fujino Y, Bezerra HG, Attizzani GF, et al. Frequency-domain optical coherence tomography assessment of unprotected left main coronary artery disease-a comparison with intravascular ultrasound. Catheter Cardiovasc Interv 2013;82(3): E173–83.

31. Hamilos M, Muller O, Cuisset T, et al. Long-term clinical outcome after fractional flow reserve-guided treatment in patients with angiographically equivocal left main coronary artery stenosis. Circulation 2009;120(15):1505–12.

32. Ragosta M, Dee S, Sarembock IJ, et al. Prevalence of unfavorable angiographic characteristics for percutaneous intervention in patients with unprotected left main coronary artery disease. Catheter Cardiovasc Interv 2006;68(3):357–62.

33. Puri R, Kapadia SR, Nicholls SJ, et al. Optimizing outcomes during left main percutaneous coronary intervention with intravascular ultrasound and fractional flow reserve: the current state of evidence. JACC Cardiovasc Interv 2012;5(7):697–707.

34. Mohr FW, Morice MC, Kappetein AP, et al. Coronary artery bypass graft surgery versus percutaneous coronary intervention in patients with three-vessel disease and left main coronary disease: 5-year follow-up of the randomised, clinical SYNTAX trial. Lancet 2013;381(9867):629–38.

35. Ahn JM, Roh JH, Kim YH, et al. Randomized trial of stents versus bypass surgery for left main coronary artery disease: five-year outcomes of the PRECOMBAT Study. J Am Coll Cardiol 2015;65(20):2198–206.

36. Yong AS, Daniels D, De Bruyne B, et al. Fractional flow reserve assessment of left main stenosis in the presence of downstream coronary stenoses. Circ Cardiovasc Interv 2013;6(2):161–5.

37. Capodanno D, Miano M, Cincotta G, et al. EuroSCORE refines the predictive ability of SYNTAX score in patients undergoing left main percutaneous coronary intervention. Am Heart J 2010; 159(1):103–9.

38. Chen SL, Chen JP, Mintz G, et al. Comparison between the NERS (New risk Stratification) score and the SYNTAX (Synergy Between Percutaneous Coronary Intervention with Taxus and Cardiac Surgery) score in outcome prediction for unprotected left main stenting. JACC Cardiovasc Interv 2010;3(6): 632–41.

39. Briguori C, Airoldi F, Chieffo A, et al. Elective versus provisional intraaortic balloon pumping in unprotected left main stenting. Am Heart J 2006;152(3): 565–72.

40. Pandya SB, Kim YH, Meyers SN, et al. Drug-eluting versus bare-metal stents in unprotected left main coronary artery stenosis a meta-analysis. JACC Cardiovasc Interv 2010;3(6):602–11.

41. Mehilli J, Kastrati A, Byrne RA, et al. Paclitaxel-versus sirolimus-eluting stents for unprotected left main coronary artery disease. J Am Coll Cardiol 2009;53(19):1760–8.

42. Mehilli J, Richardt G, Valgimigli M, et al. Zotarolimus- versus everolimus-eluting stents for unprotected left main coronary artery disease. J Am Coll Cardiol 2013;62(22):2075–82.

43. Takagi K, Ielasi A, Shannon J, et al. Clinical and procedural predictors of suboptimal outcome after the treatment of drug-eluting stent restenosis in the unprotected distal left main stem: the Milan and New-Tokyo (MITO) registry. Circ Cardiovasc Interv 2012;5(4):491–8.

44. Almudarra SS, Gale CP, Baxter PD, et al. Comparative outcomes after unprotected left main stem percutaneous coronary intervention: a national linked cohort study of 5,065 acute and elective cases from the BCIS Registry (British Cardiovascular Intervention Society). JACC Cardiovasc Interv 2014; 7(7):717–30.

45. Salvatella N, Morice MC, Darremont O, et al. Unprotected left main stenting with a second-generation drug-eluting stent: one-year outcomes of the LEMAX pilot study. EuroIntervention 2011; 7(6):689–96.

46. Bernelli C, Chieffo A, Buchanan GL, et al. New-generation drug-eluting stent experience in the percutaneous treatment of unprotected left main coronary artery disease: the NEST registry. J Invasive Cardiol 2013;25(6):269–75.

47. Baim DS, Mauri L, Cutlip DC. Drug-eluting stenting for unprotected left main coronary artery disease: are we ready to replace bypass surgery? J Am Coll Cardiol 2006;47(4):878–81.

48. Toyofuku M, Kimura T, Morimoto T, et al. Three-year outcomes after sirolimus-eluting stent implantation for unprotected left main coronary artery disease: insights from the j-Cypher registry. Circulation 2009;120(19):1866–74.

49. Palmerini T, Sangiorgi D, Marzocchi A, et al. Ostial and midshaft lesions vs. bifurcation lesions in 1111 patients with unprotected left main coronary artery stenosis treated with drug-eluting stents: results of the survey from the Italian Society of Invasive Cardiology. Eur Heart J 2009;30(17):2087–94.

50. Koh YS, Kim PJ, Chang K, et al. Long-term clinical outcomes of the one-stent technique versus the two-stent technique for non-left main true coronary bifurcation disease in the era of drug-eluting stents. J Interv Cardiol 2013;26(3):245–53.

51. Latib A, Colombo A, Sangiorgi GM. Bifurcation stenting: current strategies and new devices. Heart 2009;95(6):495–504.

52. Chevalier B, Glatt B, Royer T, et al. Placement of coronary stents in bifurcation lesions by the "culotte" technique. Am J Cardiol 1998;82(8): 943–9.

53. Colombo A, Stankovic G, Orlic D, et al. Modified T-stenting technique with crushing for bifurcation lesions: immediate results and 30-day outcome. Catheter Cardiovasc Interv 2003;60(2):145–51.

54. Galassi AR, Colombo A, Buchbinder M, et al. Long-term outcomes of bifurcation lesions after implantation of drug-eluting stents with the "mini-crush technique". Catheter Cardiovasc Interv 2007;69(7): 976–83.

55. Chen SL, Ye F, Zhang JJ, et al. DK crush technique: modified treatment of bifurcation lesions in coronary artery. Chin Med J (Engl) 2005; 118(20):1746–50 [in Chinese].

56. Parodi G, Maehara A, Giuliani G, et al. Optical coherence tomography in unprotected left main coronary artery stenting. EuroIntervention 2010; 6(1):94–9.

57. Mauri L, Kereiakes DJ, Yeh RW, et al. Twelve or 30 months of dual antiplatelet therapy after drug-eluting stents. N Engl J Med 2014;371(23):2155–66.

58. Sheiban I, Sillano D, Biondi-Zoccai G, et al. Incidence and management of restenosis after treatment of unprotected left main disease with drug-eluting stents 70 restenotic cases from a cohort of 718 patients: FAILS (Failure in Left Main Study). J Am Coll Cardiol 2009;54(13):1131–6.

Saphenous Vein Graft Interventions

Michael S. Lee, MD*, Gopi Manthripragada, MD

KEYWORDS

- Saphenous vein graft • Percutaneous coronary intervention • Distal embolization
- Embolic protection • No-reflow phenomenon • Drug-eluting stent

KEY POINTS

- Knowledge of anatomic details and appropriate patient selection based on clinical and noninvasive data are imperative.
- Percutaneous coronary intervention of saphenous vein graft is associated with worse outcomes when compared with native coronary arteries.
- An embolic protection device should be used when technically feasible.
- Smaller stent size, avoidance of predilation, and use of an embolic protection device may reduce the likelihood of distal embolization.
- Treatment of the no-reflow phenomenon includes vasodilators like adenosine, nitroprusside, and calcium channel blocker.

INTRODUCTION

Saphenous vein graft (SVG) is the most common conduit used during coronary artery bypass graft surgery (CABG). Relative to arterial graft conduits, long-term patency of SVG is adversely affected by accelerated atherosclerosis, intimal fibrosis, and thrombotic occlusion. By 18 months after CABG, SVG failure rates have been reported to be near 25%.[1–4]

Despite the increase in percutaneous coronary intervention (PCI) for select patients with unprotected left main coronary artery disease, CABG remains the gold standard for complex coronary artery disease.[5] SVG intervention will, therefore, remain an important skill set in the interventional cardiologist's armamentarium.

PATHOPHYSIOLOGY

The high rate of SVG failure compared with arterial graft conduits, specifically the left internal mammary artery, can be attributed to[6–10]

- Harvesting
  - Loss of the vasa vasorum
  - Endovascular approach, possibly from endothelial damage
- Vascular biology
  - Exposure to arterial pressure promoting accelerated atherosclerosis
  - Endothelial dysfunction due to reduced production of nitric oxide
  - Neointimal hyperplasia and thrombosis
  - Increased lesion bulk with friable fibrous caps
- Target and graft anatomy
  - Poor distal runoff
  - Pre-existing venous dysfunction
- Technical failure
  - Excessive graft length causing mechanical torsion and kinking
  - Early anastomotic occlusion
  - Longer operative duration
  - Bypass grafting of nonischemia producing coronary artery lesions

LESION SELECTION

Similar to lesions in native coronary arteries, indications to intervene include ischemia on

No conflicts of interest to report.
Cardiology Division, Department of Medicine, 100 Medical Plaza, Suite 630, Los Angeles, CA 90095, USA
* Corresponding author. 200 UCLA Medical Plaza, Suite C365, Los Angeles, CA 90095.
E-mail address: mslee@mednet.ucla.edu

Intervent Cardiol Clin 5 (2016) 135–141
http://dx.doi.org/10.1016/j.iccl.2015.12.002

noninvasive testing; patient symptoms, including in the setting of acute coronary syndrome; and angiographic evidence of a significant stenosis. Myocardial perfusion imaging (MPI) has good specificity but variable sensitivity for detecting ischemia after CABG.[11] Results should be interpreted cautiously because ischemia may be present in vascular territories not amenable to CABG or proximal to the anastomosis.

Fractional flow reserve (FFR) is widely used in native coronary arteries to assess hemodynamic significance of intermediate coronary stenosis. However, data are insufficient to guide the use in SVG intervention. In limited studies, FFR has a high specificity but low sensitivity for identifying lesions associated with ischemia on MPI.[12]

Intravascular ultrasound (IVUS) may be helpful with stent selection, particularly because balloon predilation may be detrimental.[13,14] Positive remodeling on IVUS is a strong predictor of postintervention no-reflow warranting adequate preparation with embolic protection device (EDP) and pharmacotherapy before stenting.[15]

In a substudy of the stenting of saphenous vein grafts trial, patients with an intermediate (30%–60%) lesion who were noted to have lesion progression on follow-up angiography had a high rate of acute coronary syndrome (64%) and PCI (73%).[16,17] Although it is difficult to draw conclusions because of the small number of patients in this study, FFR and IVUS have limitations in predicting SVG lesion progression.

The comparison of plaque sealing with paclitaxel-eluting stents versus medical therapy for the treatment of moderate nonsignificant SVG lesions: the Moderate Vein Graft Lesion Stenting with the Taxus Stent and Intravascular Ultrasound (VELETI) trial randomized 57 patients with moderate (30%–60%) SVG stenosis to medical therapy or revascularization with drug-eluting stents (DES).[18–20] On average, patients were 12 years after CABG. IVUS was performed during the index coronary angiogram and again at 1-year follow-up. Both minimal luminal diameter and percent stenosis were decreased in the intervention group. Major adverse cardiac events (MACE) were nonsignificantly higher in the medical therapy group (19% vs 3%, $P = .091$). Although the VELETI I trial was underpowered for clinical end points, the results suggest improved outcomes with SVG intervention of intermediate stenoses. The ongoing VELETI II trial may shed further light on the issue because the primary end point is clinical rather than angiographic.[21] Although treatment of moderately diseased SVGs remains controversial, these studies have established the very

rapid progression of intermediate lesions in SVGs.

INTERVENTION TECHNIQUE
Preparation
Knowledge of previous angiograms and details of the operative report can be very helpful, including graft location, number, and anatomy as well as any challenges encountered during CABG. On identification of appropriate patients with established ischemia, the SVG may be engaged with a variety of guide catheters, including the multipurpose catheter for right coronary graft intervention and the Judkins right catheter for left coronary graft intervention. Amplatz and left coronary bypass guide catheters are also frequently chosen for their ability to provide backup support. Right coronary grafts are best imaged in a left anterior oblique projection, whereas left coronary grafts are best viewed in a right anterior oblique projection.

Intervention of the native coronary artery should be considered whenever feasible because of the rapid progression of SVG stenoses and inferior long-term outcomes with SVG intervention.[22,23]

Predilation Versus Direct Stenting
Predilation, although frequently used as a lesion preparation strategy in non-SVG interventions, might be suboptimal in this setting. In a registry of patients who underwent SVG intervention, direct stenting was associated with a marked reduction in postprocedural myocardial infarction.[24]

Choice of Stent
The ISAR-CABG (Drug-eluting versus bare-metal stents in saphenous vein graft lesions) trial, which was the largest randomized trial comparing bare-metal stents (BMS) to DES in SVG intervention, reported a significantly lower target vessel revascularization rate in the DES group (7% vs 13%, $P = .01$).[25] The Reduction in Restenosis in Saphenous Vein Grafts with Cypher Sirolimus-Eluting Stent (RRISC) trial reported a lower rate of target lesion revascularization in patients randomized to DES at 6 months (5.3% vs 21.6%, $P = .047$) without a difference in mortality.[26] However, at the 3-year follow-up (DELAYED RRISC), the benefit in target lesion revascularization was lost, with an increase in mortality in the DES group. However, the trial was underpowered to demonstrate a difference in mortality (75 patients vs 610 in the ISAR-CABG trial).[27]

These studies were preceded by the Saphenous Vein de Novo (SAVED) trial, which demonstrated higher procedural success (92% vs 69%, P<.001) and lower MACE through 240 days (26% vs 38%, P = .04) for BMS when compared with balloon angioplasty.[28]

In a long-term comparison of first- and second-generation DES, no significant difference was noted with respect to target vessel revascularization, death, or myocardial infarction.[29]

Covered stents have been postulated to be beneficial in SVG intervention, potentially reducing distal embolization by trapping atherosclerotic debris that would otherwise extrude between stent struts. In the randomized Barrier Approach to Restenosis: Restrict Intima to Curtail Adverse Events (BARRICADE) trial, polytetrafluoroethylene (PTFE)–covered stents were associated with increased long-term target vessel failure.[30] In the Stents In Grafts (STING) trial, when compared with conventional stents, the rates of death and myocardial infarction were similar.[31] The SYMBIOT III trial comparing the self-expanding PTFE-covered Symbiot (Boston Scientific, Marlborough, MA) with BMS demonstrated no difference in clinical outcomes, although early results using alternative covered stents are promising.[32,33]

In a retrospective study of 209 patients undergoing SVG intervention, IVUS was used to determine the stent to reference vessel ratio. Increasing the stent size with respect to the reference vessel was associated with an escalating incidence of postprocedural Creatine Kinase-MB elevation, with the lowest rates seen when the stent size was less than 0.89 relative to the reference vessel.[34] Theoretically, SVG stent oversizing causes increased distal embolization akin to predilation before stenting. However, stent undersizing may lead to a higher risk of in-stent restenosis and stent thrombosis.

Embolic Protection Devices

EPDs are associated with a decreased rate of distal embolization, no-reflow phenomenon, and postprocedure myocardial infarction.[21] However, despite an IB recommendation for their use in the 2011 guidelines from the American College of Cardiology (ACCF)/American Heart Association (AHA)/Society for Cardiovascular Angiography and Interventions (SCAI), only 21.2% of SVG intervention involved the use of EPD.[35,36] Their widespread adoption has been limited by increased complexity and procedure time and lack of eligibility for either distal or proximal protection.[37] Furthermore, routine use of EPD in SVG intervention has been questioned because of improvement in outcomes in contemporary practice.[38,39] In a longitudinal cohort from the National Cardiovascular Data Registry comprising 49,325 patients, EPD use was associated with a slightly higher rate of periprocedural complications, including no-reflow (3.9% vs 2.8%, P<.001) and myocardial infarction (2.8% vs 1.8%, P<.001).[36] By 3 years, there was no significant difference in target lesion revascularization, myocardial infarction, or death between EPD and non-EPD groups. However, the use of EPD was slightly higher in higher-risk patients, such as those with acute coronary syndrome. This finding is in contrast to previous studies that showed improvement in clinical outcomes with EPD.[40] Although the registry shows real-world outcomes from EPD use, challenges with extrapolating the data include a lack of randomization and potential inclusion of operators unfamiliar with EPD use.[41]

In select patients, EPD may still play a role in decreasing distal embolization with mechanisms that include proximal occlusion, distal filter, and distal balloon occlusion.

Distal occlusion system

The PercuSurge GuardWire (Medtronic, Minneapolis, MN) was the first EPD to gain Food and Drug Administration (FDA) approval based on the results of the Saphenous Vein Graft Angioplasty Free of Emboli Randomized (SAFER) trial. Compared with no EPD, the device reduced MACE by 42% at 30 days (8.6% vs 14.7%, P = .008) and no reflow (3% vs 9% P = .02).[40] Of note, the SAFER trial was conducted from 1999 to 2000, whereas enrollment in the longitudinal cohort discussed earlier spanned procedures from 2005 to 2009 when more contemporary strategies were more likely to be used.

This technique requires an adequate (3 cm) distal landing zone where the distal balloon is deployed. Once SVG intervention is completed, debris within the blood column proximal to the balloon is aspirated. Visualization of the lesion is limited because of the presence of the stagnant blood column, which may produce ischemia while the balloon is inflated, and the balloon needs to be sized appropriately for the distal vessel.

Distal filtration system

Distal filters are the most commonly used EDP for SVG intervention. These devices permit lesion visualization as antegrade flow is preserved during intervention (**Figs. 1** and **2**). Similarly, they require an adequate distal landing zone of 3 to 4 cm, and complications may involve filter entrapment. The FilterWire EX Randomized Evaluation (FIRE) study established noninferiority of the FilterWire EX (Boston Scientific,

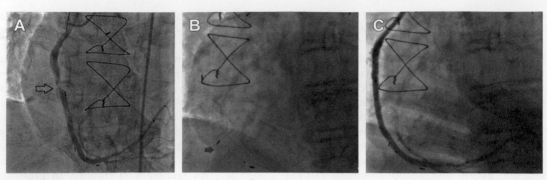

Fig. 1. (*A*) Severe stenosis (*arrow*) within the body of an SVG to right posterior descending artery. (*B*) Filtration system in place, with deployment of filter (*red arrow*) distal to the stenosis. (*C*). Poststent angiogram.

Marlborough, MA) distal filter system to the GuardWire balloon occlusion device.[42]

The FilterWire includes a microcatheter that houses the filter over a preloaded 0.014-in guidewire. The device is advanced to the distal landing zone; the microcatheter is retracted, leaving the filter and wire in place. After completion of the intervention, the filter is retrieved with a retrieval catheter.

The SpiderFX (Covidien-Ev3, Irvine, CA) catheter allows advancement over a workhorse 0.014-in guidewire. The guidewire is removed, and the capture wire is advanced. The microcatheter is retracted as described earlier, with the filter deployed in the distal landing zone. The filter is removed similarly to the FilterWire catheter.

Proximal occlusion system
The proximal occlusion device occludes the vessel proximal to the target lesion and inhibits antegrade flow. At the conclusion of the procedure, stagnant debris is then aspirated. The Proxis system (St. Jude Medical, Saint Paul, MI) is the only FDA-approved proximal occlusion device. The Proximal Protection During Saphenous Vein Graft Intervention (PROXIMAL) trial, which

randomized 594 patients, showed the Proxis device was noninferior to distal EPD (30-day MACE 9.2% versus 10.0%, $P = .006$ for noninferiority).[43] However, the Proxis is no longer commercially available.

ADJUNCTIVE PHARMACOLOGY

A pooled analysis of 5 randomized clinical trials (EPIC, EPILOG, EPISTENT, IMPACT II, and PURSUIT) showed no benefit from adjunctive glycoprotein IIb/IIIa inhibition in SVG intervention[44] and is a class III (no benefit) recommendation in the ACCF/AHA/SCAI guidelines.[35] No difference in clinical end points was seen between bivalirudin monotherapy and bivalirudin or unfractionated heparin plus a glycoprotein IIb/IIIa inhibitor in the subset of patients undergoing SVG intervention in the Acute Catheterization and Urgent Intervention Triage Strategy (ACUITY) trial.[45]

Dual antiplatelet therapy recommendations are similar to that in native coronary artery PCI.[35] In a retrospective analysis of patients who underwent SVG intervention, those who received no antiplatelet therapy before hospital admission had higher rates of MACE when

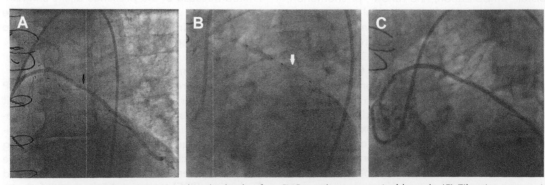

Fig. 2. (*A*) Severe stenosis (*arrow*) within the body of an SVG to obtuse marginal branch. (*B*) Filtration system in place, with deployment of filter (*white arrow*) distal to the stenosis. (*C*) Poststent angiogram.

compared with those on either aspirin or clopidogrel or dual antiplatelet therapy at both 30 days and 1 year (38.1% vs 14.9% and 13.9%, $P = .01$; 52.4% vs 29.5% and 28.3%, $P = .03$).[46]

COMPLICATIONS DURING SAPHENOUS VEIN GRAFT INTERVENTION

Vein graft plaques are bulky and friable, and the absence of side branches results in slow-flow or no-reflow phenomena when distal embolization occurs. This results in poor distal vessel opacification due to diminished antegrade blood flow in the absence of an apparent obstruction. Mechanisms involved might include neurohormonal release, platelet aggregation, and microvascular dysfunction.[23,47]

Independent predictors of slow or no-reflow in SVG intervention include

- Probable thrombus (hazard ratio [HR] 6.9; 95% confidence interval [CI] 2.1–23.9; $P = .001$)
- Acute coronary syndrome (HR 6.4; 95% CI 2.0–25.3; $P = .003$)
- Degenerated SVG (HR 5.2; 95% CI 1.7–16.6; $P = .003$)
- Lesion ulceration (HR 3.4; 95% CI 0.99–11.6; $P = .04$)[21,48]

Despite the absence of significant clinical data, vasodilators are the mainstay of therapy for no-reflow. Adenosine is very short acting and has inhibitory effects on platelet activation and aggregation but may cause profound bradycardia, although its effect is transient. Preprocedural adenosine does not seem to be beneficial, but repeated boluses of high-dose adenosine showed promising results.[49,50]

Calcium channel blockers improve no-reflow. The Vasodilator Prevention of No-Reflow (VAPOR) trial was a small study involving 22 patients but showed a significant reduction in no-reflow with prophylactic intragraft verapamil.[51]

Prophylactic nicardipine followed by direct stenting, even without the use of EPD, resulted in a low incidence of no-reflow and MACE.[52] In a study of 19 consecutive patients with impaired flow or no-reflow during revascularization, 14 had a significant improvement in flow after the administration of intracoronary nitroprusside.[53]

In a prospective analysis of 4264 patients undergoing PCI, no-reflow was observed in 3.2% of patients and associated with acute coronary syndrome and SVG intervention.[54] No-reflow was predictive of postprocedural myocardial infarction (17.7% vs 3.5% in patients without

no-reflow, $P<.001$) and death (7.4% vs 2.0%, $P<.001$) and remained a strong independent predictor of death or myocardial infarction after multivariate analysis (odds ratio 3.6, $P<.001$). The administration of intracoronary vasodilators did not impact clinical outcomes.

SUMMARY/DISCUSSION

Although optimal surgical revascularization strategies involve the use of arterial conduits, widespread use of SVG has resulted in patients with ischemia. A hybrid approach with an internal mammary artery-to-left anterior descending artery graft and PCI with DES of non-LAD vessels remains a niche procedure. SVG intervention, although technically feasible using EPDs and the strategies outlined earlier, suffers from high rates of periprocedural complications and subsequent ischemic events. Strategies and techniques to minimize these are vital to the short- and long-term success of SVG intervention.

REFERENCES

1. Fitzgibbon GM, Kafka HP, Leach AJ, et al. Coronary bypass graft fate and patient outcome: angiographic follow-up of 5,065 grafts related to survival and reoperation in 1,388 patients during 25 years. J Am Coll Cardiol 1996;28(3):616.
2. Alexander JH, Hafley G, Harrington RA, et al, for the PREVENT IV Investigators. Efficacy and safety of edifoligide, an E2F transcription factor decoy, for the prevention of vein graft failure following coronary artery bypass surgery: PREVENT IV: a randomized controlled trial. JAMA 2005;294:2446–54.
3. Hess CN, Lopes RD, Gibson CM, et al. Saphenous vein graft failure after coronary artery bypass surgery: insights from PREVENT IV. Circulation 2014; 130(17):1445.
4. Harskamp RE, Lopes RD, Baisden CE, et al. Saphenous vein graft failure after coronary artery bypass surgery: pathophysiology, management, and future directions. Ann Surg 2013;257(5):824–33.
5. Mohr FW, Morice MC, Feldman TE, et al. Coronary artery bypass graft surgery versus percutaneous coronary intervention in patients with three-vessel disease and left main coronary disease: 5-year follow-up of the randomised, clinical SYNTAX trial. Lancet 2013;381(9867):629–38.
6. Lopes RD, Hafley GE, Allen KB, et al. Endoscopic versus open vein-graft harvesting in coronary-artery bypass surgery. N Engl J Med 2009;361:235–44.
7. Desai ND, Cohen EA, Naylor CD, et al. A randomized comparison of radial-artery and saphenous-vein coronary bypass grafts. N Engl Med 2004;351:2302–9.

8. Murphy GJ, Angelini GD. Insights into the patho-genesis of vein graft disease: lessons from intravas-cular ultrasound. Cardiovasc Ultrasound 2004;2:8.

9. Cox JL, Chiasson DA, Gotlieb AI. Stranger in a strange land: the pathogenesis of saphenous vein graft stenosis with emphasis on structural and func-tional differences between veins and arteries. Prog Cardiovasc Dis 1991;34:45–68.

10. Botman CJ, Schonberger J, Koolen S, et al. Does ste-nosis severity of native vessels influence bypass graft patency? A prospective fractional flow reserve-guided study. Ann Thorac Surg 2007;83:2093–7.

11. Lakkis NM, Mahmarian JJ, Verani MS. Exercise thallium-201 single photon emission computed to-mography for evaluation of coronary artery bypass graft patency. Am J Cardiol 1995;76:107–11.

12. Aqel R, Zoghbi GJ, Hage F, et al. Hemodynamic evaluation of coronary artery bypass graft lesions using fractional flow reserve. Catheter Cardiovasc Interv 2008;72:479–85.

13. Wilson SH, Berger PB, Mathew V, et al. Immediate and late outcomes after direct stent implantation without balloon predilation. J Am Coll Cardiol 2000;4:937–43.

14. Carrozza JP Jr, Mumma M, Breall JA, et al. Randomized evaluation of the TriActiv balloon-protection flush and extraction system for the treat-ment of saphenous vein graft disease. J Am Coll Cardiol 2005;46(9):1677–83.

15. Hong YJ, Jeong MH, Ahn Y, et al. Intravascular ul-trasound analysis of plaque characteristics and postpercutaneous coronary intervention catheteri-zation outcomes according to the remodeling pattern in narrowed saphenous vein grafts. Am J Cardiol 2012;110:1290–5.

16. Abdel-Karim AR, Da Silva M, Lichtenwalter C, et al. Prevalence and outcomes of intermediate saphe-nous vein graft lesions: findings from the stenting of saphenous vein grafts randomized-controlled trial. Int J Cardiol 2013;168:2468–73.

17. Brilakis ES, Lichtenwalter C, de Lemos JA, et al. A randomized controlled trial of a paclitaxel-eluting stent versus a similar bare-metal stent in saphenous vein graft lesions the SOS (stenting of saphenous vein grafts) trial. J Am Coll Cardiol 2009;53:919–28.

18. Brilakis ES, Wang TY, Rao SV, et al. Frequency and predictors of drug-eluting stent use in saphenous vein bypass graft percutaneous coronary interven-tions: a report from the American College of Cardi-ology national cardiovascular data cathPCI registry. JACC Cardiovasc Interv 2010;3:1068–73.

19. Brodie BR, Wilson H, Stuckey T, et al. Outcomes with drug-eluting versus bare-metal stents in saphenous vein graft intervention: results fro the STENT (stra-tegic transcatheter evaluation of new therapies) group. JACC Cardiovasc Interv 2009;2:1105–12.

20. Rodés-Cabau J, Bertrand OF, Larose E, et al. Com-parison of plaque sealing with paclitaxel-eluting stents versus medical therapy for the treatment of moderate nonsignificant saphenous vein graft le-sions: the moderate vein graft lesion stenting with the taxus stent and intravascular ultrasound (VELETI) pilot trial. Circulation 2009;120:1978–86.

21. Lee MS, Park SJ, Kandzari DE, et al. Saphenous vein graft intervention. JACC Cardiovasc Interv 2011;8: 831–43.

22. Hindnavis V, Cho SH, Goldberg S. Saphenous vein graft intervention: a review. J Invasive Cardiol 2012; 24:64–71.

23. van Gaal WJ, Banning AP. Percutaneous coronary intervention and the no-reflow phenomenon. Expert Rev Cardiovasc Ther 2007;5(4):715–31.

24. Leborgne L, Cheneau E, Pichard A, et al. Effect of direct stenting on clinical outcome in patients treated with percutaneous coronary intervention on saphenous vein graft. Am Heart J 2003;146:501–6.

25. Mehilli J, Pache J, Abdel-Wahab M, et al. Drug-eluting versus bare-metal stents in saphenous vein graft lesions (ISAR-CABG): a randomised controlled superiority trial. Lancet 2011;378:1071–8.

26. Vermeersch P, Agostoni P, Verheye S, et al. Ran-domized double-blind comparison of sirolimus-eluting stent versus bare-metal stent implantation in diseased saphenous vein grafts: six-month angiographic, intravascular ultrasound, and clinical follow-up of the RRISC trial. J Am Coll Cardiol 2006;48(12):2423–31.

27. Vermeersch P, Agostoni P, Verheye S, et al. Increased late mortality after sirolimus-eluting stents versus bare-metal stents in diseased saphe-nous vein grafts: results from the randomized DELAYED RRISC trial. J Am Coll Cardiol 2007; 50(3):261–7.

28. Savage MP, Douglas JS Jr, Fischman DL, et al. Stent placement compared with balloon angio-plasty for obstructed coronary bypass grafts. Saphenous Vein de Novo trial investigators. N Engl J Med 1997;337:740–7.

29. Taniwaki M, Raber L, Magro M. Long-term compar-ison of everolimus-eluting stents with sirolimus- and paclitaxel-eluting stents for percutaneous coronary intervention of saphenous vein grafts. EuroIntervention 2014;9(12):1432–40.

30. Stone GW, Goldberg S, O'Shaughnessy C, et al. 5-year follow-up of polytetrafluoroethylene-covered stents compared with bare-metal stents in aortocoronary saphenous vein grafts. The ran-domized BARRICADE (barrier approach to resteno-sis: restrict intima to curtail adverse events) trial. JACC Cardiovasc Interv 2011;4:300–9.

31. Schachinger V, Hamm CW, Munzel T, et al, STING (STents IN Grafts) Investigators. A randomized trial of polytetrafluoroethylene-membrane-covered

stents compared with conventional stents in aorto-coronary saphenous vein grafts. J Am Coll Cardiol 2003;42(8):1360–9.

32. Turco MA, Buchbinder M, Popma JJ, et al. Pivotal, randomized U.S study of the Symbiot™ covered stent system in patients with saphenous vein graft disease: eight-month angiographic and clinical results from the Symbiot III trial. Catheter Cardiovasc Interv 2006;68(3):379–88.

33. Abizaid A, Weiner B, Bailey SR, et al. Use of a self-expanding super-elastic all-metal endoprosthesis; to treat degenerated SVG lesions: the SESAME first in man trial. Catheter Cardiovasc Interv 2010;76(6):781–6.

34. Hong YJ, Pichard AD, Mintz GS, et al. Outcome of undersized drug-eluting stents for percutaneous coronary intervention of saphenous vein graft lesions. Am J Cardiol 2010;105:179–85.

35. Levine GN, Bates ER, Blankenship JC, et al. 2011 ACCF/AHA/SCAI guideline for percutaneous coronary intervention: executive summary: a report of the American College of Cardiology Foundation/American Heart Association Task Force on Practice Guidelines and the Society for Cardiovascular Angiography and Interventions. Catheter Cardiovasc Interv 2012;79:453–95.

36. Brennan JM, Al-Hejily M, Dai D, et al. Three-year outcomes associated with embolic protection in saphenous vein graft intervention. Results in 49 325 senior patients in the Medicare-linked national cardiovascular data registry CathPCI registry. Circ Cardiovasc Interv 2015;8:e001403.

37. Webb LA, Dixon SR, Safian RD, et al. Usefulness of embolic protection devices during saphenous vein graft intervention in a nonselected population. J Interv Cardiol 2005;18:73–5.

38. Narayanan A, Abdallah M, Helmy T. Embolic protection devices in saphenous vein graft interventions: is there still a role? J Invasive Cardiol 2012;24:4.

39. Satler LF. Do we still need distal protection in the treatment of SVG disease? Catheter Cardiovasc Interv 2008;72:804–5.

40. Baim DS, Wahr D, George B, et al. Randomized trial of a distal embolic protection device during percutaneous intervention of saphenous vein aorto-coronary bypass grafts. Circulation 2002;105:1285–90.

41. Waksman R, Koifman E. Embolic protection device for saphenous vein graft intervention: too early to take off the seat belt [editorial]. Circ Cardiovasc Interv 2015;8(3):e002371.

42. Stone GW, Rogers C, Hermiller J, et al. Randomized comparison of distal filter protection with a filter-based catheter and a balloon occlusion and aspiration system during percutaneous intervention of diseased saphenous vein aorto-coronary bypass grafts. Circulation 2003;108:548–53.

43. Mauri L, Cox D, Hermiller J, et al. The PROXIMAL trial: proximal protection during saphenous vein graft intervention using the Proxis embolic protection system: a randomized, prospective, multicenter clinical trial. J Am Coll Cardiol 2007;50:1442–9.

44. Mak KH, Challapalli R, Eisenberg MJ, et al. Effect of platelet glycoprotein IIb/IIIa inhibition as adjunctive treatment for percutaneous interventions of aorto-coronary bypass grafts: a pooled analysis of five randomized clinical trials. Circulation 2002;106:3063–7.

45. Kumar D, Dangas G, Mehran R, et al. Comparison of bivalirudin versus bivalirudin plus glycoprotein IIb/IIIa inhibitor in patients with acute coronary syndromes having percutaneous intervention for narrowed saphenous vein aorto-coronary grafts (the ACUITY Trial Investigators). Am J Cardiol 2010; 106:941–5.

46. Harskamp RE, Beijk MA, Damman P, et al. Prehospitalization antiplatelet therapy and outcomes after saphenous vein graft intervention. Am J Cardiol 2013;111:153–8.

47. Kloner RA, Rude RE, Carlson N, et al. Ultrastructural evidence of microvascular damage and myocardial cell injury after coronary artery occlusion: which comes first? Circulation 1980;62(5):945–52.

48. Sdringola S, Assali AR, Ghani M, et al. Risk assessment of slow or no-reflow phenomenon in aorto-coronary vein graft percutaneous intervention. Catheter Cardiovasc Interv 2001;54:318–24.

49. Sdringola S, Assali A, Ghani M, et al. Adenosine use during aorto-coronary vein graft interventions reverses but does not prevent the slow-no reflow phenomenon. Catheter Cardiovasc Interv 2000; 51(4):394–9.

50. Fischell TA, Carter AJ, Foster MT, et al. Reversal of "no reflow" during vein graft stenting using high velocity boluses of intracoronary adenosine. Cathet Cardiovasc Diagn 1998;45(4):360–5.

51. Michaels AD, Appleby M, Otten MH, et al. Pretreatment with intragraft verapamil prior to percutaneous coronary intervention of saphenous vein graft lesions: results of the randomized, controlled vasodilator prevention on no-reflow (VAPOR) trial. J Invasive Cardiol 2002;14(6):299–302.

52. Fischell TA, Subraya RG, Ashraf K, et al. "Pharmacologic" distal protection using prophylactic intragraft nicardipine to prevent no-reflow and non-Q wave myocardial infarction during elective saphenous vein graft intervention. J Invasive Cardiol 2007;19(2):58–62.

53. Hillegass WB, Dean NA, Liao L, et al. Treatment of no-reflow and impaired flow with the nitric oxide donor nitroprusside following percutaneous coronary interventions: initial human clinical experience. J Am Coll Cardiol 2001;37(5):1335–43.

54. Resnic FS, Wainstein M, Lee M, et al. No-reflow is an independent predictor of death and myocardial infarction after percutaneous coronary intervention. Am Heart J 2003;145(1):42–6.

Atherectomy Devices for the Treatment of Calcified Coronary Lesions

Jeffrey W. Chambers, MD[a],*, Ann N. Behrens, BS[b],
Brad J. Martinsen, PhD[b]

KEYWORDS

- Atherectomy • Calcification • Coronary artery disease • Angioplasty • Coronary
- Orbital atherectomy • Percutaneous coronary intervention • Stents

---

KEY POINTS

- An indicator of advanced coronary artery disease is the presence of coronary artery calcification (CAC).
- Advanced age, diabetes mellitus, and chronic kidney disease are important risks factors for CAC.
- Calcified coronary lesions are challenging to treat and have increased acute complications and worse long-term outcomes.
- Atherectomy can be used to modify the calcified plaque to facilitate percutaneous coronary intervention.

INTRODUCTION

Coronary artery disease (CAD) affects more than 16 million subjects in the United States, making it the most common form of heart disease. An indicator of advanced CAD is the presence of coronary artery calcification (CAC) and the extent of calcification strongly correlates with the degree of atherosclerosis and, therefore, with the rate of future cardiac events.[1–3] Percutaneous coronary intervention (PCI) in severely calcified lesions is associated with lower success rates, higher complication rates, and worse long-term outcomes compared with noncalcified lesions.[4–6]

PREVALENCE OF AND RISK FACTORS FOR CORONARY ARTERY CALCIFICATION

The prevalence of moderate/severe CAC in the PCI patient population is 32%, of which 5.9% is considered severe.[4] Several health behaviors and risk factors, as well as chronic inflammatory conditions, lead to calcium deposition in the coronary arteries.[1,6–8] Key factors include:

- Smoking and tobacco use;
- Physical inactivity;
- Obesity;
- Advanced age;
- Family history;
- Hyperlipidemia;
- Hypertension;
- Diabetes mellitus;
- The metabolic syndrome; and
- Chronic kidney disease.

These conditions cause endothelial injury and subsequent cell dysfunction, escalating an inflammatory response from leukocytes and vascular smooth muscle cells which leads to

---

Conflict of Interest: J.W. Chambers receives consulting fees from Cardiovascular Systems, Inc. A.N. Behrens and B.J. Martinsen are employees of Cardiovascular Systems, Inc.
a Metropolitan Heart and Vascular Institute, The Heart Center, Mercy Hospital, Suite 120, 4040 Coon Rapids Boulevard, Minneapolis, MN 55433, USA; b Science & Research Department, Cardiovascular Systems, Inc, 1225 Old Highway 8 NW, St Paul, MN 55112, USA
* Corresponding author.
E-mail address: J.Chambers@mhvi.com

calcium deposition in the intimal and medial layers of arterial walls.[6,9,10] Many of these risks are increasing in the United States, including diabetes and obesity; therefore, CAC is becoming a greater issue for interventional cardiologists.[7]

IMPACT OF CALCIUM ON PERCUTANEOUS CORONARY INTERVENTION OUTCOMES

The presence of CAC may lead to:

- Unsuccessful PCI owing to undilatable lesions[11,12];
- Balloon ruptures[12,13];
- Coronary dissection[11];
- Coronary perforation or rupture[14,15];
- Asymmetric, malapposed, and underexpanded stents[13,16];
- Higher incidence of major adverse cardiac events (MACE)[17];
- Higher incidence of restenosis and target lesion revascularization[18];
- Higher incidence of periprocedural myocardial infarction (MI)[19]; and
- Higher incidence of stent thrombosis.[20]

Coronary perforation or rupture, albeit rare, remains one of the most serious complications in the catheterization laboratory, with multiple studies demonstrating very poor outcomes, particularly in relationship to cardiac tamponade, MI, and death.[15] In the general CAD population (all lesion types), coronary perforation has been reported in 0.1% to 3.0% of lesions treated with various interventional techniques.[15,21] Elderly, female patients and those with CAC are at greatest risk.[15]

The current standard of care for treating patients with severe and symptomatic CAD is PCI with a drug-eluting stent (DES). The use of DES in severely calcified coronary lesions results in worse outcomes compared with patients with noncalcified lesions.[4,22,23]

ATHERECTOMY TREATMENT OPTIONS FOR CALCIFIED CORONARY ARTERIES

Atherectomy devices have been used for vessel preparation before PCI in calcified coronary lesions. These devices can facilitate successful stent implantation that may otherwise not be possible. Commercially available coronary atherectomy devices currently include:

- Rotational atherectomy (RA; Rotablator, Boston Scientific, Marlborough, MA);
- Orbital atherectomy system (OAS; Diamondback 360, Cardiovascular Systems, Inc, St Paul, MN); and
- Laser atherectomy (Spectranetics, Colorado Springs, CO).

A comparison of these atherectomy devices in regards to mechanism of action, clinical indication, and technical features is shown in Table 1. We present the clinical data from a controlled literature search of the past 5 years of coronary atherectomy in de novo, severely calcified lesions.

Rotational Atherectomy

The clinical data from RA (studies with ≥150 patients) for the past 5 years are summarized in Table 2. One publication includes clinical data regarding RA from a prospective, randomized, multicenter clinical trial (Rotational Atherectomy prior to Taxus Stent Treatment for Complex Native Coronary Artery Disease [ROTAXUS]).[24] Acute gain was higher in the RA group. However, late lumen loss in the RA plus DES group was significantly higher than the DES alone group at 9 months follow-up (0.44 ± 0.58 vs 0.31 ± 0.52 mm; $P = .04$). The 12.5% crossover rate from the DES alone to RA indicates the need for atherectomy in certain complex calcified coronary lesions.

In RA studies reporting 12-month results, the MACE rates ranged from 12% to 23.5%.[25–27] One retrospective study not included in Table 2 reported on 221 consecutive patients at a single center who underwent RA and stenting to assess clinical outcomes stratifying by the age, creatinine, and ejection fraction (ACEF) and the clinical Synergy between Percutaneous Coronary Intervention with TAXUS and Cardiac Surgery (SYNTAX) score.[28] At 1 year, the MACE rate, defined as cardiac death, MI, and target vessel revascularization ranged from 9% to 24% by the ACEF score and 8% to 25% by the clinical SYNTAX score.

The current PCI guidelines state that RA is reasonable for fibrotic or heavily calcified lesions that might not be crossed by a balloon catheter or adequately dilated before stent implantation (class IIa level of evidence C).[14]

Orbital Atherectomy

Two clinical studies were performed with the coronary OAS in the past 5 years (Table 3). The pilot study to evaluate the safety and performance of the Orbital Atherectomy System in treating de novo calcified coronary lesions (ORBIT I) was a prospective, nonrandomized clinical trial that was conducted in 2 centers in India to assess the safety of using the OAS in de novo calcified coronary lesions in 50 subjects.[29] Device success (≤50% residual stenosis after

Table 1
Coronary atherectomy device comparison

Rotational Atherectomy Rotablator	Coronary Orbital Atherectomy System Diamondback 360 (Classic)	Coronary Laser Atherectomy Catheter ELCA
Mechanism of action		
Rotational	Orbital	Laser
Diamond-tipped burr spins concentrically on the wire	Eccentrically mounted diamond-coated crown uses centrifugal force to orbit	Multifiber laser catheters transmit ultraviolet energy
Atheroablation via sanding/abrasion	Atheroablation via sanding/abrasion	Photoablation (vaporization)
Clinical indication		
A sole therapy or with adjunctive balloon angioplasty is indicated in patients with coronary artery disease who are acceptable candidates for coronary artery bypass graft surgery	To facilitate stent delivery in patients with coronary artery disease who are acceptable candidates for PTCA or stenting owing to de novo, severely calcified coronary artery lesions OAS is approved by the US FDA for the treatment of de novo, severely calcified lesions in the coronary arteries	A standalone modality or in conjunction with PTCA in patients who are acceptable candidates for coronary artery bypass graft surgery o Moderately calcified lesions o In-stent restenosis of stainless steel stents
Technical features		
Front-cutting, monodirectional burr	Diamond coated crown, bidirectional treatment	Over the wire and rapid exchange catheters
Multiple burr sizes (8) 1.25–2.5 mm	1.25 mm classic crown orbits to treat larger diameter	Available with concentric and eccentric tip designs
0.009″/0.014″ tip RotaWire guide wires	0.012″/0.014″ tip ViperWire advance coronary guide wire	0.014″ guidewire
Power source: pneumatic system, requires console, foot pedal and compressed gas supply; nitrogen tank or room air	Power source: electronic system able to be placed on the operating field connects to a specialized saline pump	Power source: Spectranetics CVX-300 requires console and foot pedal
Speed: 140–180 krpm during treatment	Speeds: 80 and 120 krpm	Adjustable laser energy settings

Abbreviations: FDA, Food and Drug Administration; OAS, orbital atherectomy system; PTCA, percutaneous transluminal coronary angioplasty.

OAS treatment) occurred in 98% of patients. Angiographic complications included 6 dissections (types A–C) and 1 perforation. The MACE rates at 30-days and 6 months were 6% and 8%, respectively. Long-term follow-up was collected at a single center (n = 33). The MACE rates at 3 and 5 years were 18.2% and 21.2%, respectively.[30,31]

The ORBIT II trial evaluated the use of the coronary OAS to prepare de novo, severely calcified coronary lesions for stent placement (see Table 3). It was a prospective, single-arm, multicenter clinical trial which prospectively enrolled 443 consecutive patients at 49 US sites from May 25, 2010 to November 26, 2012. Stents were successfully delivered 97.7% of the time.[32] The primary safety endpoint was freedom from MACE at 30 days, which occurred in 89.6% of patients compared with the performance goal of 83% (95% CI, 86.7%–92.5%).[32] The 1-year MACE rate was 16.4%, including cardiac death (3.0%), MI (9.7%), and target vessel revascularization (5.9%). The 1-year target lesion revascularization rate was 4.7%, and stent thrombosis occurred in 1 patient (0.2%)[33] (Table 4).

Table 2
Recent Rotablator clinical study evidence

Publication	Couper et al[25] 2015	Jinnouchi et al[26] 2015	Nishida et al[44] 2013	Jiang et al[45] 2012	Naito et al[46] 2012		Abdel-Wahab et al[47] 2013	Abdel-Wahab et al[24] 2013	Mangiacapra et al[27] 2012		Dardas et al[48] 2011	Schwartz et al[49] 2011
Treatment	RA + stent	RA + DES	RA + DES	RA + DES	RA + SES	RA + PES	RA + DES	RA + DES	RA + BMS	RA + DES	RA + DES	RA + stent
No. of patients	167	252	268[a]	115[b]	179	54	205	120	83	104	184	158
Dissection (%)	6.1	2.6	—	1.2	2.2	0	—	3.3	—	—	—	4.2
No reflow/slow flow (%)	4.4	1.5	—	2.0	—	—	1.9	0	—	—	—	2.1
Perforation (%)	0	1.8	—	0.8	0.6	0	—	1.7	—	—	—	0.8
In-hospital MACE (%)	4.8	—	—	—	—	—	4.4	4.2	—	—	—	5.7
Death (%)	1.8	—	—	0.8	—	—	—	1.7	—	—	—	3.2
MI (%)	1.8	2.2	—	1.2	0.6	3.7	—	1.7	—	—	—	1.9
TVR (%)	0	—	—	0	—	—	—	0.8	—	—	—	0.6 (CABG)
Long-term follow-up	12 mo	12 mo	5 y	3 y	630 d	625 d	15 mo	9 mo	12 mo	12 mo	49 mo	—
MACE at follow-up (%)	15.6	16.4	22.2	67.9	14.8	13.7	17.7	24.2	23.5	12	14.85	—
Death (%)	6.6	6.7	2.9	17.3	7.4	3.9	4.4	5.0	—	—	3.8	—
MI (%)	4.2	1.2	—	—	2.5	2.0	3.4	6.7	—	—	3.2	—
TVR (%)	7.8	21.3	17.7 (TLR)	54.7 (TLR)	6.8	11.8	9.9	16.7	12.3	5	3.25	—
Stent thrombosis at follow-up (%)	—	2.1	2.1	6.2	1.9	—	0.5	0.8	4.9	3	—	—

Based on studies with >150 patients during the past 5 years.
Data not reported (—).
Abbreviations: BMS, bare metal stent; CABG, coronary artery bypass graft; DES, drug eluting stent; MACE, major adverse cardiac events; MI, myocardial infarction; PES, paclitaxel eluting stent; RA, rotational atherectomy; SES, sirolimus eluting stent; TLR, target lesion revascularization; TVR, target vessel revascularization.
[a] Nonhemodialysis patients.
[b] Hemodialysis patients.
Data from Refs.[24–27,44–49]

Table 3
Orbital atherectomy clinical study evidence

Publication	Parikh et al,[29] 2013	ORBIT I		ORBIT II	
		Bhatt et al,[30] 2014	Bhatt et al,[31] 2015	Chambers et al,[32] 2014	Genereux et al,[33] 2015
Treatment	OAS + DES	OAS + DES	OAS + DES	OAS + BMS/DES	OAS + BMS/DES
No. of patients	50	33[a]	33[a]	443	443
Dissection (%)	12[b]	—	—	3.4[c]	—
No reflow/slow flow (%)	0	—	—	0.9	—
Perforation (%)	2	—	—	1.8	—
In-hospital MACE (%)	4	6.1	6.1	9.8	—
Cardiac death (%)	0	0	0	0.2	—
MI (%)	4	6.1	6.1	9.3	—
TVR (%)	—	—	—	0.7	—
Long-term follow-up	6 mo	3 y	5 y	30 d	1 y
MACE at follow-up (%)	8	18.2	21.2	10.4	16.4
Cardiac death (%)	2	9.1	12.1	0.2	3.0
MI (%)	6	6.1	6.1	9.7	9.7
TVR/TLR (%)	—	—	—	1.4	5.9
TLR (%)	2	3	3	0.7	4.7

Data not reported (—).

Abbreviations: BMS, bare metal stent; DES, drug eluting stent; MACE, major adverse cardiac events; MI, myocardial infarction; ORBIT, Evaluate the Safety and Efficacy of OAS in Treating Severely Calcified Coronary Lesions; TLR, target lesion revascularization; TVR, target vessel revascularization.

[a] Patients enrolled at single-center in ORBIT I study.
[b] Dissection type A–C.
[c] Dissection type C–F.
Data from Refs.[29–33]

Table 4
ORBIT II 1-year revascularization rates compared with drug-eluting stent literature

Stent Type	1-y TLR	TVR
ORBIT II–all stent types[33]	4.7%	1.9%[a]
ORBIT II–DES only[33]	3.4%	1.6%[a]
ROTAXUS–RA + DES[24]	11.7%[b]	16.7%[b]
DES randomized trials including severe calcium	0.0%–7.8%[50–66]	0.7%–7.6%[50–62]

Note: Based on literature review from 2003/07/01 to 2013/06/27.
  Abbreviations: DES, drug eluting stent; ORBIT, Evaluate the Safety and Efficacy of OAS in Treating Severely Calcified Coronary Lesions; RA, rotational atherectomy; TLR, target lesion revascularization; TVR, target vessel revascularization.
  [a] TVR remote (TVR non-TLR).
  [b] Rate at 9 months.

Laser Atherectomy

Early studies reported inconsistent results when laser atherectomy was used to treat CAC. The majority of studies demonstrated a higher incidence of complications including dissection and perforation and no difference in the clinic outcomes.[34–43] Two studies found increased restenosis or target lesion revascularization in calcified lesions.[35,42]

In the controlled literature search of the past 5 years of coronary atherectomy in de novo, severely calcified lesions, 1 study of laser atherectomy in severely calcified lesions was identified. In a retrospective, single-center study of excimer laser coronary atherectomy treatment followed by DES in 25 patients with de novo, severely calcified coronary lesions, procedural complications included no reflow (8.0%) and perforation (4.0%).[43] No patient experienced a dissection, thrombus, major bleeding, or periprocedural MI. The angiographic success rate was 84%, defined as less than 50% final residual stenosis.

One of the current applications of laser atherectomy is to ablate calcium beneath underexpanded stents to allow complete expansion.[37]

SUMMARY

The presence of moderate and severe CAC is associated with higher rates of angiographic complications during PCI, as well as higher MACE rates compared with noncalcified lesions. There are clearly situations where PCI is not feasible in heavily calcified lesions owing to the inability to deliver or fully expand the stent. Appropriate identification of CAC and use of atherectomy may improve procedural outcomes especially in those with severe CAC. Additional randomized trials are needed to further clarify which patients will benefit from plaque modification with atherectomy.

REFERENCES

1. Lee MS, Shah N. The impact and pathophysiologic consequences of coronary artery calcium deposition in percutaneous coronary interventions. J Invasive Cardiol 2015. [Epub ahead of print].
2. Mintz GS. Intravascular imaging of coronary calcification and its clinical implications. JACC Cardiovasc Imaging 2015;8:461–71.
3. Polonsky TS, McClelland RL, Jorgensen NW, et al. Coronary artery calcium score and risk classification for coronary heart disease prediction. JAMA 2010; 303:1610–6.
4. Genereux P, Madhavan MV, Mintz GS, et al. Ischemic outcomes after coronary intervention of calcified vessels in acute coronary syndromes: pooled analysis from the HORIZONS-AMI (Harmonizing Outcomes with Revascularization and Stents in Acute Myocardial Infarction) and ACUITY (Acute Catheterization and Urgent Intervention Triage Strategy) trials. J Am Coll Cardiol 2014;63:1845–54.
5. Chambers JW, Diage T. Evaluation of the diamondback 360 coronary orbital atherectomy system for treating de novo, severely calcified lesions. Expert Rev Med Devices 2014;11(5):457–66.
6. Leopold JA. Vascular calcification: mechanisms of vascular smooth muscle cell calcification. Trends Cardiovasc Med 2015;25:267–74.
7. Mozaffarian D, Benjamin EJ, Go AS, et al, American Heart Association Statistics Committee and Stroke Statistics Subcommittee. Heart disease and stroke statistics–2015 update: a report from the American Heart Association. Circulation 2015;131:e29–322.
8. Madhavan MV, Tarigopula M, Mintz GS, et al. Coronary artery calcification: pathogenesis and prognostic implications. J Am Coll Cardiol 2014; 63:1703–14.
9. Bentzon JF, Otsuka F, Virmani R, et al. Mechanisms of plaque formation and rupture. Circ Res 2014; 114:1852–66.
10. Otsuka F, Sakakura K, Yahagi K, et al. Has our understanding of calcification in human coronary

atherosclerosis progressed? Arterioscler Thromb Vasc Biol 2014;34:724–36.

11. Schlüter M, Cosgrave J, Tübler T, et al. Rotational atherectomy to enable sirolimus-eluting stent implantation in calcified, nondilatable de novo coronary artery lesions. Vasc Dis Manag 2007;4:63–9.

12. Cavusoglu E, Kini AS, Marmur JD, et al. Current status of rotational atherectomy. Catheter Cardiovasc Interv 2004;62:485–98.

13. Moussa I, Di Mario C, Moses J, et al. Coronary stenting after rotational atherectomy in calcified and complex lesions. Angiographic and clinical follow-up results. Circulation 1997;96:128–36.

14. Levine GN, Bates ER, Blankenship JC, et al. 2011 ACCF/AHA/SCAI guideline for percutaneous coronary intervention. A report of the American College of Cardiology Foundation/American Heart Association Task Force on Practice Guidelines and the Society for Cardiovascular Angiography and Interventions. J Am Coll Cardiol 2011;58:e44–122.

15. Colombo A, Stankovic G. Coronary perforations: old screenplay, new actors! J Invasive Cardiol 2004;16:302–3.

16. Moussa I, Ellis SG, Jones M, et al. Impact of coronary culprit lesion calcium in patients undergoing paclitaxel-eluting stent implantation (a TAXUS-IV sub study). Am J Cardiol 2005;96:1242–7.

17. Mosseri M, Satler LF, Pichard AD, et al. Impact of vessel calcification on outcomes after coronary stenting. Cardiovasc Revasc Med 2005;6:147–53.

18. Onuma Y, Tanimoto S, Ruygrok P, et al. Efficacy of everolimus eluting stent implantation in patients with calcified coronary culprit lesions: two-year angiographic and three-year clinical results from the SPIRIT II study. Catheter Cardiovasc Interv 2010;76:634–42.

19. Clavijo LC, Steinberg DH, Torguson R, et al. Sirolimus-eluting stents and calcified coronary lesions: clinical outcomes of patients treated with and without rotational atherectomy. Catheter Cardiovasc Interv 2006;68:873–8.

20. Benezet J, Diaz de la Llera LS, Cubero JM, et al. Drug-eluting stents following rotational atherectomy for heavily calcified coronary lesions: long-term clinical outcomes. J Invasive Cardiol 2011;23:28–32.

21. Rogers JH, Lasala JM. Coronary artery dissection and perforation complicating percutaneous coronary intervention. J Invasive Cardiol 2004;16:493–9.

22. Serruys PW, van Hout B, Bonnier H, et al. Randomised comparison of implantation of heparin-coated stents with balloon angioplasty in selected patients with coronary artery disease (Benestent II). Lancet 1998;352:673–81.

23. Pinto DS, Stone GW, Ellis SG, et al. Impact of routine angiographic follow-up on the clinical benefits of paclitaxel-eluting stents: results from the TAXUS-IV trial. J Am Coll Cardiol 2006;48:32–6.

24. Abdel-Wahab M, Richardt G, Joachim Buttner H, et al. High-speed rotational atherectomy before paclitaxel-eluting stent implantation in complex calcified coronary lesions: the randomized ROTAXUS (Rotational Atherectomy prior to Taxus Stent Treatment for Complex Native Coronary Artery Disease) trial. JACC Cardiovasc Interv 2013;6:10–9.

25. Couper LT, Loane P, Andrianopoulos N, et al, Melbourne Interventional Group (MIG) Investigators. Utility of rotational atherectomy and outcomes over an eight-year period. Catheter Cardiovasc Interv 2015;86(4):626–31.

26. Jinnouchi H, Kuramitsu S, Shinozaki T, et al. Two-year clinical outcomes of newer-generation drug-eluting stent implantation following rotational atherectomy for heavily calcified lesions. Circ J 2015;79(9):1938–43.

27. Mangiacapra F, Heyndrickx GR, Puymirat E, et al. Comparison of drug-eluting versus bare-metal stents after rotational atherectomy for the treatment of calcified coronary lesions. Int J Cardiol 2012;154:373–6.

28. Pyxaras SA, Mangiacapra F, Wijns W, et al. ACEF and clinical SYNTAX score in the risk stratification of patients with heavily calcified coronary stenosis undergoing rotational atherectomy with stent implantation. Catheter Cardiovasc Interv 2014;83:1067–73.

29. Parikh K, Chandra P, Choksi N, et al. Safety and feasibility of orbital atherectomy for the treatment of calcified coronary lesions: the ORBIT I trial. Catheter Cardiovasc Interv 2013;81:1134–9.

30. Bhatt P, Parikh P, Patel A, et al. Orbital atherectomy system in treating calcified coronary lesions: 3-year follow-up in first human use study (ORBIT I Trial). Cardiovasc Revasc Med 2014;15(4):204–8.

31. Bhatt P, Parikh P, Patel A, et al. Long-term safety and performance of the orbital atherectomy system for treating calcified coronary artery lesions: 5-year follow-up in the ORBIT I trial. Cardiovasc Revasc Med 2015;16:213–6.

32. Chambers JW, Feldman RL, Himmelstein SI, et al. Pivotal trial to evaluate the safety and efficacy of the orbital atherectomy system in treating de novo, severely calcified coronary lesions (ORBIT II). JACC Cardiovasc Interv 2014;7:510–8.

33. Généreux P, Lee AC, Kim CY, et al. Orbital atherectomy for treating de novo severely calcified coronary narrowing (1-year results from the pivotal ORBIT II trial). Am J Cardiol 2015;115:1685–90.

34. Topaz O. Plaque removal and thrombus dissolution with the photoacoustic energy of pulsed-wave lasers-biotissue interactions and their clinical manifestations. Cardiology 1996;87:384–91.

35. Bittl JA, Sanborn TA, Tcheng JE, et al. Clinical success, complications and restenosis rates with excimer laser coronary angioplasty. The percutaneous excimer laser coronary angioplasty registry. Am J Cardiol 1992;70:1533–9.

36. Mintz GS, Kovach JA, Javier SP, et al. Mechanisms of lumen enlargement after excimer laser coronary angioplasty. An intravascular ultrasound study. Circulation 1995;92:3408–14.

37. Fernandez JP, Hobson AR, McKenzie D, et al. Beyond the balloon: excimer coronary laser atherectomy used alone or in combination with rotational atherectomy in the treatment of chronic total occlusions, non-crossable and non-expansible coronary lesions. EuroIntervention 2013;9:243–50.

38. Ghazzal ZM, Hearn JA, Litvack F, et al. Morphological predictors of acute complications after percutaneous excimer laser coronary angioplasty. Results of a comprehensive angiographic analysis: importance of the eccentricity index. Circulation 1992; 86:820–7.

39. Baumbach A, Oswald H, Kvasnicka J, et al. Clinical results of coronary excimer laser angioplasty: report from the European coronary excimer laser angioplasty registry. Eur Heart J 1994;15:89–96.

40. Reifart N, Vandormael M, Krajcar M, et al. Randomized comparison of angioplasty of complex coronary lesions at a single center. Excimer laser, rotational atherectomy, and balloon angioplasty comparison (ERBAC) study. Circulation 1997;96:91–8.

41. Stone GW, de Marchena E, Dageforde D, et al. Prospective, randomized, multicenter comparison of laser-facilitated balloon angioplasty versus stand-alone balloon angioplasty in patients with obstructive coronary artery disease. The laser angioplasty versus angioplasty (LAVA) trial investigators. J Am Coll Cardiol 1997;30:1714–21.

42. Appelman YE, Piek JJ, Redekop WK, et al. Clinical events following excimer laser angioplasty or balloon angioplasty for complex coronary lesions: subanalysis of a randomised trial. Heart 1998;79:34–8.

43. Badr S, Ben-Dor I, Dvir D, et al. The state of the excimer laser for coronary intervention in the drug-eluting stent era. Cardiovasc Revasc Med 2013;14:93–8.

44. Nishida K, Kimura T, Kawai K, et al. Comparison of outcomes using the sirolimus-eluting stent in calcified versus non-calcified native coronary lesions in patients on- versus not on-chronic hemodialysis (from the j-cypher registry). Am J Cardiol 2013;112:647–55.

45. Jiang J, Sun Y, Xiang M, et al. Complex coronary lesions and rotational atherectomy: one hospital's experience. J Zhejiang Univ Sci B 2012;13:645–51.

46. Naito R, Sakakura K, Wada H, et al. Comparison of long-term clinical outcomes between sirolimus-eluting stents and paclitaxel-eluting stents following rotational atherectomy. Int Heart J 2012;53:149–53.

47. Abdel-Wahab M, Baev R, Dieker P, et al. Long-term clinical outcome of rotational atherectomy followed by drug-eluting stent implantation in complex calcified coronary lesions. Catheter Cardiovasc Interv 2013;81:285–91.

48. Dardas P, Mezilis N, Ninios V, et al. The use of rotational atherectomy and drug-eluting stents in the treatment of heavily calcified coronary lesions. Hellenic J Cardiol 2011;52:399–406.

49. Schwartz BG, Mayeda GS, Economides C, et al. Rotational atherectomy in the drug-eluting stent era: a single-center experience. J Invasive Cardiol 2011;23:133–9.

50. Kedhi E, Joesoef KS, McFadden E, et al. Second-generation everolimus-eluting and paclitaxel-eluting stents in real-life practice (COMPARE): a randomised trial. Lancet 2010;375:201–9.

51. Maresta A, Varani E, Balducelli M, et al, DESSERT Investigators. Comparison of effectiveness and safety of sirolimus-eluting stents versus bare-metal stents in patients with diabetes mellitus (from the Italian multicenter randomized DESSERT Study). Am J Cardiol 2008;101:1560–6.

52. Kim W-J, Lee S-W, Park S-W, et al, ESSENCE-DIABETES Study Investigators. Randomized comparison of everolimus-eluting stent versus sirolimus-eluting stent implantation for de novo coronary artery disease in patients with diabetes mellitus (ESSENCE-DIABETES): results from the ESSENCE-DIABETES trial. Circulation 2011;124: 886–92.

53. Sabate M, Cequier A, Iñiguez A, et al. Everolimus-eluting stent versus bare-metal stent in ST-segment elevation myocardial infarction (EXAMINATION): 1 year results of a randomised controlled trial. Lancet 2012;380:1482–90.

54. Park KW, Chae I-H, Lim D-S, et al. Everolimus-eluting versus sirolimus-eluting stents in patients undergoing percutaneous coronary intervention: the EXCELLENT (efficacy of xience/promus versus cypher to reduce late loss after stenting) randomized trial. J Am Coll Cardiol 2011;58: 1844–54.

55. Park D-W, Kim Y-H, Song H-G, et al. Comparison of everolimus- and sirolimus-eluting stents in patients with long coronary artery lesions: a randomized LONG-DES-III (percutaneous treatment of LONG native coronary lesions with drug-eluting stent-III) Trial. JACC Cardiovasc Interv 2011;4: 1096–103.

56. Atary JZ, van der Hoeven BL, Liem SS, et al. Three-year outcome of sirolimus-eluting versus bare-metal stents for the treatment of ST-segment elevation myocardial infarction (from the MISSION! intervention study). Am J Cardiol 2010;106:4–12.

57. Suttorp MJ, Laarman GJ, Rahel BM, et al. Primary Stenting of totally occluded native coronary arteries II (PRISON II): a randomized comparison of bare metal stent implantation with sirolimus-eluting stent implantation for the treatment of total coronary occlusions. Circulation 2006;114: 921–8.

58. Kimura T, Morimoto T, Natsuaki M, et al, RESET Investigators. Comparison of everolimus-eluting and sirolimus-eluting coronary stents: 1-year outcomes from the randomized evaluation of sirolimus-eluting versus everolimus-eluting stent trial (RESET). Circulation 2012;126:1225–36.

59. Stefanini GG, Serruys PW, Silber S, et al. The impact of patient and lesion complexity on clinical and angiographic outcomes after revascularization with zotarolimus- and everolimus-eluting stents: a substudy of the RESOLUTE all comers trial (a randomized comparison of a zotarolimus-eluting stent with an everolimus-eluting stent for percutaneous coronary intervention). J Am Coll Cardiol 2011;57:2221–32.

60. Menichelli M, Parma A, Pucci E, et al. Randomized trial of sirolimus-eluting stent versus bare-metal stent in acute myocardial infarction (SESAMI). J Am Coll Cardiol 2007;49:1924–30.

61. von Birgelen C, Basalus MWZ, Tandjung K, et al. A randomized controlled trial in second-generation zotarolimus-eluting resolute stents versus everolimus-eluting xience V stents in real-world patients: the TWENTE trial. J Am Coll Cardiol 2012;59:1350–61.

62. Park D-W, Kim Y-H, Yun S-C, et al. Comparison of zotarolimus-eluting stents with sirolimus- and paclitaxel-eluting stents for coronary revascularization: the ZEST (comparison of the efficacy and safety of zotarolimus-eluting stent with sirolimus-eluting and paclitaxel-eluting stent for coronary lesions) randomized trial. J Am Coll Cardiol 2010;56:1187–95.

63. Mehilli J, Kastrati A, Byrne RA, et al, LEFT-MAIN Intracoronary Stenting and Angiographic Results: Drug-Eluting Stents for Unprotected Coronary Left Main Lesions Study Investigators. Paclitaxel- versus sirolimus-eluting stents for unprotected left main coronary artery disease. J Am Coll Cardiol 2009;53:1760–8.

64. Kang WC, Ahn T, Lee K, et al. Comparison of zotarolimus-eluting stents versus sirolimus-eluting stents versus paclitaxel-eluting stents for primary percutaneous coronary intervention in patients with ST-elevation myocardial infarction: results from the Korean multicentre endeavor (KOMER) acute myocardial infarction (AMI) trial. EuroIntervention 2011;7:936–43.

65. Di Lorenzo E, De Luca G, Sauro R, et al. The PASEO (paclitaxel or sirolimus-eluting stent versus bare metal stent in primary angioplasty) randomized trial. JACC Cardiovasc Interv 2009;2:515–23.

66. Lee J-H, Kim H-S, Lee S-W, et al. Prospective randomized comparison of sirolimus- versus paclitaxel-eluting stents for the treatment of acute ST-elevation myocardial infarction: pROSIT trial. Catheter Cardiovasc Interv 2008;72:25–32.

Percutaneous Coronary Intervention for Bifurcation Lesions

Björn Redfors, MD, PhD[a,b], Philippe Généreux, MD[a,c,*]

KEYWORDS

- Percutaneous coronary intervention • Bifurcation • Coronary artery disease

---

KEY POINTS

- Bifurcation lesions are common (approximately 20% of all lesions treated with percutaneous coronary intervention [PCI]).
- Bifurcation PCI is associated with higher risk of complications.
- Careful assessment of the bifurcation lesion by invasive and noninvasive testing is important.
- The provisional 1-stent technique, that is, stenting of the main vessel (MV) with balloon dilatation of the side branch (SB), is preferred when possible.
- Two-stent techniques are necessary in up to 25% of cases and should be mastered.

 Video content accompanies this article at http://www.interventional.theclinics.com/

INTRODUCTION

More than 3 million PCIs are performed each year. Up to 20% of these procedures include a bifurcation lesion. Bifurcation lesions remain one of the most difficult lesion types to treat, and bifurcation PCI is associated with lower procedural success rates and a higher risk of adverse cardiac events.[1] The optimal management of bifurcation lesions remains a matter of considerable debate. This article summarizes current knowledge of bifurcation lesions and techniques used to treat these lesions.

DEFINITION AND CLASSIFICATIONS
Definition of Coronary Bifurcation Lesions
A coronary bifurcation lesion is defined as a narrowing (usually ≥50% angiographic diameter

stenosis) at, or adjacent (3–5 mm) to, the origin of a significant SB.[2] A significant SB can be defined by different criteria, including reference vessel diameter (ie, ≥2.5 mm by visual assessment) or subjectively as a branch that an operator does not want to compromise or lose, taking into consideration factors, such as myocardial area at risk, ischemia location, myocardial viability, patients symptoms, and so forth.

Classification of Coronary Bifurcation Lesions
Coronary bifurcation lesions are anatomically heterogenous and complex. An ideal classification system should be easy to remember, should reflect prognosis and technical difficulty of treating the lesion, and should differentiate between optimal treatment options. Several classifications have been developed for bifurcation lesions.

Disclosures: Institutional research grant from TRYTON medical, Cardiovascular System Inc, Boston Scientific; Consultant fees from Cardiovascular System Inc and Abbott Vascular (P. Généreux).
[a] Clinical Trial Center, Cardiovascular Research Foundation, 111 East 59th Street, New York, NY 10022, USA;
[b] Department of Cardiology, Sahlgrenska University Hospital, Bruna Straket 16, 413 45 Gothenburg, Sweden;
[c] Department of Cardiology, Hôpital du Sacré-Coeur de Montréal, Université de Montréal, 5400, boul. Gouin Ouest, Montréal, Québec H4J 1C5, Canada
* Corresponding author. Cardiovascular Research Foundation, 111 East 59th Street, 12th Floor, New York, NY 10022.
E-mail address: pgenereux@crf.org

Intervent Cardiol Clin 5 (2016) 153–175
http://dx.doi.org/10.1016/j.iccl.2015.12.011
2211-7458/16/$ – see front matter © 2016 Elsevier Inc. All rights reserved.

These include the Sanborn, Lefèvre, Safian, Duke, Medina, and Movahed classifications.[3–5] None of these classifications fully captures the nature of bifurcation lesions and none has gained full acceptance. The Medina classification is simple and has been the most widely adopted.[6] It assigns a binary score (1 if presence of lesion with ≥50% diameter stenosis [percent diameter stenosis (% DS)] and 0 if not) to each component of the bifurcation lesion in the following order: proximal segment, main distal segment, and SB.[7] The values are separated by commas (Fig. 1). A true bifurcation lesion is defined as any lesion involving both the MV, proximal or distal, and the ostium of the SB.[8] This corresponds to Medina classifications 1,1,1; 1,0,1; and 0,1,1.

The Medina classification is criticized for being too simple. Important parameters that are not captured by the Medina classification include vessel diameter, angulation, Thrombolysis In Myocardial Infarction (TIMI) flow grade, degree of calcification, and plaque distribution. In addition, adjunctive imaging and physiology diagnostic modalities, such as intravascular ultrasound (IVUS), optical coherence tomography (OCT), and fractional flow reserve (FFR), can add additional information.

The relationship between the diameters of the proximal MV, the distal MV, and the SB vessel is important when choosing stent size and/or type. The Huo and Kassab model has been shown to hold true for all bifurcation types (Table 1). This model is particularly useful when, for any reason, the reference diameter of 1 of the 3 vessel branches cannot be estimated directly.[9,10]

Anatomic characteristics of bifurcation lesions are incorporated into the Synergy Between PCI with Taxus and Cardiac Surgery (SYNTAX) score. The SYNTAX score was developed to characterize and objectively quantify the severity of coronary artery disease.[11–13] Bifurcation lesion is considered when all segments involved are of at least 1.5-mm vessel diameter and may involve the proximal MV, the distal MV, and the SB according to the Medina classification. Clinicians should score only the SYNTAX coronary segment numbers of the bifurcation that have a greater than or equal to 50% DS in direct contact with the bifurcation. The smaller of the 2 daughter branches should be designated as the SB. In cases of the main stem, either the left circumflex artery (LCX) or the left anterior descending coronary artery (LAD) can be designated as the SB depending on its respective calibers. A bifurcation where the SB has no lesion greater than or equal to 50% (ie, 1,0,0; 1,1,0; and 0,1,0) adds 1 point to the SYNTAX score; bifurcation with involvement of the SB (0,0,1; 0,1,1; 1,0,1; and 1,1,1) adds 2 points. Also included in the SYNTAX score for bifurcation is the presence of bifurcation angle less than 70°, which, if present, adds 1 additional point.

Classification of Stenting Techniques
Many stenting strategies and techniques exist for treating bifurcation lesions, and more are being

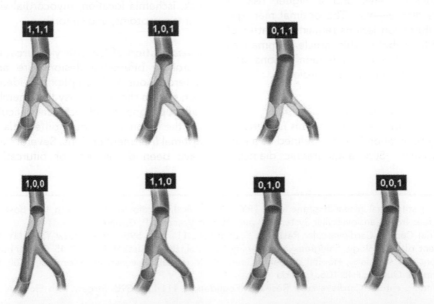

Fig. 1. Medina classification. Each segment is given a binary score depending on the presence (1) or absence (0) of a greater than 50% luminal stenosis. The mother segment is presented first, followed by the distal MV and then the SB.

Table 1
The Huo and Kassab model for determination of vessel diameter

Diameter of Smaller Daughter Vessel	Diameter of Larger Daughter Vessel							
(mm)	2.25	2.50	2.75	3.00	3.25	3.50	3.75	4.00
2.25	3.03	3.20	3.39	3.58	3.78	3.99	4.20	4.42
	Δ=0.78	Δ=0.70	0.64	Δ=0.53	Δ=0.49	Δ=0.45	Δ=0.42	Δ=0.42
2.50		3.36	3.54	3.72	3.91	4.11	4.32	4.53
		Δ=0.86	Δ=0.79	Δ=0.72	Δ=0.66	Δ=0.61	Δ=0.57	Δ=0.53
2.75			3.70	3.87	4.06	4.25	4.44	4.64
			Δ=0.95	Δ=0.87	Δ=0.81	Δ=0.75	Δ=0.69	Δ=0.64
3.00				4.04	4.21	4.39	4.58	4.77
				Δ=1.04	Δ=0.96	Δ=0.89	Δ=0.83	Δ=0.77
3.25					4.37	4.5	4.73	4.91
					Δ=1.12	Δ=1.05	Δ=0.98	Δ=0.91
3.50						4.71	4.88	5.06
						Δ=1.21	Δ=1.13	Δ=1.06
3.75							5.05	5.22
							Δ=1.30	Δ=1.22
4.00								5.38
								Δ=1.38

Blue and red colors represent the diameter of the mother segment and the stepwise difference.
The Huo and Kassab relationship between the diameters of the mother vessel segment, larger daughter vessel, and smaller daughter vessel for selected daughter vessel sizes (based on stent sizes in use).

developed. These are discussed later. Few classifications of these techniques have been published. The European Bifurcation Club endorses the main, across, distal, side (MADS) classification. The MADS classification, similar to the Medina classification, is easy to memorize.[14] It is based on the order of implantation and position of the stent(s) within the bifurcation (Fig. 2). Each stenting technique is grouped into any of 4 categories according to whether it begins with a stent in the proximal main segment (M); a stent in the MV, which extends beyond the bifurcation (A); stents in both the MV branch and the SB (double [D]); or a stent in the SB (S). The MADS classification does not describe balloon or wire techniques.

LESION CHARACTERISTICS AS PREDICTORS OF ADVERSE OUTCOME
Procedural Complications
Procedural complications are more common in patients with true bifurcation lesions (Medina 1,1,1; 1,0,1; or 0,1,1) than in patients with other types of bifurcation lesions.[15,16] Several other vessel characteristics have been postulated to influence the risk of SB occlusion in bifurcation PCI. These include preprocedural %DS of the SB, preprocedure %DS of the proximal MV, length of the

SB, and bifurcation angle. Clinical presentation (ie, acute coronary syndrome vs stable coronary artery disease) has also been shown to influence the risk of SB occlusion.[16,17] Dou and colleagues[18] recently developed the Risk prEdiction of Side branch OccLusion in coronary bifurcation interVEntion (RESOLVE) score for predicting the risk of periprocedural SB occlusion. The investigators identified 6 parameters that independently predicted SB occlusion: (1) plaque distribution; (2) TIMI flow in the MV prior to the intervention; (3) preprocedural %DS of the bifurcation core; (4) bifurcation angle; (5) diameter ratio between the MV and the SB; and (6) preprocedural %DS of the SB before stenting of the MV. Based on these parameters, they assigned each lesion a score of 0 to 43. They used the majority of their data set for constructing the score and subsequently validated the score in an independent smaller subset.[18] Flow can be restored in the majority of occluded SBs but up to one-third may remain occluded. Placing a wire in the SB facilitates recovery if it occludes.[16]

Long-term Adverse Events
Occlusion of large SBs (≥2.3 mm) is associated with higher risk of subsequent adverse events.[16]

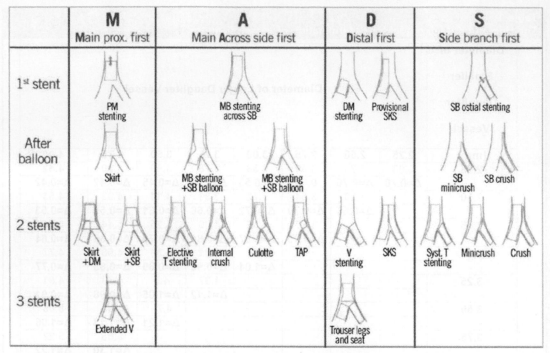

Fig. 2. MADS classification. Each treatment strategy is classified according to which segment is stented first and how many stents are used. Prox, proximal; Syst, systematic. (*From* Louvard Y, Thomas M, Dzavik V, et al. Classification of coronary artery bifurcation lesions and treatments: time for a consensus! Catheter Cardiovasc Interv 2008;71(2):175–83; with permission.)

In the Coronary Bifurcation Stenting (COBIS) registry, SB occlusion (including cases of flow subsequently restored) was associated with higher risk of cardiac death, stent thrombosis, and major adverse cardiac events (MACEs).[16] Data are inconclusive regarding the risk of occlusion of SBs with a diameter less than 2.3 mm due to low number of patients in these studies.[17,19]

Most studies that compared true bifurcation lesions to nontrue bifurcation lesions have not been powered for clinical events, but a recent nonrandomized observational study showed that treatment of true bifurcation lesions was associated with an increased risk of stent thrombosis, myocardial infarction, target vessel revascularization, and MACEs.[20] Death rate was also higher among patients with true bifurcation lesions. The groups were fairly well balanced regarding cardiovascular risk factors. Patients with true bifurcation lesions were more likely to have 3-vessel disease but were less likely to have left main (LM) lesions.[20]

The SYNTAX score, which incorporates information on the complexity of coronary lesions including bifurcation lesions, predicts the risk of MACEs in patients who undergo PCI or who are treated conservatively, regardless of clinical presentation.[12,21,22] The combination of the anatomic SYNTAX score with clinical parameters

(ie, the clinical SYNTAX score, logistic clinical SYNTAX score, or SYNTAX score II) further improves prediction of adverse events.[23–26]

TREATMENT OPTIONS

Randomized studies that have compared different treatment strategies for coronary bifurcation lesions are summarized in Table 2. This table also includes pivotal nonrandomized studies.

Main Vessel Stenting with Provisional Stenting of the Side Branch Versus Systematic Two-vessel Stenting

Several randomized controlled trials have compared MV stenting with systematic 2-vessel stenting in bifurcation lesions.[27–36] Most of these trials used first-generation drug-eluting stents (DESs). These trials, as well as analyses that pooled several trials, have shown superiority of the 1-stent provisional approach over systematic 2-vessel stenting,[37,38] with myocardial infarction and target vessel revascularizations more common with the systematic 2-vessel approach. Therefore, current guidelines recommend the 1-stent provisional approach as the initial approach in bifurcation PCI (class I, level of evidence A according to American College of

Table 2
Randomized trials and pivotal studies comparing treatment strategies in bifurcation percutaneous coronary intervention

Study, Year, Patients	Type	Months Clinical Follow-up/ Angiographic Follow-up	Stent Technique	Device	Primary Outcome	Primary Angiographic Outcome	Side Branch Reference Vessel Diameter (mm)	Minimal Luminal Diameter (mm)	In-stent Diameter Stenosis (%)	Late Loss (mm)
Colombo et al,[27] 2004, N = 85	RCT	6/6	2-Stent vs provisional	SES	Restenosis 28.0% vs 18.7%	—	2.1 vs 2.1	1.59 vs 1.42	29.4 vs 32.0	—
Pan et al,[28] 2004, N = 91	RCT	11/6	2-Stent vs provisional	RES	MACE	—	2.5 vs 2.5	1.73 vs 1.78	23 vs 18	—
Nordic,[29] 2006, N = 413	RCT	6/8	2-Stent vs provisional	SES	MACE/ST 3.5% vs 2.9%, P = NS	MV DS >50% and SB 100% 5.1% vs 5.3%, P = NS	2.6 vs 2.6	1.86 vs 1.52 P<.001	24 vs 31 P<.002	0.20 vs −0.04 P<.001
SCANDSTENT,[82] 2006, N = 126	RCT	6/6	2-Stent	SES vs BMS	—	MLD	2.2 vs 2.2	1.70 vs 1.19 P<.001	28.0 vs 45.1 P<.001	0.03 vs 0.56 P<.001
Adriaenssens et al,[83] 2008, N = 132	Obs	12/12	Culotte stenting	DES	MACE 26.5%	—	2.50	1.81	28.0	0.30
Ferenc et al,[31] 2008, N = 202	RCT	12/9	2-Stent vs provisional	SES	TVR 8.9% vs 10.9%	In-segment %DS 27.7 vs 23.0	—	1.98 vs 1.98 P = .65	23.4 vs 18.3 P = .15	0.32 vs 0.03 P = .005
DKCRUSH-1,[42] 2008, N = 311	RCT	8/8	DK crush vs crush	DES	MACE 24.4% vs 11.4, P = .02	—	2.45 vs 2.49 P<.5	0.83 vs 0.88 P = .4	22.6 vs 15.5 P = .04	36.6 vs 20.9 P = .01
CACTUS,[30] 2009, N = 350	RCT	6/6	Crush vs provisional	SES	MACE 15.8% vs 15% P = NS	In-segment restenosis 13.2% vs 14.7%, P = NS	2.30 vs 2.16 P<.05	1.66 vs 1.52 P<.05	30 vs 31 P = NS	0.29 vs 0.13 P = NS
BBC ONE,[32] 2010, N = 500	RCT	9	2-Stent vs provisional	PES	MACE 15.2% vs 8.0%	—	—	—	—	—

(continued on next page)

Study, Year, Patients	Type	Months Clinical Follow-up/ Angiographic Follow-up	Stent Technique	Device	Primary Outcome	Primary Angiographic Outcome	Side Branch Reference Vessel Diameter (mm)	Minimal Luminal Diameter (mm)	In-stent Diameter Stenosis (%)	Late Loss (mm)
NORDIC II,[73] 2009, N = 424	RCT	6/8	Crush vs culotte	SES	MACE/ST 4.3% vs 3.7%, P = .87	In-stent restenosis 10.5% vs 4.5%, P = .046	2.39 vs 2.38 P = .93	2.04 vs 2.08 P = .57	20.4 vs 17.3 P = .14	0.21 vs 0.20
NORDIC III,[53] 2011, N = 477	RCT	6/8	Final kiss vs no kiss	—	MACE/ST 2.1% vs 2.5%, P = 1.0	Binary restenosis rate 11.0% vs 17.3%, P = .11	2.31 vs 2.35 P = .59	1.74 vs 1.63 P = .06	25 vs 30 P = .009	−0.13 vs −0.10
DKCRUSH-II,[33] 2011, N = 370	RCT	12/8	DK crush vs provisional	—	MACE 10.3% vs 17.3%, P = .07	Angiorestenosis 4.9% vs 22.2%, P<.001	2.38 vs 2.29 P = .33	1.85 vs 1.43 P = .002	22.9 vs 32.2 P = .01	0.22 vs 0.18 P = .49
Garg et al,[84] 2011, N = 497	Post hoc	12/0	Variable	BES vs SES	MACE 12.8% vs 16.3%, P = .31	—	—	—	—	—
PEPCAD V,[85] 2011, N = 28	RCT	9/9	—	DEB	—	—	—	1.7	23	0.21
Pan et al,[86] 2012, N = 293	RCT	—	Provisional	SES vs EES	MACE 6.2% vs 6.1%, P = NS	—	2.4 vs 2.4	—	—	—

Trial	Design	Follow-up (mo)	Stent	Technique	Clinical outcome	Angiographic restenosis				
SMART-STRATEGY,[34] 2012, N = 258	RCT	12/9	SES and EES	2-Stent vs provisional	MACE 9.2% vs 9.4%, P = .97	—	2.49 vs 2.46 P = .64	1.57 vs 1.34 P = .004	37.0 vs 45.0 P = .001	0.23 vs 0.13 P = .08
NORDIC: 5 year,[35] 2013, N = 404	RCT	60/—	SES	2-Stent vs provisional	MACE 15.8% vs 21.8%, P = .15	—	—	—	—	—
DKCRUSH-III,[43] 2013, N = 419	RCT	12/8	DES	DK crush vs culotte	MACE 6.2% vs 16.3%, P<.05	In-stent restenosis 6.8% vs 12.6%, P = .04	—	—	—	—
Nordic Stent Technique,[44] 2013, N = 424	RCT	36/—	DES	Culotte vs crush	MACE 20.6% vs 16.7%, P = .32	—	2.77 vs 2.78 P = .77	—	—	—
COBIS registry,[87] 2014, N = 2044, non-LM cohort	Obs	36/—	DES	2-Stent vs provisional	TVF 8.0% vs 12.2%, P = .01	—	2.4 vs 2.4 P<.01	0.9 vs 0.9 P<.01	—	—
Tryton,[36] 2015, N = 704	RCT	9/9	BMS	Provisional vs Tryton bifurcation stent	TVF 17.4% vs 12.8%, P = .11	%DS 31.6% vs 38.6%, P = .002	2.25 vs 2.21 P = .09	0.95 vs 1.02 P<.01	31.6 vs 38.6 P<.01	0.48 vs 0.20

Late loss and binary restenosis are measured at follow-up.

Abbreviations: BES, biolimus-eluting stent; BMS, bare metal stent; DEB, drug-eluting balloon; DS, diameter stenosis; EES, everolimus-eluting stent; NS, Non-significent; Obs, observational; PES, paclitaxel-eluting stent; Post hoc, post hoc analysis of RCT data; RCT, randomized controlled trial; RES, rapamycin-eluting stent; SES, sirolimus-eluting stent; ST, stent thrombosis; TVF, target vessel failure; TVR, target vessel revascularization.

Data from Refs.[27–36,42–44,53,73,82–87]

Cardiology Foundation/American Heart Association/Society for Cardiovascular Angiography and Interventions 2011; and class IIB, level of evidence A in European Society of Cardiology/European Association for Cardio-Thoracic Surgery 2014).[39,40]

The superiority of the provisional 1-stent technique (Fig. 3) over systematic 2-vessel stenting is more evident with first-generation DESs than with second-generation DESs. Increasingly sophisticated stent designs, including thinner stent struts, may improve the results of 2-vessel

A

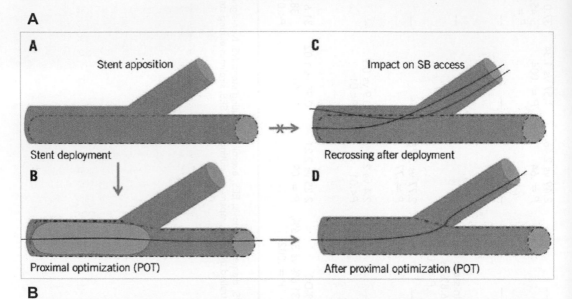

B

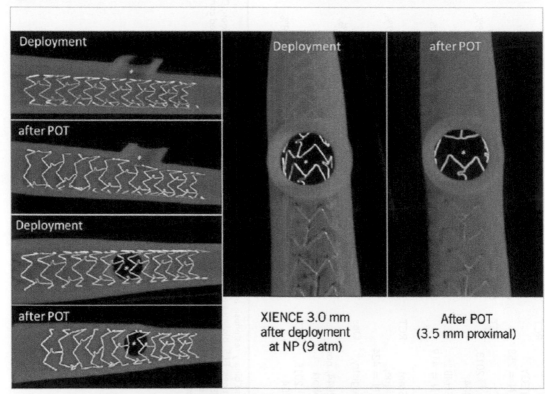

Fig. 3. The POT. (*A*) By expanding the proximal portion of the stent and creating an oblique angle to the SB, the POT facilitates SB access. (*B*) Illustration of the impact of the POT on stent apposition and SB access. (*Adapted from* Foin N, Sen S, Allegria E et al. Maximal expansion capacity with current DES platforms: a critical factor for stent selection in the treatment of left main bifurcations? EuroIntervention 2013;8:1315–25.)

stenting techniques. Recently, a dedicated stent specifically designed for bifurcation SB stenting (Fig. 4) was compared with the provisional 1-stent approach in a randomized trial. Similar to earlier trials, stenting of the SB was associated with higher risk of adverse events[36]; however, a subgroup analysis revealed that the dedicated Tryton bare metal stent was noninferior to the provisional approach in terms of adverse clinical events, with superior angiographic results in vessels with a diameter greater than or equal to 2.25 mm.[41] Hence, vessel characteristics influence the relative efficacy of provisional versus 2-vessel stenting approaches. Although dedicated bifurcation stent seems an attractive option for treating complex bifurcation involving large SB, provisional stenting should be the preferred approach for simple bifurcation lesion, especially when involving smaller SB.

Three randomized trials have compared different 2-vessel stenting techniques head to head. The Double-kissing double-crush (DKCRUSH-1) trial demonstrated superiority of the double kissing, double crush (DK crush) technique compared with the classic crush technique.[42] The DKCRUSH-III trial subsequently showed that the DK crush technique was superior

to the culotte technique for second-generation DES PCI of unprotected LM lesions.[43] The Nordic Stent Technique Study demonstrated similar outcomes with the classical crush technique and the culotte technique.[44] Given the heterogeneity and complexity of coronary bifurcation lesions, it is reasonable to assume that no 1-stenting technique is consistently superior for all types of bifurcation lesions.[6] Operator experience, accessibility of the SBs, and other factors should be considered when choosing between stenting techniques.[6] The different stent techniques are discussed later.

Bioresorbable Scaffolds

Bioresorbable scaffolds (BRSs) can restore vessel patency without implanting a permanent prosthesis.[45] This is an advantage over other stent types that may be particularly valuable in bifurcation lesions. An important drawback with current BRS designs is that they are thick and bulky.[45] This may counteract the potential benefits associated with BRSs in bifurcation PCI. Unfortunately, completed randomized trials of BRSs have excluded bifurcation lesions involving SB greater than or equal to 2 mm in diameter.[46] Data on BRSs in bifurcation lesions are, therefore, restricted to observational studies and

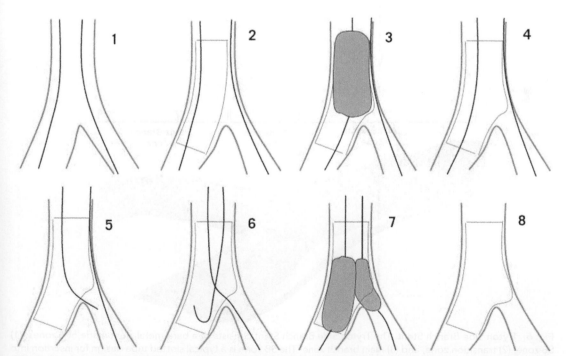

Fig. 4. Provisional stent technique. 1. Wiring of both the MV branch and the SB; 2. predilatation and stenting of the main branch; 3. POT; 4. stent apposition; 5. recrossing of the main branch guide wire through the most distal stent strut; 6. removing the jailed wire from the SB and placing it in the main branch with a loop; 7. final kissing balloon; and 8. end result. (*Adapted from* Louvard Y, Medina A. Definitions and classifications of bifurcation lesions and treatment. EuroIntervention 2015;11 Suppl V:V23–6.)

experimental data; however, these data are promising.[47] In their latest report, the European Bifurcation Club provided some guidance on the use of BRSs in bifurcation lesions but recognized the need for dedicated randomized trials.[6]

Dedicated Bifurcation Stents

Conventional stents are suboptimal for bifurcation PCI. Dedicated bifurcation stents aim to overcome shortcomings of conventional stents, including difficulties in maintaining access to the SB and risk of distortion of the MV stent with SB balloon dilation. Dedicated MV stents as well as SB stents have been developed. Observational data support the feasibility and efficacy of these dedicated stents[48,49]; however, only the Tryton Side Branch dedicated stent has been compared head to head with conventional therapy in a large randomized trial[36,41] (Fig. 5).

Kissing Balloon

Postimplantation kissing balloon inflation (ie, inflation of balloons in both the MV and the SB so that the proximal portions "kiss" at the bifurcation) has been commonly applied with the 1-stent provisional technique. The potential benefits of kissing balloon inflation include (1)

customizing the stent to the proximal MV (the proximal and distal portion of the MV have different dimensions, as illustrated by the Huo and Kassab model, discussed previously); (2) counteracting the shift of the carina toward the MV and distortion of the MV stent, which occurs with SB balloon dilation; and (3) improvement in postprocedural FFR.[50,51] Potential disadvantages include SB dissection and accidental stent crush.[52] Two randomized trials have compared postimplantation kissing balloon inflation to no kissing balloon inflation. Kissing balloon inflation in these trials did not improve outcomes.[53,54] These results led the European Bifurcation Club to recommend postimplantation kissing balloon inflation only for angiographically significant SB lesions (>75% DS or TIMI flow <3).[6] If, on the other hand, a 2-stent strategy is chosen, then postimplantation kissing balloon inflation is considered mandatory.[6]

The Proximal Optimization Technique

The proximal optimization technique (POT) uses a short oversized balloon to expand the proximal portion (almost up to the carina) of the MV stent.[55] This improves stent apposition in the MV and is particularly useful if the difference

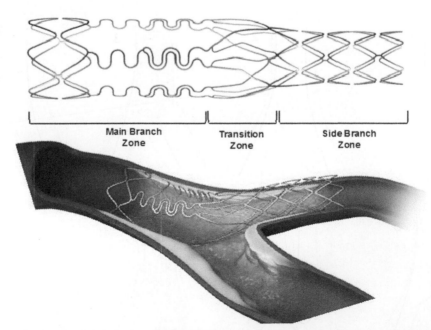

Fig. 5. Tryton Side Branch Stent. The Tryton Side Branch Stent consists of a bare metal stent made of 3 zones: (1) SB zone, (2) transition zone, and (3) main branch zone. The SB zone is a typical slotted tube design for insertion into the SB; the transition zone is composed of undulating struts designed to provide adequate radial strength and coverage throughout the carina; and the main branch zone has a minimal metal-to-artery ratio intended as an open path for a main branch stent. The implantation technique involves lesion preparation (predilatation of both main branch and SB), placement of the Tryton Side Branch Stent into the SB, and placement of a standard metallic DES (or BRS) within the main branch. Simultaneous or sequential final kissing balloon inflations are then performed.

between the proximal and distal reference vessel diameters is large. POT also facilitates SB access because of its oblique angle to the SB (see Fig. 3). It is, therefore, a useful technique when rewiring of the SB is difficult.[56] There is currently no consensus on whether POT should be part of routine bifurcation PCI but the European Bifurcation Cub recommends POT when (1) proximal and distal reference vessel diameters differ considerably and (2) when recrossing the wire into the SB is difficult. Use of the POT is also illustrated in Fig. 4, step 3.

Fractional Flow Reserve

FFR is increasingly used as an adjunctive diagnostic method to guide PCI and is recommended for patients with stable coronary artery disease who do not display objective evidence of ischemia.[57–59] It is reasonable to extrapolate these recommendations to the MV in bifurcation PCI. Routine FFR of the SB is more controversial. Studies using SB FFR have improved understanding of the relationship between a lesion's angiographic appearance and physiologic consequence[60,61]; however, for an individual, patient safety concerns may be too high and the interpretability of SB FFR recordings after MV stenting can be affected by local edema, plaque debris, and distal embolization.[50,62]

Quantitative Coronary Analysis and Intracoronary Imaging

Advances in quantitative coronary analysis (QCA), IVUS, and OCT may translate to better clinical outcomes after bifurcation PCI. Dedicated 2-D bifurcation QCA software improves measurement of vessel angulations.[63] 3-D QCA increases the accuracy of lumen measurement and allows for calculation of the optimal projection angle[64,65]; however, use of real-time QCA for guiding bifurcation PCI has not been studied.

Both IVUS and OCT can detect stent underexpansion, dissection, or malapposition. IVUS use has been shown to improve postimplantation lumen diameters in both the MV and the SB and has been associated with lower rates of myocardial infarction and cardiac death.[66] Routine OCT after bifurcation PCI detected at least 1 complication in each of 55 bifurcation lesions[67]; however, IVUS and/or OCT catheters may cause complications, including stent distortion or fracture. In a jailed SB, this risk may be considerable.[68] No randomized trial has compared OCT or IVUS to angiography alone in bifurcation PCI. Judicious use of IVUS or OCT for bifurcation PCI is recommended by the European Bifurcation Club for (1) assessment

of the SB ostium when segments are overlapping on angiography, (2) evaluation of wire positions, and (3) evaluation of optimal vessel and stent dimensions.[6]

STENTING TECHNIQUES

As discussed previously, the provisional 1-stent technique is associated with lower rates of adverse events than systematic 2-stent techniques. When 2-vessel stenting is necessary, the most appropriate technique varies depending on factors, such as plaque distribution (Medina classification), lesion location (ostium, midshaft, or distal involving bifurcation), bifurcation angulation, and operator experience and expertise. This section reviews the most commonly used techniques.

Provisional Stent Technique

The provisional stent technique involves the initial placement of a single stent in the MV[69] (see Fig. 4; Fig. 6, Videos 1–6).

The steps are as follows (see Fig. 4):

1. Wiring the MV and SB
2. Balloon predilatation of the MV and SB (SB optional)
3. Stenting MV with both wires in place
4. Assessment of SB integrity: consider whether balloon angioplasty or stenting is required. If the stenosis is less than 50%, without good flow and without dissection, SB treatment may be deferred. Otherwise, intervention is usually performed, most frequently balloon angioplasty first to achieve an acceptable result. Stenting may be required in approximately 20% of cases (although the threshold varies by operator from <10% to >30%) if TIMI flow is less than 3 or there is severe ostial compromise (>80% stenosis), threatened SB closure, dissection type greater than or equal to B, or FFR less than 0.75. Placement of a second stent in the SB may be done by T stent, T-stenting and small protrusion (TAP) technique, reverse crush, or culotte approach.
5. Rewiring the SB and final kissing balloon inflation (per operator discretion if an SB stent is not placed; mandatory if 2-stent approach)

Positioning of a wire in the SB until MV stenting and/or postdilatation is complete, especially in the presence of complex anatomy (tortuosity, acute angle, severe stenosis, or presence of heavily calcification), is an important step and facilitates SB access in cases of SB closure or

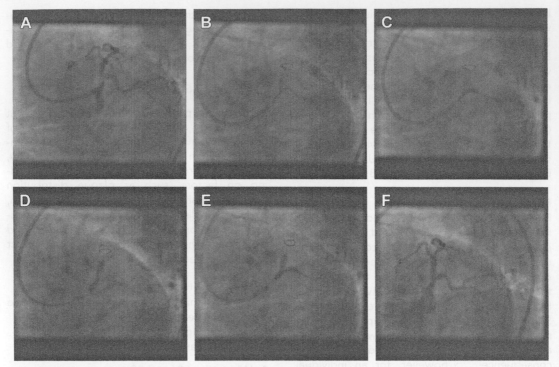

Fig. 6. LM PCI using a 1-stent provisional approach with final kissing. (A) Baseline angiogram showing severe distal LM disease with involvement of the proximal LAD and an intermediate lesion of the LCX. (B) Predilatation of LM and LAD. (C) Predilatation of LCX. (D) Stent implantation in the LM-LAD axis. (E) After removal and rewiring of the LCX, simultaneous final kissing. (F) Final angiogram showing an excellent result.

significant compromise. The temporary jailed wire can usually be retrieved easily. A jacketed polymer-coated wire should not be used for this purpose, because the polymer may be stripped off during retrieval of the jailed wire; however, polymer-coated wires may be used effectively for recrossing the stent into the SB. Postdilatation of the proximal MV stent after stent implantation before kissing balloon inflation and placement of a second stent (POT) are strongly recommended to optimize final geometry of the bifurcation and facilitates SB accessibility through the distal side cell of the MV stent.[55,70,71]

Two-stent Techniques

Various 2-stent techniques have been described. Selection of a particular technique should be based on bifurcation characteristics, operator preference, and experience. The following general principles should be considered when selecting the most appropriate technique for a given patient.

Size of side branch

If a significant discrepancy in vessel diameter exists between the SB and the MV (ie, SB considerably smaller than MV), the culotte stenting technique may be problematic and should be avoided. T-stenting, the crush technique, or a DK crush should be favored in this situation.

Lesion length in side branch

Focal lesions less than 5 mm, even if angiographically severe, are rarely physiologically significant and should usually be treated initially with a provisional approach, followed by an FFR-guided assessment and management, and optimized with or without final kissing inflation. If a significant lesion extends several millimeters (>5 mm) into the SB, however, especially if angulated or calcified, a 2-stent approach should be considered.

Bifurcation angulation

For angles less than 70° or Y-shaped morphology, SB access may be more easily performed; however, plaque shift (or carina shift) may still occur and be severe. In lesions with angles greater than or equal to 70° or T-shaped morphology, SB access is difficult but plaque shift is less pronounced. For bifurcation lesions requiring a 2-stent technique with SB angulation greater than or equal to 70°, a T-stent, modified

T-stent, or TAP technique is usually performed.[72] If the SB angulation is less than 70°, the crush, DK crush, or culotte technique is usually preferred.

Calcification severity and extent

Calcification severity and extent is underestimated by angiography compared with IVUS. If at least moderate calcification is present, plaque modification, with either a cutting or scoring balloon, or atherectomy is recommended. Although the necessity to perform atherectomy does not mandate a 2-stent technique, patients with at least moderate coronary calcification often have diffuse atherosclerotic disease, increasing the likelihood to benefit from an upfront 2-stent approach.

DESCRIPTION OF TWO-STENT TECHNIQUES

Culotte Technique

The culotte technique uses 2 stents and results in full coverage of the bifurcation area (especially the carina and SB ostium), although with 2 layers of metal in the proximal MV (**Fig. 7**, Videos 7–17). The steps described were used in Nordic Stent Technique Study[73]:

1. Wiring of both MV and SB
2. Predilatation of MV and/or SB (optional but recommended)
3. Stenting of the MV
4. Rewiring SB through MV stent and removal of jailed wire in SB
5. Dilatation of SB through MV stent
6. Stenting proximal MV and SB through MV stent
7. Rewiring MV through SB stent
8. Final kissing balloon inflation

Typically, the first stent should be placed in the branch with the most angulated entry, whether the MB or SB. To allow full opening of the SB and preservation of the SB stent architecture, an open-cell design stent, rather than a closed-cell design, should be used when performing culotte stenting. This technique should not be used if a large difference (≥1.5 mm) in vessel diameter between the MV and SB exists.[74]

Crush Techniques

The crush technique was first described by Colombo and colleagues[75,76] and has been revised several times (**Figs. 8** and **9**, Videos 18–41):

1. Wiring of both MV and SB
2. Predilatation of MV and/or SB (optional but recommended)

3. Stenting of the SB first, with an uninflated stent (or balloon) positioned in the MV. The proximal end of the SB stent should be several millimeters in the MV, but the proximal edge of the uninflated MV stent (or balloon) must be proximal to the proximal edge of the SB stent
4. Assess patency and flow in the SB to ensure an additional SB stent or immediate balloon angioplasty is not required.
5. SB wire and stent balloon are removed.
6. Crushing the SB stent with MV stent or balloon inflation (followed by MV stent)
7. Rewiring the SB through MV stent
8. High-pressure inflation of SB (optional)
9. Final kissing balloon inflation (mandatory)

Some variants of this technique have been described. Today, most operators try to minimize the length (2–3 mm) of the SB stent within the MV to reduce the multiple layers of crumpled stent (minicrush technique).[72,77] If the SB stent is crushed within the MV stent, it is called internal or reverse crush technique. In another variant, the MV stent is crushed by the SB stent (inverted crush technique).[78] Another variant was developed to make this technique feasible by radial approach using a 6F catheter. In this technique, the balloon is used to crush the SB stent, and the 2 stents are advanced and deployed sequentially (step crush or modified balloon crush technique). Disadvantages of the crush technique include difficulty in SB rewiring for final kissing inflation and the presence of multiple layers of crumpled stent at the SB ostium, substantially increasing the rate of SB ostial in-stent restenosis. In cases of difficult rewiring with conventional wire, a hydrophilic wire may be helpful in crossing into the SB. The most recent variation of this technique is the DK crush.[43,79] It involves 2 instances of balloon kissing, the first after the SB stent is crushed (facilitating rewiring for final kissing) and the second (final kiss) after deployment of the MV stent (see **Fig. 9**).

T-Stent Techniques

T-stent techniques are used when SB stenting is required after a suboptimal result with provisional stenting or in a planned 2-stent approach when the angle into the SB is greater than or equal to 70 but less than or equal to 100 (**Fig. 10**, Videos 42–50).

1. Wiring of MV and SB
2. MV and/or SB dilatation (recommended but optional)

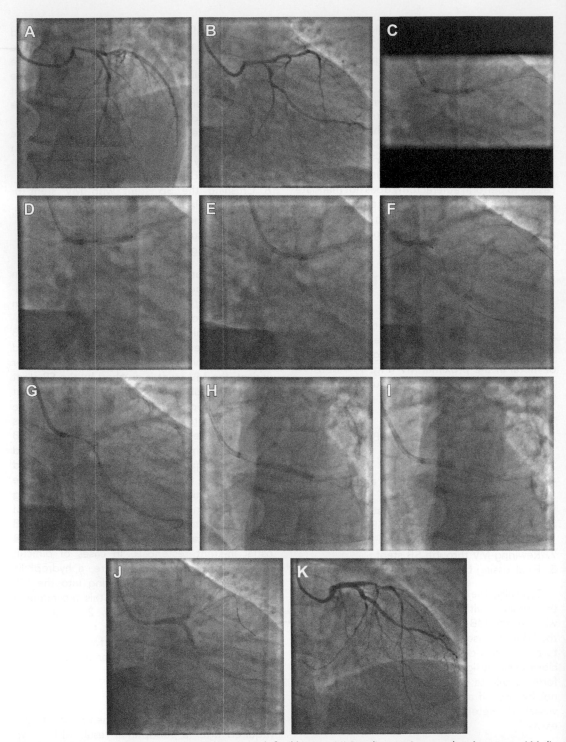

Fig. 7. LM PCI using a 2-stent culotte technique with final kissing. (*A*) Baseline angiogram showing severe LM disease with involvement of the proximal LAD and (*B*) an intermediate lesion of the ostial LCX and more severe lesion of the proximal LCX. (*C*) Predilatation of the LM and LAD. (*D*) Stent implantation in the LM-LAD axis. (*E*) Balloon inflation of the LM segment of the previously deployed stent, just proximal to the LCX ostium, using a short noncompliant balloon (POT). (*F*) After removal of the LCX wire and rewiring of the LCX, predilatation of the ostial LCX through the LM stent. (*G*) After removal of the wire in the LAD, stent placement of the LM-LCX stent, through the first deployed LM-LAD stent. (*H*) Stent implantation in the LM-LCX axis. (*I*) Balloon inflation of the LM segment of the previously deployed stent, just proximal to the LAD ostium, using a short noncompliant balloon (POT). (*J*) After rewiring of the LAD, simultaneous final kissing. (*K*) Final angiogram showing an excellent result.

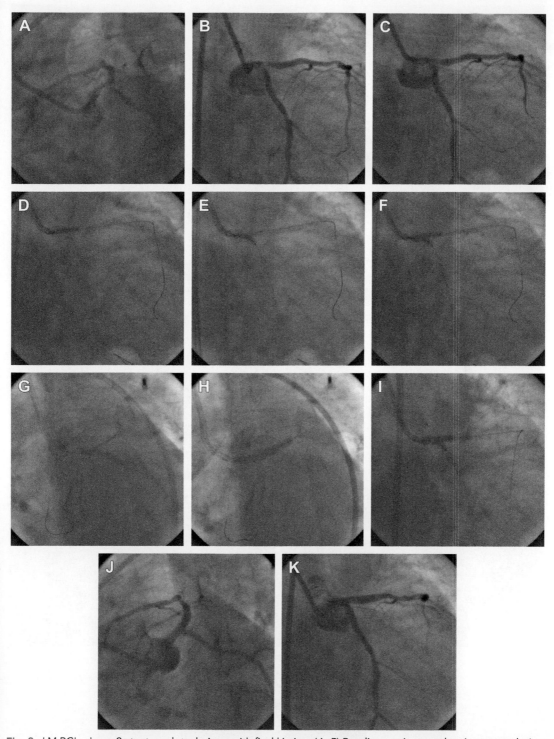

Fig. 8. LM PCI using a 2-stent crush technique with final kissing. (*A, B*) Baseline angiogram showing severe lesions involving the distal LM, the ostial LAD, and the ostial LCX (Medina bifurcation 1,1,1). (*C*) Wiring of the 2 branches. (*D*) Predilatation of the LAD. (*E*) Predilatation of the LCX. (*F*) Simultaneous kissing predilatation. (*G*) Two stents are simultaneously positioned in the bifurcation lesion: the eventually crushed stent (LCX) is positioned in the LCX, with minimal (approximately 2–3 mm) protrusion in the LM; the crushing stent is positioned in the LM-LAD axis. The LCX stent is deployed first, with the LM-LAD stent in place but not deployed. (*H*) After removal of the LCX stent balloon and wire, deployment of the LM-LAD stent, crushing the LM and carina portion of the previously deployed LCX stent. (*I*) After rewiring of the LCX through the crushed stent, final kissing inflation. (*J, K*) An excellent final result.

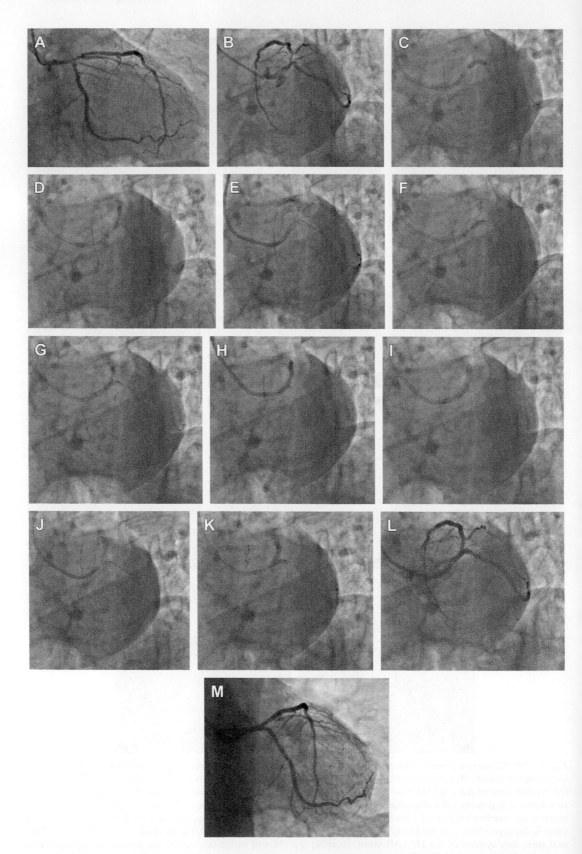

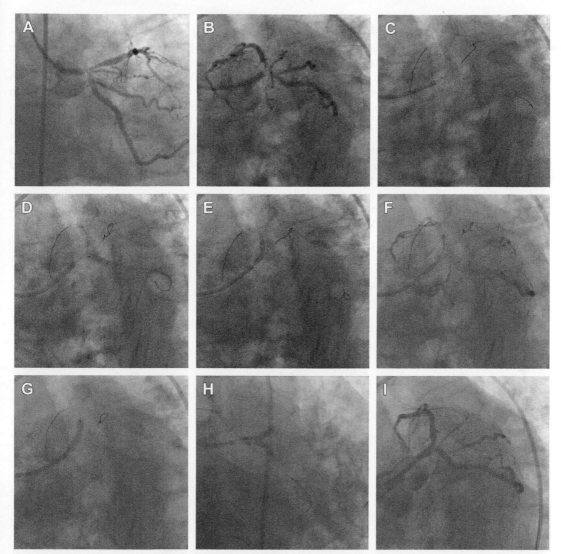

Fig. 10. LM PCI using a 2-stent T-stent technique. (*A*, *B*) Baseline angiogram showing a trifurcation lesion involving the distal LM, the LAD, LCX, and ramus. A sharp angle (approximately 90°) is present between the LM and the LCX, making this favorable for a T-stent technique. (*C*) Predilatation of the LCX. (*D*) Stent implantation in the LCX with minimal protrusion of the LCX stent in the LM. Note the wire in the LAD and ramus helping to position the stent in the LCX. (*E*) Predilatation of the LAD after LCX stent deployment. If LCX struts were protruding in the LM, they would have been crushed, facilitating stent passage into the LAD. (*F*) Stent placement in the LM-LAD axis. (*G*) Stent deployment in the LM-LAD axis. (*H*) After removal and rewiring of the LCX, final kissing inflation. (*I*) Final angiogram showing an excellent result.

Fig. 9. LM PCI using the DK crush technique. (*A*, *B*) Baseline angiograms showing LM bifurcation (Medina bifurcation 1,1,1) with involvement of LAD (distal main branch) and LCX (SB). (*C*) After predilatation of both branches, implantation of the first stent in the SB (LCX) with a balloon already in place in the distal main branch (LAD) (*D*) After removal of the stent balloon in the LCX, inflation of the balloon in the LM-LAD to crush the portion of LCX stent protruding in the LM. (*E*) After removal of the LAD balloon, removal of the LCX guide wire and rewire of the LCX. Performance of the first kissing inflation with (*F*) dilatation of the ostium of the LCX followed by (*G*) the simultaneous kissing. (*H*) Stenting of the LM-LAD, (*I*) followed by postdilation of the proximal LM stent, with the distal portion of the balloon in front of the LCX ostium (POT). (*J*) Removal of the guidewire in the LCX and rewire of the LCX. (*K*) Second kissing simultaneous inflation. (*L*, *M*) Angiogram of the final result.

3. Stenting MV with wire in place in SB (alternatively SB may be stented first)
4. Rewiring SB and removal of jailed wire
5. Dilatation of SB though MV stent
6. Stenting SB though MV stent with no stent protrusion in MV (or placement of the MV stent if the SB was stented first)
7. Final kissing balloon inflation

The main disadvantage of this technique is the high rate of ostial restenosis of the SB due to suboptimal stent coverage in the bifurcation area, particularly the ostium; however, full coverage is possible with this technique if the angle into the SB from the MV is near 90°.

Alternatively, the TAP technique, with intentional minimal protrusion of the SB stent within the MV, may be performed when dealing with bifurcation angle greater than 70°. After stenting of the MV, the SB stent is positioned in the SB with minimal protrusion in the MV, with a deflated balloon concurrently positioned in the MV. After inflation of the SB stent, the stent balloon is removed from the SB and the MV balloon is inflated. After rewiring of the SB, a final kissing inflation is performed. If performed correctly, this technique increases the likelihood of complete coverage of the ostium without deformation of the stent or malapposed struts.

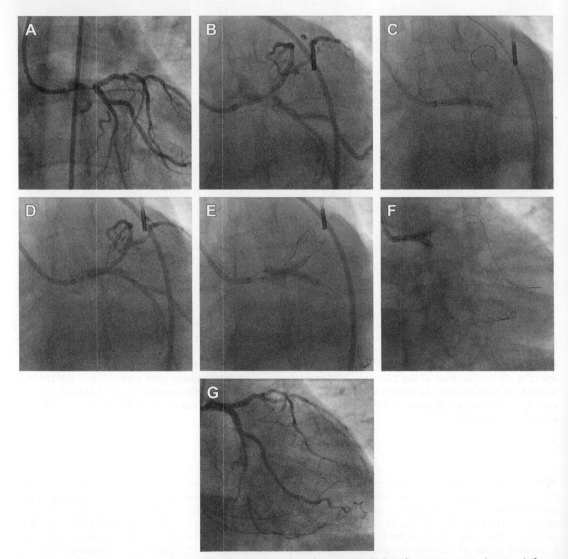

Fig. 11. LM PCI using a 2-stent V-stenting (double-barrel) technique. (A, B) Baseline angiogram showing bifurcation lesion involving the distal LM, the ostial LAD and the ostial LCX (Medina bifurcation 1,1,1). (C) Balloon predilatation of the LCX. (D) Simultaneous stent placement. (E) Simultaneous stent deployment. (F) Simultaneous postdilatation (without removing the wires). (G) Final angiogram showing an excellent result.

V-Stent Technique

In the V-stent technique, both MV and SB are stented simultaneously (**Fig. 11**, Videos 51–57). It is mainly used for distal LM disease bifurcations (Medina 0,1,1).

1. Wiring of MV and SB
2. Predilatation of MV and SB
3. Placement of stents in both branches with minimal proximal protrusion in MV
4. Placement of balloons in both branches and simultaneous (or sequential) deployment of stents
5. Final kissing balloon inflation

In cases of involvement of MV and SB (ie, Medina 1,1,1), both stents are lined up in the MV, creating a new carina—this approach is called the Y technique, simultaneous kissing stents, or double-barrel technique. In another variant of this technique for cases of extensive proximal disease in the MV, a proximal stent is first implanted before the bifurcation stenting—this is termed the skirt or extended Y technique. Y-stenting is rarely used, because the new carina is often eccentric and difficult to rewire in cases of in-stent restenosis, and if a proximal dissection develops it must be converted to a crush or culotte, a complex procedure. MACE rates have also been reported to be high after Y-stenting.[80,81] Y-stenting may be useful, however, in patients with hemodynamic instability in whom rapid stabilization of a high-grade LM stenosis is the main priority.

SUMMARY

Bifurcation lesions are frequent in clinical practice, representing approximately 20% of lesions treated by PCI. Revascularization decisions for patients with bifurcation lesions are complex and should take into consideration many factors, such as the complexity of bifurcation lesion, vessel diameter of the SB, and the area of myocardium at risk. Adequate lesion assessment from noninvasive and invasive testing is crucial if optimal results after bifurcation PCI are to be achieved. Although a 1-stent provisional approach should be considered as the default approach when facing most of the bifurcation lesions, the need for treating the SB is necessary in up to a quarter of the patients. Therefore, 2-stents techniques and dedicated bifurcation stent strategies should be mastered to insure adequate treatment of complex bifurcation involving large SB that supply a large myocardium area.

SUPPLEMENTARY DATA

Videos related to this article can be found on-line at http://dx.doi.org/10.1016/j.iccl.2015.12.011.

REFERENCES

1. Gao XF, Zhang YJ, Tian NL, et al. Stenting strategy for coronary artery bifurcation with drug-eluting stents: a meta-analysis of nine randomised trials and systematic review. EuroIntervention 2014;10: 561–9.
2. Louvard Y, Thomas M, Dzavik V, et al. Classification of coronary artery bifurcation lesions and treatments: time for a consensus! Catheter Cardiovasc Interv 2008;71:175–83.
3. Movahed MR, Stinis CT. A new proposed simplified classification of coronary artery bifurcation lesions and bifurcation interventional techniques. J Invasive Cardiol 2006;18:199–204.
4. Louvard Y, Lefevre T, Morice MC. Percutaneous coronary intervention for bifurcation coronary disease. Heart 2004;90:713–22.
5. Y-Hassan S, Lindroos MC, Sylven C. A novel descriptive, intelligible and ordered (DINO) classification of coronary bifurcation lesions. Review of current classifications. Circ J 2011;75:299–305.
6. Lassen JF, Holm NR, Stankovic G, et al. Percutaneous coronary intervention for coronary bifurcation disease: consensus from the first 10 years of the European bifurcation club meetings. EuroIntervention 2014;10:545–60.
7. Medina A, Suarez de Lezo J, Pan M. A new classification of coronary bifurcation lesions. Rev Esp Cardiol 2006;59:183 [in Spanish].
8. Thomas M, Hildick-Smith D, Louvard Y, et al. Percutaneous coronary intervention for bifurcation disease. A consensus view from the first meeting of the European bifurcation club. EuroIntervention 2006;2:149–53.
9. Huo Y, Kassab GS. A scaling law of vascular volume. Biophys J 2009;96:347–53.
10. Huo Y, Finet G, Lefevre T, et al. Optimal diameter of diseased bifurcation segment: a practical rule for percutaneous coronary intervention. EuroIntervention 2012;7:1310–6.
11. Sianos G, Morel MA, Kappetein AP, et al. The SYNTAX Score: an angiographic tool grading the complexity of coronary artery disease. EuroIntervention 2005;1:219–27.
12. Serruys PW, Morice MC, Kappetein AP, et al. Percutaneous coronary intervention versus coronary-artery bypass grafting for severe coronary artery disease. N Engl J Med 2009;360:961–72.
13. Capodanno D, Capranzano P, Di Salvo ME, et al. Usefulness of SYNTAX score to select patients with left main coronary artery disease to be treated

with coronary artery bypass graft. JACC Cardiovasc Interv 2009;2:731–8.

14. Louvard Y, Medina A. Definitions and classifications of bifurcation lesions and treatment. EuroIntervention 2015;11(Suppl V):V23–6.

15. Al Suwaidi J, Berger PB, Rihal CS, et al. Immediate and long-term outcome of intracoronary stent implantation for true bifurcation lesions. J Am Coll Cardiol 2000;35:929–36.

16. Hahn JY, Chun WJ, Kim JH, et al. Predictors and outcomes of side branch occlusion after main vessel stenting in coronary bifurcation lesions: results from the COBIS II Registry (COronary BIfurcation Stenting). J Am Coll Cardiol 2013;62:1654–9.

17. Kralev S, Poerner TC, Basorth D, et al. Side branch occlusion after coronary stent implantation in patients presenting with ST-elevation myocardial infarction: clinical impact and angiographic predictors. Am Heart J 2006;151:153–7.

18. Dou K, Zhang D, Xu B, et al. An angiographic tool for risk prediction of side branch occlusion in coronary bifurcation intervention: the RESOLVE score system (risk prediction of side branch occlusion in coronary bifurcation intervention). JACC Cardiovasc Interv 2015;8:39–46.

19. Fischman DL, Savage MP, Leon MB, et al. Fate of lesion-related side branches after coronary artery stenting. J Am Coll Cardiol 1993;22:1641–6.

20. Park TK, Park YH, Song YB, et al. Long-term clinical outcomes of true and non-true bifurcation lesions according to medina classification- results from the COBIS (COronary BIfurcation Stent) II registry. Circ J 2015;79:1954–62.

21. Palmerini T, Genereux P, Caixeta A, et al. Prognostic value of the SYNTAX score in patients with acute coronary syndromes undergoing percutaneous coronary intervention: analysis from the ACUITY (acute catheterization and urgent intervention triage strategy) trial. J Am Coll Cardiol 2011;57: 2389–97.

22. Garg S, Sarno G, Serruys PW, et al. Prediction of 1-year clinical outcomes using the SYNTAX score in patients with acute ST-segment elevation myocardial infarction undergoing primary percutaneous coronary intervention: a substudy of the STRATEGY (single high-dose bolus tirofiban and sirolimus-eluting stent versus abciximab and bare-metal stent in acute myocardial infarction) and MULTISTRATEGY (multicenter evaluation of single high-dose bolus tirofiban versus abciximab with sirolimus-eluting stent or bare-metal stent in acute myocardial infarction study) trials. JACC Cardiovasc Interv 2011;4:66–75.

23. Garg S, Sarno G, Garcia-Garcia HM, et al. A new tool for the risk stratification of patients with complex coronary artery disease: the clinical SYNTAX score. Circ Cardiovasc Interv 2010;3:317–26.

24. Farooq V, Vergouwe Y, Raber L, et al. Combined anatomical and clinical factors for the long-term risk stratification of patients undergoing percutaneous coronary intervention: the logistic clinical SYNTAX score. Eur Heart J 2012;33:3098–104.

25. Farooq V, Vergouwe Y, Genereux P, et al. Prediction of 1-year mortality in patients with acute coronary syndromes undergoing percutaneous coronary intervention: validation of the logistic clinical SYNTAX (synergy between percutaneous coronary interventions with taxus and cardiac surgery) score. JACC Cardiovasc Interv 2013;6:737–45.

26. Farooq V, van Klaveren D, Steyerberg EW, et al. Anatomical and clinical characteristics to guide decision making between coronary artery bypass surgery and percutaneous coronary intervention for individual patients: development and validation of SYNTAX score II. Lancet 2013;381:639–50.

27. Colombo A, Moses JW, Morice MC, et al. Randomized study to evaluate sirolimus-eluting stents implanted at coronary bifurcation lesions. Circulation 2004;109:1244–9.

28. Pan M, de Lezo JS, Medina A, et al. Rapamycin-eluting stents for the treatment of bifurcated coronary lesions: a randomized comparison of a simple versus complex strategy. Am Heart J 2004;148:857–64.

29. Steigen TK, Maeng M, Wiseth R, et al. Randomized study on simple versus complex stenting of coronary artery bifurcation lesions: the Nordic bifurcation study. Circulation 2006;114:1955–61.

30. Colombo A, Bramucci E, Sacca S, et al. Randomized study of the crush technique versus provisional side-branch stenting in true coronary bifurcations: the CACTUS (coronary bifurcations: application of the crushing technique using sirolimus-eluting stents) Study. Circulation 2009;119:71–8.

31. Ferenc M, Gick M, Kienzle RP, et al. Randomized trial on routine vs. provisional T-stenting in the treatment of de novo coronary bifurcation lesions. Eur Heart J 2008;29:2859–67.

32. Hildick-Smith D, de Belder AJ, Cooter N, et al. Randomized trial of simple versus complex drug-eluting stenting for bifurcation lesions: the British bifurcation coronary study: old, new, and evolving strategies. Circulation 2010;121:1235–43.

33. Chen SL, Santoso T, Zhang JJ, et al. A randomized clinical study comparing double kissing crush with provisional stenting for treatment of coronary bifurcation lesions: results from the DKCRUSH-II (double kissing crush versus provisional stenting technique for treatment of coronary bifurcation lesions) trial. J Am Coll Cardiol 2011;57:914–20.

34. Song YB, Hahn JY, Song PS, et al. Randomized comparison of conservative versus aggressive strategy for provisional side branch intervention in coronary bifurcation lesions: results from the SMART-STRATEGY (smart angioplasty research team-optimal strategy

for side branch intervention in coronary bifurcation lesions) randomized trial. JACC Cardiovasc Interv 2012; 5:1133–40.

35. Maeng M, Holm NR, Erglis A, et al. Long-term results after simple versus complex stenting of coronary artery bifurcation lesions: nordic bifurcation study 5-year follow-up results. J Am Coll Cardiol 2013;62:30–4.

36. Genereux P, Kumsars I, Lesiak M, et al. A randomized trial of a dedicated bifurcation stent versus provisional stenting in the treatment of coronary bifurcation lesions. J Am Coll Cardiol 2015; 65:533–43.

37. Behan MW, Holm NR, Curzen NP, et al. Simple or complex stenting for bifurcation coronary lesions: a patient-level pooled-analysis of the nordic bifurcation study and the British bifurcation coronary study. Circ Cardiovasc Interv 2011;4:57–64.

38. Zhang F, Dong L, Ge J. Simple versus complex stenting strategy for coronary artery bifurcation lesions in the drug-eluting stent era: a meta-analysis of randomised trials. Heart 2009;95:1676–81.

39. Windecker S, Kolh P, Alfonso F, et al. 2014 ESC/EACTS guidelines on myocardial revascularization: the task force on myocardial revascularization of the European society of cardiology (ESC) and the European association for cardio-thoracic surgery (EACTS)developed with the special contribution of the European association of percutaneous cardiovascular interventions (EAPCI). Eur Heart J 2014;35:2541–619.

40. Levine GN, Bates ER, Blankenship JC, et al. 2011 ACCF/AHA/SCAI guideline for percutaneous coronary intervention. A report of the American college of cardiology foundation/American heart association task force on practice guidelines and the society for cardiovascular angiography and interventions. J Am Coll Cardiol 2011;58:e44–122.

41. Genereux P, Kini A, Lesiak M, et al. Outcomes of a dedicated stent in coronary bifurcations with large side branches: a subanalysis of the randomized TRYTON bifurcation study. Catheter Cardiovasc Interv 2015. [Epub ahead of print].

42. Chen SL, Zhang JJ, Ye F, et al. Study comparing the double kissing (DK) crush with classical crush for the treatment of coronary bifurcation lesions: the DKCRUSH-1 bifurcation study with drug-eluting stents. Eur J Clin Invest 2008;38:361–71.

43. Chen SL, Xu B, Han YL, et al. Comparison of double kissing crush versus culotte stenting for unprotected distal left main bifurcation lesions: results from a multicenter, randomized, prospective DKCRUSH-III study. J Am Coll Cardiol 2013;61: 1482–8.

44. Kervinen K, Niemela M, Romppanen H, et al. Clinical outcome after crush versus culotte stenting of coronary artery bifurcation lesions: the nordic stent technique study 36-month follow-up results. JACC Cardiovasc Interv 2013;6:1160–5.

45. Verheye S, Ormiston JA, Stewart J, et al. A next-generation bioresorbable coronary scaffold system: from bench to first clinical evaluation: 6- and 12-month clinical and multimodality imaging results. JACC Cardiovasc Interv 2014;7:89–99.

46. Ellis SG, Kereiakes DJ, Metzger DC, et al. Everolimus-eluting bioresorbable scaffolds for coronary artery disease. N Engl J Med 2015;373(20):1905–15.

47. Capodanno D, Gori T, Nef H, et al. Percutaneous coronary intervention with everolimus-eluting bioresorbable vascular scaffolds in routine clinical practice: early and midterm outcomes from the European multicentre GHOST-EU registry. EuroIntervention 2015;10:1144–53.

48. Grundeken MJ, Asgedom S, Damman P, et al. Six-month and one-year clinical outcomes after placement of a dedicated coronary bifurcation stent: a patient-level pooled analysis of eight registry studies. EuroIntervention 2013;9:195–203.

49. Buysschaert I, Dubois CL, Dens J, et al. Three-year clinical results of the axxess biolimus A9 eluting bifurcation stent system: the DIVERGE study. EuroIntervention 2013;9:573–81.

50. Kumsars I, Narbute I, Thuesen L, et al. Side branch fractional flow reserve measurements after main vessel stenting: a nordic-baltic bifurcation study III substudy. EuroIntervention 2012;7:1155–61.

51. Foin N, Torii R, Mortier P, et al. Kissing balloon or sequential dilation of the side branch and main vessel for provisional stenting of bifurcations: lessons from micro-computed tomography and computational simulations. JACC Cardiovasc Interv 2012;5:47–56.

52. Foin N, Torii R, Alegria E, et al. Location of side branch access critically affects results in bifurcation stenting: insights from bench modeling and computational flow simulation. Int J Cardiol 2013; 168:3623–8.

53. Niemela M, Kervinen K, Erglis A, et al. Randomized comparison of final kissing balloon dilatation versus no final kissing balloon dilatation in patients with coronary bifurcation lesions treated with main vessel stenting: the nordic-baltic bifurcation study III. Circulation 2011;123:79–86.

54. Korn HV, Yu J, Ohlow MA, et al. Interventional therapy of bifurcation lesions: a TIMI flow-guided concept to treat side branches in bifurcation lesions–a prospective randomized clinical study (thueringer bifurcation study, THUEBIS study as pilot trial). Circ Cardiovasc Interv 2009;2:535–42.

55. Hildick-Smith D, Lassen JF, Albiero R, et al. Consensus from the 5th European bifurcation club meeting. EuroIntervention 2010;6:34–8.

56. Foin N, Secco GG, Ghilencea L, et al. Final proximal post-dilatation is necessary after kissing

balloon in bifurcation stenting. EuroIntervention 2011;7:597–604.

57. Montalescot G, Sechtem U, Achenbach S, et al. 2013 ESC guidelines on the management of stable coronary artery disease: the task force on the management of stable coronary artery disease of the European society of cardiology. Eur Heart J 2013; 34:2949–3003.

58. Fihn SD, Blankenship JC, Alexander KP, et al. 2014 ACC/AHA/AATS/PCNA/SCAI/STS focused update of the guideline for the diagnosis and management of patients with stable ischemic heart disease: a report of the American college of cardiology/ American heart association task force on practice guidelines, and the American association for thoracic surgery, preventive cardiovascular nurses association, society for cardiovascular angiography and interventions, and society of thoracic surgeons. J Am Coll Cardiol 2014;64:1929–49.

59. Fihn SD, Gardin JM, Abrams J, et al. 2012 ACCF/ AHA/ACP/AATS/PCNA/SCAI/STS guideline for the diagnosis and management of patients with stable ischemic heart disease: a report of the American college of cardiology foundation/American heart association task force on practice guidelines, and the American college of physicians, American association for thoracic surgery, preventive cardiovascular nurses association, society for cardiovascular angiography and interventions, and society of thoracic surgeons. Circulation 2012;126:e354–471.

60. Koo BK, Park KW, Kang HJ, et al. Physiological evaluation of the provisional side-branch intervention strategy for bifurcation lesions using fractional flow reserve. Eur Heart J 2008;29:726–32.

61. Koo BK, Kang HJ, Youn TJ, et al. Physiologic assessment of jailed side branch lesions using fractional flow reserve. J Am Coll Cardiol 2005;46:633–7.

62. Ahn JM, Lee JY, Kang SJ, et al. Functional assessment of jailed side branches in coronary bifurcation lesions using fractional flow reserve. JACC Cardiovasc Interv 2012;5:155–61.

63. Goktekin O, Kaplan S, Dimopoulos K, et al. A new quantitative analysis system for the evaluation of coronary bifurcation lesions: comparison with current conventional methods. Catheter Cardiovasc Interv 2007;69:172–80.

64. Tu S, Jing J, Holm NR, et al. In vivo assessment of bifurcation optimal viewing angles and bifurcation angles by three-dimensional (3D) quantitative coronary angiography. Int J Cardiovasc Imaging 2012; 28:1617–25.

65. Girasis C, Schuurbiers JC, Muramatsu T, et al. Advanced three-dimensional quantitative coronary angiographic assessment of bifurcation lesions: methodology and phantom validation. EuroIntervention 2013;8:1451–60.

66. Kim JS, Hong MK, Ko YG, et al. Impact of intravascular ultrasound guidance on long-term clinical outcomes in patients treated with drug-eluting stent for bifurcation lesions: data from a Korean multicenter bifurcation registry. Am Heart J 2011;161:180–7.

67. Burzotta F, Brancati MF, Trani C, et al. Impact of drug-eluting balloon (pre- or post-) dilation on neointima formation in de novo lesions treated by bare-metal stent: the IN-PACT CORO trial. Heart Vessels 2015. [Epub ahead of print].

68. Sato K, Panoulas VF, Naganuma T, et al. Bioresorbable vascular scaffold strut disruption after crossing with an optical coherence tomography imaging catheter. Int J Cardiol 2014;174:e116–9.

69. Louvard Y, Lefevre T. Tools & techniques: PCI in coronary bifurcations lesions. EuroIntervention 2011;7:160–3.

70. Mylotte D, Routledge H, Harb T, et al. Provisional side branch-stenting for coronary bifurcation lesions: evidence of improving procedural and clinical outcomes with contemporary techniques. Catheter Cardiovasc Interv 2013;82:E437–45.

71. Stankovic G, Lefevre T, Chieffo A, et al. Consensus from the 7th European bifurcation club meeting. EuroIntervention 2013;9:36–45.

72. Burzotta F, Gwon HC, Hahn JY, et al. Modified T-stenting with intentional protrusion of the side-branch stent within the main vessel stent to ensure ostial coverage and facilitate final kissing balloon: the T-stenting and small protrusion technique (TAP-stenting). Report of bench testing and first clinical Italian-Korean two-centre experience. Catheter Cardiovasc Interv 2007;70:75–82.

73. Erglis A, Kumsars I, Niemela M, et al. Randomized comparison of coronary bifurcation stenting with the crush versus the culotte technique using sirolimus eluting stents: the nordic stent technique study. Circ Cardiovasc Interv 2009;2:27–34.

74. Foin N, Sen S, Allegria E, et al. Maximal expansion capacity with current DES platforms: a critical factor for stent selection in the treatment of left main bifurcations? EuroIntervention 2013;8:1315–25.

75. Colombo A. Balloon crush: new tool in bifurcation treatment armamentarium. Catheter Cardiovasc Interv 2004;63:417–8.

76. Colombo A, Stankovic G, Orlic D, et al. Modified T-stenting technique with crushing for bifurcation lesions: immediate results and 30-day outcome. Catheter Cardiovasc Interv 2003;60:145–51.

77. Galassi AR, Colombo A, Buchbinder M, et al. Long-term outcomes of bifurcation lesions after implantation of drug-eluting stents with the "mini-crush technique". Catheter Cardiovasc Interv 2007;69: 976–83.

78. Furuichi S, Airoldi F, Colombo A. Rescue inverse crush: a way of get out of trouble. Catheter Cardiovasc Interv 2007;70:708–12.

79. Chen S, Zhang J, Ye F, et al. DK crush (double-kissing and double-crush) technique for treatment of true coronary bifurcation lesions: illustration and comparison with classic crush. J Invasive Cardiol 2007;19:189–93.

80. Siotia A, Morton AC, Malkin CJ, et al. Simultaneous kissing drug-eluting stents to treat unprotected left main stem bifurcation disease: medium term outcome in 150 consecutive patients. EuroIntervention 2012;8:691–700.

81. Stinis CT, Hu SP, Price MJ, et al. Three-year outcome of drug-eluting stent implantation for coronary artery bifurcation lesions. Catheter Cardiovasc Interv 2010;75:309–14.

82. Kelbaek H, Thuesen L, Helqvist S, et al. The stenting coronary arteries in non-stress/benestent disease (SCANDSTENT) trial. J Am Coll Cardiol 2006;47:449–55.

83. Adriaenssens T, Byrne RA, Dibra A, et al. Culotte stenting technique in coronary bifurcation disease: angiographic follow-up using dedicated quantitative coronary angiographic analysis and 12-month clinical outcomes. Eur Heart J 2008;29:2868–76.

84. Garg S, Wykrzykowska J, Serruys PW, et al. The outcome of bifurcation lesion stenting using a biolimus-eluting stent with a bio-degradable polymer compared to a sirolimus-eluting stent with a durable polymer. EuroIntervention 2011;6: 928–35.

85. Mathey DG, Wendig I, Boxberger M, et al. Treatment of bifurcation lesions with a drug-eluting balloon: the PEPCAD V (paclitaxel eluting PTCA balloon in coronary artery disease) trial. EuroIntervention 2011;7(Suppl K):K61–5.

86. Pan M, Medina A, Suarez de Lezo J, et al. Randomized study comparing everolimus- and sirolimus-eluting stents in patients with bifurcation lesions treated by provisional side-branch stenting. Catheter Cardiovasc Interv 2012;80:1165–70.

87. Song YB, Hahn JY, Yang JH, et al. Differential prognostic impact of treatment strategy among patients with left main versus non-left main bifurcation lesions undergoing percutaneous coronary intervention: results from the COBIS (coronary bifurcation stenting) registry II. JACC Cardiovasc Interv 2014; 7:255–63.

Update on Coronary Chronic Total Occlusion Percutaneous Coronary Intervention

Emmanouil S. Brilakis, MD, PhD[a],*,
Dimitri Karmpaliotis, MD[b], Minh N. Vo, MD[c],
Mauro Carlino, MD[d], Alfredo R. Galassi, MD[e,f],
Marouane Boukhris, MD[e,g], Khaldoon Alaswad, MD[h],
Leszek Bryniarski, MD[i], William L. Lombardi, MD[j],
Subhash Banerjee, MD[a]

KEYWORDS

- Chronic total occlusion • Coronary revascularization • Percutaneous coronary intervention
- Techniques • Outcomes

KEY POINTS

- Chronic total occlusions (CTOs) are common and can be treated with high success rates at experienced centers using a variety of crossing techniques and equipment.
- Several observational studies suggest clinical benefit with CTO percutaneous coronary intervention.
- Performance of randomized clinical trials is critical for further expansion and refinement of the procedure.

INTRODUCTION

Coronary chronic total occlusions (CTOs) are lesions with thrombolysis in myocardial infarction 0 flow with an estimated or known occlusion duration of 3 months or more.[1] Coronary CTOs are commonly encountered in patients with coronary artery disease undergoing coronary angiography (13.3%–52.0%).[2–6] Successful

Conflict of Interest Disclosures Related to this article: Dr E.S. Brilakis: consulting/speaker honoraria from St. Jude Medical, Terumo, Somahlution, Elsevier, Asahi, Abbott Vascular, Boston Scientific; research support from InfraRedx and Boston Scientific; spouse is an employee of Medtronic; Dr D. Karmpaliotis: speaker bureau, Abbott Vascular, Medtronic, Boston Scientific; Dr M.N. Vo: Consultant, Boston Scientific; Dr M. Carlino, Dr A.R. Galassi, Dr M. Boukhris: Dr L. Bryniarski: none; Dr K. Alaswad: consulting fees from Terumo and Boston Scientific; consultant, no financial, Abbott Laboratories. Dr W.W. Lombardi: equity with Bridgepoint Medical; Dr S. Banerjee: research grants from Gilead and the Medicines Company; consultant/speaker honoraria from Covidien and Medtronic; ownership in MDCARE Global (spouse); intellectual property in HygeiaTel.

[a] Department of Cardiovascular Diseases, VA North Texas Healthcare System, University of Texas Southwestern Medical Center at Dallas, Dallas, TX, USA; [b] Department of Cardiovascular Diseases, NYP Columbia University, New York, NY, USA; [c] St Boniface Hospital Cardiac Science Program, University of Manitoba, Winnipeg, Canada; [d] Department of Cardiovascular Diseases, San Raffaele Scientific Institute, Milan, Italy; [e] Department of Clinical and Experimental Medicine, University of Catania, Catania, Italy; [f] Department of Cardiovascular Diseases, University of Zurich, Zurich, Switzerland; [g] Faculty of Medicine of Tunis, University of Tunis El Manar, Tunis, Tunisia; [h] Department of Cardiovascular Diseases, Henry Ford Hospital, Detroit, MI, USA; [i] Department of Cardiology and Hypertension, Jagiellonian University Medical College, Krakow, Poland; [j] University of Washington, Seattle, WA, USA

* Corresponding author. Dallas VA Medical Center (111A), 4500 South Lancaster Road, Dallas, TX 75216.
E-mail address: esbrilakis@gmail.com

CTO percutaneous coronary intervention (PCI) can provide significant clinical benefits, but can also be technically challenging, requiring specialized equipment and techniques. With rapid improvement in equipment and techniques, greater than 90% success rates can be achieved in a variety of settings by experienced operators.[7,8]

The goal of this review was to summarize the clinical evidence and technical evolution of CTO PCI, with emphasis on more recent developments.

SUCCESS RATES IN CHRONIC TOTAL OCCLUSION PERCUTANEOUS CORONARY INTERVENTION

Historically, due to technical complexity and limited availability of advanced equipment and techniques, success rates have been low (approximately 70%–80%). Patel and colleagues[9] performed a systematic review and meta-analysis of 65 studies published between 2000 and 2011, including 18,061 patients: angiographic success was 77% with low incidence of major complications: death 0.2%; emergent coronary artery bypass graft surgery (CABG) 0.1%; stroke less than 0.01%; myocardial infarction 2.5%; and tamponade 0.3%. However, when complications occurred, patients had worse outcomes, as described in another meta-analysis by Khan and colleagues.[10] Procedural success

increased over time, whereas the incidence of complications decreased.[9] More recently, technical success has further increased to more than 90% at experienced centers[7] (Fig. 1), even among complex patient and lesion subgroups, such as patients with prior CABG[11] in whom success rates had been significantly lower in the past.[12,13]

These improved outcomes are likely the result of significant evolution in equipment and techniques. Consistent implementation of basic principles of CTO PCI, such as use of dual injection[14] and use of microcatheters to support guidewires, is likely responsible for a large part of the improvement in outcomes. In addition to antegrade wire escalation that has traditionally been the preferred (or only) crossing strategy for many operators,[15] the development of the retrograde approach[16-18] and antegrade dissection/reentry[19-21] have revolutionized the field by providing multiple crossing options for previously "impossible" cases.

ANTEGRADE WIRE ESCALATION

Antegrade wire escalation remains the most commonly used CTO crossing technique[7] and is highly successful in simple occlusions, but often fails in more complex lesions[22] (Fig. 2). A microcatheter is advanced to the proximal cap, followed by insertion of various guidewires in an effort to penetrate and cross the occluded

PROspective Global REgiStry for the Study of CTO interventions

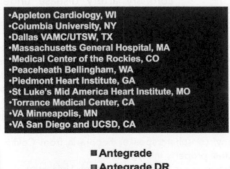

- Appleton Cardiology, WI
- Columbia University, NY
- Dallas VAMC/UTSW, TX
- Massachusetts General Hospital, MA
- Medical Center of the Rockies, CO
- Peaceheath Bellingham, WA
- Piedmont Heart Institute, GA
- St Luke's Mid America Heart Institute, MO
- Torrance Medical Center, CA
- VA Minneapolis, MN
- VA San Diego and UCSD, CA

1/2012 to 3/2015
11 centers, 1,036 lesions
Technical success: 91%
Major complications: 1.7%

Successful technique

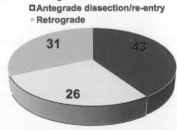

Fig. 1. Outcomes of CTO PCI in a contemporary US registry. (*From* Christopoulos G, Karmpaliotis D, Alaswad K, et al. Application and outcomes of a hybrid approach to chronic total occlusion percutaneous coronary intervention in a contemporary multicenter US registry. Int J Cardiol 2015;198:225.)

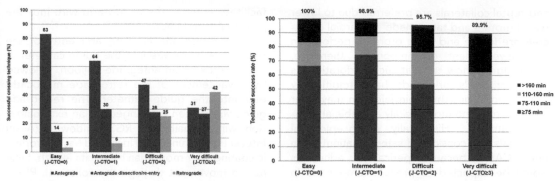

Fig. 2. Impact of J-CTO score on use of various crossing strategies, technical success and procedure time. (*From* Christopoulos G, Wyman RM, Alaswad K, et al. Clinical utility of the Japan-chronic total occlusion score in coronary chronic total occlusion interventions: results from a multicenter registry. Circ Cardiovasc Interv 2015;8(7):e002171.)

segment. A microcatheter is important to enhance the penetrating power of the guidewires and to facilitate wire exchanges. In contrast to small balloons that have a radiopaque marker in the middle, microcatheters have the radiopaque marker at the tip, facilitating recognition of their position. They are also more flexible and less likely to kink. Microcatheters with braided bodies (Corsair, Asahi Intecc, Naichi, Japan; and Turnpike, Vascular Solutions, Minneapolis, MI) also increase the penetration power of the guidewire, as compared with over-the-wire balloons. Excellent support is crucial for antegrade wire escalation and any type of CTO crossing and can be achieved using various techniques, such as guide catheter extensions,[23] side-branch anchor, or support catheters.[24] The choice of guidewire and guidewire manipulation technique remains highly variable; however, there is an increasing trend among expert operators to decrease procedural time and facilitate education by reducing the number of guidewire options for antegrade wiring. Traditionally, initial crossing attempts were performed with a tapered, low tip-load polymer-jacketed guidewire, followed by progressively stiffer guidewires (stiff, tapered when the vessel course is well understood or stiff, polymer-jacketed if the vessel course is ambiguous).[25,26] With increasing experience and the introduction of composite-core guidewires (consisting of stainless steel tube rope coil with traditional spring-coil on the outside),[27–29] many operators currently start with either a stiff, polymer-jacketed guidewire (such as the Pilot 200, Abbott Vascular Santa Clara, CA) or with a stiff, composite-core, tapered-tip guidewire (such as the Gaia 2nd, Asahi Intecc). In case of unintentional subintimal guidewire entry, there remains a divergence of opinion regarding the optimal course of action: some operators perform parallel wire technique by leaving the

initial subintimal guidewire in place and advancing a second guidewire "parallel" to the first until true lumen entry is achieved; other operators convert the case to dissection/reentry with the aim to optimize efficiency while still minimizing the length of dissection.

The Retrograde Approach

The retrograde approach involves advancement of a guidewire and a microcatheter through a collateral vessel into the distal true lumen, followed by occluded segment crossing and subsequent antegrade or retrograde wire true lumen placement with various subintimal tracking techniques (controlled antegrade and retrograde subintimal tracking [CART], reverse CART), or wiring techniques (marker wire, kissing wire). Pathology studies have demonstrated that the distal cap is usually tapered and is also softer than the proximal cap, making crossing easier.[30] The retrograde approach is used in many cases after antegrade failure, but is increasingly being used as a frontline technique in complex lesions such as those with ambiguous proximal cap, ostial occlusions,[31,32] occlusions with diffusely diseased distal vessel, or with an important bifurcation at the distal cap.[1] In the European Registry of CTOs (ERCTO), Galassi and colleagues[33] reported that retrograde strategy as first approach was more successful than immediately after a failed antegrade attempt (82.2% vs 53.1%, respectively; *P*<.001). This might be because a first antegrade failure could lead to operator/patient fatigue, increased contrast and radiation consumption, and extensive dissections, thus compromising the success of a retrograde bailout attempt.

Collateral channels used for the retrograde approach include septal and epicardial collaterals as well as bypass grafts. Bypass grafts and septal collaterals are preferred due to lower risk of rupture and tamponade. Epicardial collaterals are fragile and more prone to perforation and development of tamponade, therefore, knowledge of how to treat such perforations is important; coils or beads have traditionally been used,[34] but thrombin injection may offer a satisfactory and more readily available alternative treatment.[35] Historically, wiring epicardial collaterals was considered safer in patients with prior CABG because pericardial adhesions would be expected to prevent tamponade in case of perforation. However, several case reports of localized tamponade (for example, left atrial compression) have been reported in these patients[36,37] and may be very challenging to drain percutaneously, often requiring emergency surgery and/or leading to death. Many CTO experts advise extreme caution when crossing epicardial collaterals in patients with prior CABG and recommend immediate treatment should a perforation occur.

Collateral channel crossing is currently performed with composite-core guidewires (usually Sion, Asahi Intecc) advanced through a microcatheter, such as Corsair (Asahi Intecc), Turnpike (Vascular Solutions), and Finecross (Terumo, Warren, NJ). After successful guidewire crossing, a microcatheter is advanced through the collateral vessel, followed by retrograde crossing of the CTO, which is usually achieved using the reverse CART technique[38]: a balloon (usually of large size, often guided by intravascular ultrasonography) is inflated over an antegrade guidewire that has been advanced adjacent to the retrograde guidewire to create a space for the retrograde guidewire to advance into the antegrade guide. A variation of this technique is the "guide catheter extension reverse CART" in which a guide catheter extension is advanced over the antegrade guidewire creating a target for the retrograde guidewire to enter.[39] Another variation is the "contemporary reverse CART," in which the antegrade balloon is inflated more proximal to the retrograde wire before any retrograde wiring to prevent creation of a large retrograde dissection plane, which can hinder retrograde wire manipulation. Keeping the retrograde subintimal space small and limited allows easier control of a highly torquable composite core guidewire (usually from the Gaia family) for more efficient retrograde wire crossing into the proximal true lumen. Finally, laser atherectomy over the antegrade wire has been used to ablate the tissue between the antegrade and retrograde wire to facilitate entry of the retrograde wire into the proximal true lumen.

After retrograde crossing and entry of the retrograde guidewire into the guide catheter, it is trapped with an antegrade balloon, followed by advancement of the retrograde microcatheter into the guide catheter. The retrograde guidewire is then exchanged for an externalization wire, usually the RG3 guidewire (Asahi Intecc) that is thin (0.010 inch) and has hydrophilic coating over more than half of its length, facilitating movement through the collateral. PCI is then performed in a standard antegrade fashion by loading balloons and stents on the externalized part of the wire, followed by its removal after ascertaining that the collateral vessel is intact.

The retrograde approach has been one of the main reasons why CTO PCI success rates have been increasing,[38,40–43] and was recently shown to significantly improve quality of life during long-term follow-up in the large European CTO registry.[33] Moreover, encouraging results were seen in the J-Proctor study, in which the retrograde approach was associated with more frequent subintimal crossing as compared with the antegrade approach, but had similar clinical outcomes at 12-month follow-up.[44] However, some concerns remain; the retrograde approach carries significantly higher risk for periprocedural myocardial infarction as compared with antegrade crossing techniques,[45,46] and may also carry increased risk for other complications. In a meta-analysis of 3426 patients from 26 studies, procedural success was 83% with relatively high complication rates as compared with non-CTO PCI: death 0.7%; urgent CABG 0.7%; tamponade 1.4%; donor vessel dissection 2%; stroke 0.5%; and myocardial infarction 3.1%.[47] To minimize the risk of complications, particular attention should be paid to guide catheter position, especially during wire externalization and removal, to avoid deep intubation and vessel dissection. The activated clotting time is usually kept at more than 350 seconds to minimize the risk of donor vessel thrombosis.

ANTEGRADE DISSECTION AND REENTRY

The third CTO crossing technique, antegrade dissection and reentry, has also significantly evolved over the past few years. It is now well established that extensive dissection/reentry techniques, such as the subintimal tracking and reentry (STAR) technique,[48] have high rates of restenosis and reocclusion,[49] hence, should only be used as a last resort. However, encouraging results were observed with limited antegrade dissection and reentry that had similar restenosis rates as compared with standard antegrade approach in 2 studies.[50,51]

A common challenge with subintimal techniques is the formation of large subintimal hematomas that may hinder reentry into the distal true lumen. Several techniques have been described for this clinical scenario. The subintimal transcatheter withdrawal (STRAW) technique involves aspiration of the hematoma either through a Stingray balloon (Boston Scientific, Natick, MA) or through a separate inflated over-the-wire balloon, allowing reexpansion of the lumen.[52] An alternative strategy is the "double-blind stick-and-swap" technique, in which the Stingray wire is advanced through both exit ports of the Stingray balloon followed by a Pilot 200 guidewire[53] until true lumen entry is achieved. When all else fails, retrograde crossing can provide a solution to large subintimal hematomas by ensuring true lumen wire position through a collateral vessel.[54] Overall, use of antegrade dissection/reentry can be a very time-efficient technique, but also has a steep learning curve to achieve optimal results.

In addition, the mini-STAR technique, using a soft polymeric guidewire with minimal force at the distal end (differently shaped than traditional STAR technique) and supported by a microcatheter,[55] was reported to have a high success rate and good long-term outcomes.[56]

OPTIMAL CHOICE OF CROSSING STRATEGY

Selecting the optimal technique for each CTO lesion remains controversial, with many operators having strong personal preferences; yet, everyone agrees on the importance of carefully studying the lesion and customizing the crossing approach to the anatomy of the target lesion. All crossing strategies have advantages and disadvantages; therefore, flexibility is key for maximizing success, which is prompt change of strategy if no significant progress is achieved with the initial selected strategy.[26] The hybrid crossing algorithm (Fig. 3) is one such algorithm commonly used to provide guidance on how to approach a CTO based on 4 key angiographic characteristics: (1) proximal cap (ambiguous or clear, with or without side branches), (2) length of the occlusion; (3) quality of the distal vessel (size, presence of calcification, and bifurcations, especially at the distal cap), and (4) presence of "interventional collaterals," that is, collateral channels that appear suitable for retrograde crossing.

CLINICAL BENEFITS WITH CHRONIC TOTAL OCCLUSION PERCUTANEOUS CORONARY INTERVENTION

A major limitation in the field of CTO PCI is the lack of randomized controlled trials comparing CTO PCI versus medical therapy. There is, however, ample indirect evidence that CTO PCI provides clinical benefits. In a meta-analysis of 25 studies comparing successful versus failed CTO PCI in 28,486 patients, procedural success was 71%; and during a mean follow-up of 3.11 years, successful CTO PCI was associated with lower mortality (odds ratio [OR] 0.52), less residual angina (OR 0.38), lower risk for stroke (OR 0.72), and less need for subsequent CABG (OR 0.18).[57] In another meta-analysis of 7 studies of patients who presented with ST-segment elevation acute myocardial infarction, the presence of a non–infarct-related artery CTO (present in 11.7% of patients) was associated with increased

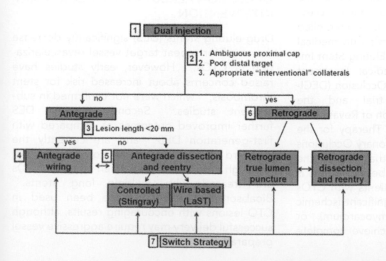

Fig. 3. Overview of the hybrid algorithm for crossing chronic total occlusions. The first step is dual coronary injection allowing assessment of 4 angiographic parameters: 1. proximal cap ambiguity, 2. length of occlusion, 3. distal vessel, and 4. interventional collaterals. Based on those parameters an initial and subsequent crossing strategy is selected. (*From* Brilakis ES, Grantham JA, Rinfret S, et al. A percutaneous treatment algorithm for crossing coronary chronic total occlusions. JACC Cardiovasc Interv 2012;5: 373; with permission.)

incidence of all-cause mortality at a median follow-up of 25.2 months (OR 2.90, *P* <.0001).[58] Although this does not prove that prophylactic CTO PCI improves outcomes in patients who subsequently developed acute coronary syndromes, it is certainly suggestive.

Successful CTO PCI improves quality of life,[59] exercise capacity,[60] and left ventricular systolic function.[61–70] A study of patients with ischemic cardiomyopathy with implantable cardioverter/defibrillators demonstrated that patients with CTOs had higher risk for appropriate shocks and higher mortality,[71] although this association was not confirmed in a second, larger study.[72] Successful CTO PCI can however, be effective in stopping a ventricular tachycardic storm.[73] In 2 recent observational studies of patients found to have CTO on diagnostic angiography, CTO PCI was associated with better outcomes as compared with medical therapy, even after multivariable adjustment.[6,74]

The first randomized controlled trial of CTO PCI versus no CTO PCI is the Evaluating Xience V and left ventricular function in Percutaneous coronary intervention on occLusiOns afteR ST-Elevation myocardial infarction (EXPLORE) trial, in which patients who underwent primary PCI for ST-segment elevation acute myocardial infarction and were found to have a CTO in a non–infarct-related artery were randomized to either elective CTO PCI within 7 days or standard medical treatment.[75] The study results were presented at the 2015 Transcatheter Cardiovascular Therapeutics meeting. At 4 months the mean ejection fraction was similar in the CTO-PCI and the no CTO-PCI arm (44.1±12·2% vs 44.9±12·1%, p=0.55). On subgroup analysis, CTO PCI appeared to be beneficial in patients with left anterior descending artery CTOs, but not among those with right coronary or circumflex CTOs (Fig. 1B). However, the core laboratory adjudicated procedural success was 72%. Two other randomized controlled clinical trials comparing CTO PCI with medical therapy are ongoing: the Drug-Eluting Stent Implantation versus Optimal Medical Treatment in Patients With Chronic Total Occlusion (DECI-SION-CTO, NCT01078051) trial and the European Study on the Utilization of Revascularization versus Optimal Medical Therapy for the Treatment of Chronic Total Coronary Occlusions (EURO-CTO, NCT01760083) trial. Given the current body of evidence, we believe that it is reasonable to revascularize patients with CTOs who are symptomatic, have significant ischemic burden (≥10% jeopardized myocardium), or have multivessel disease, to achieve complete revascularization.

SCORES FOR CHRONIC TOTAL OCCLUSION PERCUTANEOUS CORONARY INTERVENTION

Predicting the likelihood for success and efficiency of CTO PCI can be facilitated by various scores, such as the Multicenter CTO Registry of Japan (J-CTO) score and the Progress CTO score. The J-CTO score is calculated by assigning 1 point for each of 5 parameters: calcification, tortuosity, blunt stump, occlusion length of 20 mm or more, and previously failed lesion.[76] The J-CTO score stratifies CTOs into 4 difficulty groups: easy (score of 0), intermediate (score of 1), difficult (score of 2), and very difficult (score of ≥3). The J-CTO score can help predict the likelihood of guidewire crossing within 30 minutes,[76] but also the likelihood of procedural success in some, but not all,[77] series. In some centers, overall procedural success for CTO PCI appeared to remain stagnant over time,[77] but on more detailed evaluation, the reason was an increasing complexity of CTO lesions treated, as reflected by higher J-CTO scores.[78]

A variation of the angiographic J-CTO score is the coronary computed tomography CTO score (J-CTO$_{CT}$).[79] Compared with J-CTO, J-CTO$_{CT}$ yielded shorter occlusion length, but overall correlated closely with J-CTO score with similar predictive value. Finally, the Progress CTO score is calculated by assigning 1 point for each of 4 parameters: proximal cap ambiguity, lack of interventional collaterals, moderate/severe tortuosity, and circumflex CTO target vessel.[80] These scores can be useful for lesion selection, especially in early stages of CTO PCI program development.

STENT SELECTION FOR CHRONIC TOTAL OCCLUSION PERCUTANEOUS CORONARY INTERVENTION

Drug-eluting stents (DES) significantly decrease the need for repeat target vessel revascularization in CTOs.[81] However, early studies have raised concerns about increased risk for stent thrombosis,[82] which were not confirmed in subsequent studies.[83] Second-generation DES further improved outcomes as compared with first-generation DES[84] and are currently the standard of care for these complex lesions, although concerns remain when complex CTOs are treated with multiple long stents.[85] Bioabsorbable scaffolds have been used in CTO lesions with encouraging results, although successful delivery may require aggressive vessel preparation.

SUMMARY

In summary, CTOs are common and can be treated with high success rates at experienced centers using a variety of crossing techniques and equipment. Several observational studies suggest clinical benefit with CTO PCI, yet performance of randomized clinical trials is critical for further expansion of the procedure.

REFERENCES

1. Brilakis ES, editor. Manual of coronary chronic total occlusion interventions. A step-by-step approach. Waltham (MA): Elsevier; 2013.
2. Fefer P, Knudtson ML, Cheema AN, et al. Current perspectives on coronary chronic total occlusions: the Canadian multicenter chronic total occlusions registry. J Am Coll Cardiol 2012;59:991–7.
3. Christofferson RD, Lehmann KG, Martin GV, et al. Effect of chronic total coronary occlusion on treatment strategy. Am J Cardiol 2005;95:1088–91.
4. Werner GS, Gitt AK, Zeymer U, et al. Chronic total coronary occlusions in patients with stable angina pectoris: impact on therapy and outcome in present day clinical practice. Clin Res Cardiol 2009; 98:435–41.
5. Jeroudi OM, Alomar ME, Michael TT, et al. Prevalence and management of coronary chronic total occlusions in a tertiary Veterans Affairs hospital. Catheter Cardiovasc Interv 2014;84:637–43.
6. Tomasello SD, Boukhris M, Giubilato S, et al. Management strategies in patients affected by chronic total occlusions: results from the Italian registry of chronic total occlusions. Eur Heart J 2015;36: 3189–98.
7. Christopoulos G, Karmpaliotis D, Alaswad K, et al. Application and outcomes of a hybrid approach to chronic total occlusion percutaneous coronary intervention in a contemporary multicenter US registry. Int J Cardiol 2015;198:222–8.
8. Vo MN, McCabe JM, Lombardi WL, et al. Adoption of the hybrid CTO approach by a single non-CTO operator: procedural and clinical outcomes. J Invasive Cardiol 2015;27:139–44.
9. Patel VG, Brayton KM, Tamayo A, et al. Angiographic success and procedural complications in patients undergoing percutaneous coronary chronic total occlusion interventions: a weighted meta-analysis of 18,061 patients from 65 studies. JACC Cardiovasc Interv 2013;6:128–36.
10. Khan MF, Wendel CS, Thai HM, et al. Effects of percutaneous revascularization of chronic total occlusions on clinical outcomes: a meta-analysis comparing successful versus failed percutaneous intervention for chronic total occlusion. Catheter Cardiovasc Interv 2013;82:95–107.
11. Christopoulos G, Menon RV, Karmpaliotis D, et al. Application of the "hybrid approach" to chronic total occlusions in patients with previous coronary artery bypass graft surgery (from a contemporary multicenter US registry). Am J Cardiol 2014;113: 1990–4.
12. Teramoto T, Tsuchikane E, Matsuo H, et al. Initial success rate of percutaneous coronary intervention for chronic total occlusion in a native coronary artery is decreased in patients who underwent previous coronary artery bypass graft surgery. JACC Cardiovasc Interv 2014;7:39–46.
13. Michael TT, Karmpaliotis D, Brilakis ES, et al. Impact of prior coronary artery bypass graft surgery on chronic total occlusion revascularisation: insights from a multicentre US registry. Heart 2013; 99:1515–8.
14. Singh M, Bell MR, Berger PB, et al. Utility of bilateral coronary injections during complex coronary angioplasty. J Invasive Cardiol 1999;11:70–4.
15. Rinfret S, Joyal D, Spratt JC, et al. Chronic total occlusion percutaneous coronary intervention case selection and techniques for the antegrade-only operator. Catheter Cardiovasc Interv 2014;85(3): 408–15.
16. Ozawa N. A new understanding of chronic total occlusion from a novel PCI technique that involves a retrograde approach to the right coronary artery via a septal branch and passing of the guidewire to a guiding catheter on the other side of the lesion. Catheter Cardiovasc Interv 2006;68:907–13.
17. Surmely JF, Tsuchikane E, Katoh O, et al. New concept for CTO recanalization using controlled antegrade and retrograde subintimal tracking: the CART technique. J Invasive Cardiol 2006;18:334–8.
18. Brilakis ES, Grantham JA, Thompson CA, et al. The retrograde approach to coronary artery chronic total occlusions: a practical approach. Catheter Cardiovasc Interv 2012;79:3–19.
19. Whitlow PL, Burke MN, Lombardi WL, et al. Use of a novel crossing and re-entry system in coronary chronic total occlusions that have failed standard crossing techniques: results of the FAST-CTOs (facilitated antegrade steering technique in chronic total occlusions) trial. JACC Cardiovasc Interv 2012; 5:393–401.
20. Michael TT, Papayannis AC, Banerjee S, et al. Subintimal dissection/reentry strategies in coronary chronic total occlusion interventions. Circ Cardiovasc Interv 2012;5:729–38.
21. Wosik J, Shorrock D, Christopoulos G, et al. Systematic review of the bridgepoint system for crossing coronary and peripheral chronic total occlusions. J Invasive Cardiol 2015;27:269–76.
22. Christopoulos G, Wyman RM, Alaswad K, et al. Clinical utility of the Japan-chronic total occlusion score in coronary chronic total occlusion

interventions: results from a multicenter registry. Circ Cardiovasc Interv 2015;8(7):e002171.

23. Luna M, Papayannis A, Holper EM, et al. Transfemoral use of the GuideLiner catheter in complex coronary and bypass graft interventions. Catheter Cardiovasc Interv 2012;80:437–46.

24. Di Mario C, Ramasami N. Techniques to enhance guide catheter support. Catheter Cardiovasc Interv 2008;72:505–12.

25. Sianos G, Werner GS, Galassi AR, et al. Recanalisation of chronic total coronary occlusions: 2012 consensus document from the EuroCTO club. EuroIntervention 2012;8:139–45.

26. Brilakis ES, Grantham JA, Rinfret S, et al. A percutaneous treatment algorithm for crossing coronary chronic total occlusions. JACC Cardiovasc Interv 2012;5:367–79.

27. Tomasello SD, Giudice P, Attisano T, et al. The innovation of composite core dual coil coronary guide-wire technology: a didactic coronary chronic total occlusion revascularization case report. J Saudi Heart Assoc 2014;26:222–5.

28. Galassi AR, Ganyukov V, Tomasello SD, et al. Successful antegrade revascularization by the innovation of composite core dual coil in a three-vessel total occlusive disease for cardiac arrest patient using extracorporeal membrane oxygenation. Eur Heart J 2014;35:2009.

29. Khalili H, Vo M, Brilakis ES. Initial experience with the Gaia composite core guidewires in coronary chronic total occlusion crossing. J Invasive Cardiol, in press.

30. Sakakura K, Nakano M, Otsuka F, et al. Comparison of pathology of chronic total occlusion with and without coronary artery bypass graft. Eur Heart J 2014;35:1683–93.

31. Fang HY, Wu CC, Wu CJ. Successful transradial antegrade coronary intervention of a rare right coronary artery high anterior downward takeoff anomalous chronic total occlusion by double-anchoring technique and retrograde guidance. Int Heart J 2009;50:531–8.

32. Nombela-Franco L, Werner GS. Retrograde recanalization of a chronic ostial occlusion of the left anterior descending artery: how to manage extreme takeoff angles. J Invasive Cardiol 2010; 22:E7–12.

33. Galassi AR, Sianos G, Werner GS, et al. Retrograde recanalization of chronic total occlusions in Europe: procedural, in-hospital, and long-term outcomes from the multicenter ERCTO registry. J Am Coll Cardiol 2015;65:2388–400.

34. Boukhris M, Tomasello SD, Azzarelli S, et al. Coronary perforation with tamponade successfully managed by retrograde and antegrade coil embolization. J Saudi Heart Assoc 2015;27: 216–21.

35. Kotsia AP, Brilakis ES, Karmpaliotis D. Thrombin injection for sealing epicardial collateral perforation during chronic total occlusion percutaneous coronary interventions. J Invasive Cardiol 2014;26: E124–6.

36. Wilson WM, Spratt JC, Lombardi WL. Cardiovascular collapse post chronic total occlusion percutaneous coronary intervention due to a compressive left atrial haematoma managed with percutaneous drainage. Catheter Cardiovasc Interv 2015;86:407–11.

37. Aggarwal C, Varghese J, Uretsky BF. Left atrial inflow and outflow obstruction as a complication of retrograde approach for chronic total occlusion: report of a case and literature review of left atrial hematoma after percutaneous coronary intervention. Catheter Cardiovasc Interv 2013;82:770–5.

38. Tsuchikane E, Yamane M, Mutoh M, et al. Japanese multicenter registry evaluating the retrograde approach for chronic coronary total occlusion. Catheter Cardiovasc Interv 2013;82:E654–61.

39. Mozid AM, Davies JR, Spratt JC. The utility of a guideliner catheter in retrograde percutaneous coronary intervention of a chronic total occlusion with reverse cart-the "capture" technique. Catheter Cardiovasc Interv 2014;83:929–32.

40. Thompson CA, Jayne JE, Robb JF, et al. Retrograde techniques and the impact of operator volume on percutaneous intervention for coronary chronic total occlusions an early U.S. experience. JACC Cardiovasc Interv 2009;2:834–42.

41. Karmpaliotis D, Michael TT, Brilakis ES, et al. Retrograde coronary chronic total occlusion revascularization: procedural and in-hospital outcomes from a multicenter registry in the United States. JACC Cardiovasc Interv 2012;5:1273–9.

42. Rathore S, Katoh O, Matsuo H, et al. Retrograde percutaneous recanalization of chronic total occlusion of the coronary arteries: procedural outcomes and predictors of success in contemporary practice. Circ Cardiovasc Interv 2009;2:124–32.

43. Rathore S, Matsuo H, Terashima M, et al. Procedural and in-hospital outcomes after percutaneous coronary intervention for chronic total occlusions of coronary arteries 2002 to 2008: impact of novel guidewire techniques. JACC Cardiovasc Interv 2009;2:489–97.

44. Muramatsu T, Tsuchikane E, Oikawa Y, et al. Incidence and impact on midterm outcome of controlled subintimal tracking in patients with successful recanalisation of chronic total occlusions: J-PROCTOR registry. EuroIntervention 2014;10: 681–8.

45. Lo N, Michael TT, Moin D, et al. Periprocedural myocardial injury in chronic total occlusion percutaneous interventions: a systematic cardiac biomarker evaluation study. JACC Cardiovasc Interv 2014;7: 47–54.

46. Werner GS, Coenen A, Tischer KH. Periprocedural ischaemia during recanalisation of chronic total coronary occlusions: the influence of the transcollateral retrograde approach. EuroIntervention 2014;10:799–805.
47. El Sabbagh A, Patel VG, Jeroudi OM, et al. Angiographic success and procedural complications in patients undergoing retrograde percutaneous coronary chronic total occlusion interventions: a weighted meta-analysis of 3,482 patients from 26 studies. Int J Cardiol 2014;174:243–8.
48. Colombo A, Mikhail GW, Michev I, et al. Treating chronic total occlusions using subintimal tracking and reentry: the STAR technique. Catheter Cardiovasc Interv 2005;64:407–11 [discussion: 412].
49. Valenti R, Vergara R, Migliorini A, et al. Predictors of reocclusion after successful drug-eluting stent-supported percutaneous coronary intervention of chronic total occlusion. J Am Coll Cardiol 2013;61:545–50.
50. Mogabgab O, Patel VG, Michael TT, et al. Long-term outcomes with use of the crossboss and stingray coronary CTO crossing and re-entry devices. J Invasive Cardiol 2013;25:579–85.
51. Rinfret S, Ribeiro HB, Nguyen CM, et al. Dissection and re-entry techniques and longer-term outcomes following successful percutaneous coronary intervention of chronic total occlusion. Am J Cardiol 2014;114:1354–60.
52. Smith EJ, Di Mario C, Spratt JC, et al. Subintimal TRAnscatheter Withdrawal (STRAW) of hematomas compressing the distal true lumen: a novel technique to facilitate distal reentry during recanalization of chronic total occlusion (CTO). J Invasive Cardiol 2015;27:E1–4.
53. Chiristopoulos G, Kotsia AP, Brilakis ES. The "double blind stick-and-swap" technique for true lumen re-entry after subintimal crossing of coronary chronic total occlusions. J Invasive Cardiol 2015;27:E199–202, in press.
54. Latif F, Brilakis ES, Exaire JE. Retrograde approach to successfully treat antegrade failure due to subintimal hematoma of a right coronary artery chronic total occlusion. Interv Cardiol 2015;7:229–33.
55. Galassi AR, Tomasello SD, Costanzo L, et al. Mini-STAR as bail-out strategy for percutaneous coronary intervention of chronic total occlusion. Catheter Cardiovasc Interv 2012;79:30–40.
56. Galassi AR, Boukhris M, Tomasello SD, et al. Long-term clinical and angiographic outcomes of the mini-STAR technique as a bailout strategy for percutaneous coronary intervention of chronic total occlusion. Can J Cardiol 2014;30:1400–6.
57. Christakopoulos GE, Christopoulos G, Carlino M, et al. Meta-analysis of clinical outcomes of patients who underwent percutaneous coronary interventions for chronic total occlusions. Am J Cardiol 2015;115:1367–75.
58. O'Connor SA, Garot P, Sanguineti F, et al. Meta-analysis of the impact on mortality of noninfarct-related artery coronary chronic total occlusion in patients presenting with ST-segment elevation myocardial infarction. Am J Cardiol 2015;116:8–14.
59. Safley DM, Grantham JA, Hatch J, et al. Quality of life benefits of percutaneous coronary intervention for chronic occlusions. Catheter Cardiovasc Interv 2014;84:629–34.
60. Olivari Z, Rubartelli P, Piscione F, et al. Immediate results and one-year clinical outcome after percutaneous coronary interventions in chronic total occlusions: data from a multicenter, prospective, observational study (TOAST-GISE). J Am Coll Cardiol 2003;41:1672–8.
61. Melchior JP, Doriot PA, Chatelain P, et al. Improvement of left ventricular contraction and relaxation synchronism after recanalization of chronic total coronary occlusion by angioplasty. J Am Coll Cardiol 1987;9:763–8.
62. Danchin N, Angioi M, Cador R, et al. Effect of late percutaneous angioplastic recanalization of total coronary artery occlusion on left ventricular remodeling, ejection fraction, and regional wall motion. Am J Cardiol 1996;78:729–35.
63. Van Belle E, Blouard P, McFadden EP, et al. Effects of stenting of recent or chronic coronary occlusions on late vessel patency and left ventricular function. Am J Cardiol 1997;80:1150–4.
64. Sirnes PA, Myreng Y, Molstad P, et al. Improvement in left ventricular ejection fraction and wall motion after successful recanalization of chronic coronary occlusions. Eur Heart J 1998;19:273–81.
65. Piscione F, Galasso G, De Luca G, et al. Late reopening of an occluded infarct related artery improves left ventricular function and long term clinical outcome. Heart 2005;91:646–51.
66. Baks T, van Geuns RJ, Duncker DJ, et al. Prediction of left ventricular function after drug-eluting stent implantation for chronic total coronary occlusions. J Am Coll Cardiol 2006;47:721–5.
67. Kirschbaum SW, Baks T, van den Ent M, et al. Evaluation of left ventricular function three years after percutaneous recanalization of chronic total coronary occlusions. Am J Cardiol 2008;101:179–85.
68. Cheng AS, Selvanayagam JB, Jerosch-Herold M, et al. Percutaneous treatment of chronic total coronary occlusions improves regional hyperemic myocardial blood flow and contractility: insights from quantitative cardiovascular magnetic resonance imaging. JACC Cardiovasc Interv 2008;1:44–53.
69. Werner GS, Surber R, Kuethe F, et al. Collaterals and the recovery of left ventricular function after recanalization of a chronic total coronary occlusion. Am Heart J 2005;149:129–37.

70. Yamamoto Y, de Silva R, Rhodes CG, et al. A new strategy for the assessment of viable myocardium and regional myocardial blood flow using 15O-water and dynamic positron emission tomography. Circulation 1992;86:167–78.

71. Nombela-Franco L, Mitroi CD, Fernandez-Lozano I, et al. Ventricular arrhythmias among implantable cardioverter-defibrillator recipients for primary prevention: impact of chronic total coronary occlusion (VACTO primary study). Circ Arrhythm Electrophysiol 2012;5:147–54.

72. Raja V, Wiegn P, Obel O, et al. Impact of chronic total occlusions and coronary revascularization on all-cause mortality and the incidence of ventricular arrhythmias in patients with ischemic cardiomyopathy. Am J Cardiol 2015;116(9):1358–62.

73. Mixon TA. Ventricular tachycardic storm with a chronic total coronary artery occlusion treated with percutaneous coronary intervention. Proc (Bayl Univ Med Cent) 2015;28:196–9.

74. Jang WJ, Yang JH, Choi SH, et al. Long-term survival benefit of revascularization compared with medical therapy in patients with coronary chronic total occlusion and well-developed collateral circulation. JACC Cardiovasc Interv 2015;8:271–9.

75. van der Schaaf RJ, Claessen BE, Hoebers LP, et al. Rationale and design of EXPLORE: a randomized, prospective, multicenter trial investigating the impact of recanalization of a chronic total occlusion on left ventricular function in patients after primary percutaneous coronary intervention for acute ST-elevation myocardial infarction. Trials 2010;11:89.

76. Morino Y, Abe M, Morimoto T, et al. Predicting successful guidewire crossing through chronic total occlusion of native coronary lesions within 30 minutes: the J-CTO (Multicenter CTO Registry in Japan) score as a difficulty grading and time assessment tool. JACC Cardiovasc Interv 2011;4:213–21.

77. Nombela-Franco L, Urena M, Jerez-Valero M, et al. Validation of the J-chronic total occlusion score for chronic total occlusion percutaneous coronary intervention in an independent contemporary cohort. Circ Cardiovasc Interv 2013;6:635–43.

78. Syrseloudis D, Secco GG, Barrero EA, et al. Increase in J-CTO lesion complexity score explains the disparity between recanalisation success and evolution of chronic total occlusion strategies: insights from a single-centre 10-year experience. Heart 2013;99:474–9.

79. Li Y, Xu N, Zhang J, et al. Procedural success of CTO recanalization: comparison of the J-CTO score determined by coronary CT angiography to invasive angiography. J Cardiovasc Comput Tomogr 2015;9:578–84.

80. Christopoulos G, Kandzari D, Yeh RW, et al. Development and validation of a novel scoring system for predicting technical success of chronic total occlusion percutaneous coronary interventions: the prospective global registry for the study of chronic total occlusion intervention (PROGRESS CTO) score. JACC Cardiovasc Interv, in press.

81. Brilakis ES, Kotsia A, Luna M, et al. The role of drug-eluting stents for the treatment of coronary chronic total occlusions. Expert Rev Cardiovasc Ther 2013;11:1349–58.

82. Colmenarez HJ, Escaned J, Fernandez C, et al. Efficacy and safety of drug-eluting stents in chronic total coronary occlusion recanalization: a systematic review and meta-analysis. J Am Coll Cardiol 2010;55:1854–66.

83. Saeed B, Kandzari DE, Agostoni P, et al. Use of drug-eluting stents for chronic total occlusions: a systematic review and meta-analysis. Catheter Cardiovasc Interv 2011;77:315–32.

84. Lanka V, Patel VG, Saeed B, et al. Outcomes with first- versus second-generation drug-eluting stents in coronary chronic total occlusions (CTOs): a systematic review and meta-analysis. J Invasive Cardiol 2014;26:304–10.

85. Kotsia A, Navara R, Michael TT, et al. The angiographic evaluation of the everolimus-eluting stent in chronic total occlusion (ACE-CTO) study. J Invasive Cardiol 2015;27:393–400.

Hemodynamic Support Devices for Complex Percutaneous Coronary Intervention

Basil Alkhatib, MD[a], Laura Wolfe, DO[a],
Srihari S. Naidu, MD, FSCAI[b],*

KEYWORDS

- Ventricular assist devices • Complex coronary intervention • PCI • High risk • Support devices

---

KEY POINTS

- Increasing complexity of percutaneous coronary intervention (PCI) and high-risk subsets have led to the development and incorporation of hemodynamic support devices to minimize periprocedural risk and improve clinical outcomes, both short term and long term.
- Various hemodynamic support devices for high-risk PCI are currently available, including the intra-aortic balloon pump (IABP), ventricular assist device (VAD), and enhanced extracorporeal membrane oxygenation (ECMO), each with its own inherent risks and benefits as well as technical requirements.
- Data to support high-risk PCIs are available and continue to evolve, and current consensus documents and guidelines support high-risk PCI in unique patient populations.

INTRODUCTION

The field of interventional cardiology has seen rapid advances in technology that have led to the treatment of high-risk patients and complex coronary lesions. These advances include devices that directly aid in the treatment of complex coronary lesions, such as atherectomy devices and advanced guide wires, catheters and further iterations of balloons and stents, and indirect assistance in the form of cardiac assist (hemodynamic support) devices.

Cardiac assist devices can be used in various situations, such as percutaneous valvular procedures, cardiogenic shock, and acute decompensated heart failure; as a bridge to complete circulatory support; and during treatment of elective or urgent high-risk PCI. The focus of this article is on the latter.

Historically, the IABP has been the mainstay cardiac assist device due to its ease of use and wide familiarity and availability. Over the past decade, however, the category of percutaneous assist devices has blossomed to also include Impella 2.5, Impella 5.0, Impella CP, and Impella RP (Abiomed, Danvers, Massachusetts), TandemHeart (Cardiac Assist, Pittsburgh, Pennsylvania) and ECMO. Currently, there is no single unifying definition of high-risk PCI but variables that contribute to elevated risk of adverse outcomes during PCI are well established and can be divided into 3 categories: (1) patient-specific variables, (2) lesion-specific variables, and (3) the clinical setting leading to PCI.

Conflict of Interest: S.S. Naidu serves on the advisory board of Abiomed and Maquet (modest). Remaining authors cite no conflict of interest.
[a] Division of Cardiology, Winthrop University Hospital, 120 Mineola Boulevard, Suite 500, Mineola NY 11501, USA;
[b] Cardiac Catheterization Laboratory, Division of Cardiology, Winthrop University Hospital, 120 Mineola Boulevard, Suite 500, Mineola, NY 11501, USA
* Corresponding author.
E-mail address: SSNaidu@Winthrop.org

This article focuses on defining high-risk patients who may benefit from percutaneous assist devices during elective or urgent PCI. For each available percutaneous assist device, the mechanism of action and how it differs from other devices, the clinical data supporting its use, the practical implications for each device, and the current consensus opinion and guidelines for percutaneous assist device utilization are discussed.

DEVICES FOR HIGH-RISK PERCUTANEOUS CORONARY INTERVENTION

During high-risk PCI, the need to maintain hemodynamic stability is of utmost importance, because the device is used to maintain a stable hemodynamic state through a complex procedure with risk of significant ischemia in the setting of baseline cardiac dysfunction. Each device comes with a different mechanism of action and magnitude of hemodynamic support as well as procedural risk, and a proper understanding of each of these is important to guide device selection and anticipate safety and clinical outcomes (Table 1).

While performing high-risk PCI, hemodynamic measurements are essential to guiding management. Particular attention is paid to mean arterial pressure (MAP), cardiac output (CO), and pulmonary capillary wedge pressure. Coronary blood flow (CBF) is dependent on pressure difference across the vascular bed and reciprocally related to resistance to blood flow distally, which correlates with wall tension or left ventricular end-diastolic pressure (LVEDP).[1] Because coronary perfusion occurs during diastole, it is calculated as the pressure difference between the diastolic blood pressure (DBP) and the pressure in the peripheral vascular bed. The following formulae describe these relationships:

Coronary perfusion pressure (CPP) =
DBP − LVEDP

CBF = CPP/wall tension (or LVEDP)

LVEDP is also directly proportional to myocardial wall tension. Therefore, any mechanism that can increase DBP, decrease resistance to blood flow, and/or decrease myocardial wall stress/tension increases CBF. An ideal assist device is able to accomplish all of these goals.

Recently, a hemodynamic measurement of cardiac support, namely cardiac power output (CPO), measured in watts, has been discussed for its potential utility in these patients. CPO is MAP multiplied by CO and divided by a constant of 451.[1] This applies the concept that the CO parameter alone is insufficient in predicting sufficient tissue perfusion and blood pressure support. The incorporation of MAP allows better prediction of cardiac decompensation and tissue perfusion and aligns with mortality in patients with cardiogenic shock.[1]

Although supporting systemic and coronary perfusion is an important element of assist devices, these devices also reduce myocardial oxygen demand. Fig. 1 demonstrates the pressure-volume loop of the cardiac cycle, which is helpful in understanding these dynamics. It is bordered inferiorly by the end-diastolic pressure-volume relationship (EDPVR) and superiorly by the end-systolic pressure-volume relationship (ESPVR). Normal hemodynamics dictate that the area within the pressure-volume loop tracks with stroke work (SW), and the area before the flow loop tracks with potential energy (PE) stored in cardiac myocytes. Pressure-volume area (PVA), therefore, is the SW plus the PE and has recently emerged as a potent indicator of myocardial oxygen consumption on a beat-to-beat basis.[1]

PVA = SW + PE

To reduce myocardial oxygen demand, a therapy must move the pressure-volume loop down and to the left (see Fig. 1). Devices, therefore, are measured on whether they move the loop to the left, thereby reducing myocardial oxygen consumption, while at the same time providing optimal CPO and CBF.[2] In this way both the heart and the peripheral organs are prioritized simultaneously during high-risk PCI, minimizing the potential for ischemia by targeting both the supply and demand elements of ischemia and avoiding the downward cycle in contractility and ventricular function that might otherwise occur during unassisted high-risk PCI.

Extracorporeal Membrane Oxygenation
Extracorporal bypass with membrane oxygenator was the first form of mechanical assist device developed. It has the capacity to support a large volume of blood flow. It is, however, greatly hindered by the requirement for a surgical cutdown due to the large size of the arterial and femoral cannulae (20F venous and 17F arterial).[3] First approved in the 1950s for use during cardiac surgery for only several hours, ECMO has evolved over the past decades to become a well utilized option for patients with severe pulmonary and/or cardiac failure.

ECMO is divided into 2 types: venovenous (V-V) or venoarterial (V-A). V-V ECMO is used

Table 1
Various hemodynamic support devices for high-risk percutaneous coronary intervention

	Mechanism of Action	Cardiac Power Output	Myocardial O₂ Demand	Coronary Blood Flow	Complications	Ease of Use	Familiarity	Contraindications
IABP	Counterpulsation via balloon inflation in the aorta	↑	↓	↑	Limb ischemia/ bleeding	Quick insertion	Widespread use	Aortic insufficiency/ aortic disease
TandemHeart	Extracorporeal pump from LA to iliofemoral arterial system	↑	↓	↑	Pericardial tamponade/aortic puncture/limb ischemia	Large arterial cannulaes/ transseptal puncture/2 access sites	Requires an experienced center	VSD/PAD/RV failure
	Extracorporeal pump with oxygenation capacity and bypass of cardiopulmonary system	↑	↑	—	Bleeding/ thromboembolic events/hemolysis	Large cannulaes/ experienced staff	Requires an experienced center	Aortic insufficiency/ PAD
Impella	Nonpulsatile axial flow Archimedes-screw pump	↑	↓	↑	Limb ischemia/ bleeding	Single cannula with relatively quick insertion	Becoming more well known	LV thrombus/ severe AS/RV failure

Abbreviations: AS, aortic stenosis; LA, left atrium; PAD, peripheral arterial disease; VSD, ventricular septal defect.

for severe respiratory or right heart failure with no or minimal ability for effective gas exchange. V-A ECMO has the capacity to provide systemic hemodynamic support with upwards of 5 L/min, whereas the addition of a membrane oxygenator provides complete cardiopulmonary support.[2]

V-A ECMO usually requires a cannula inserted into the femoral vein and the femoral artery with the tip of the venous (inflow) cannula placed at the border of the inferior vena cava and the right atrium. Blood is removed from the inferior vena cava, oxygenated externally, and returned to the femoral artery/aorta, thus creating flow from the right atrium to the aorta and bypassing the heart and lungs. This circuit allows for retrograde flow to the heart and brain, but it does not provide any significant unloading of the left ventricle (LV). Accordingly, ECMO increases afterload more than other devices due to the high flows and consequent blood pressure. As a result, ECMO increases myocardial oxygen demand secondary to high filling pressures and volume, even if SW is markedly reduced (PVA high due to large PE component). The increase in myocardial oxygen demand is potentially deleterious by lowering the ischemic threshold during a high-risk PCI. This increase in wall tension and oxygen demand can be offset, however, by unloading of the ventricle by an additional support device, such as an Impella or IABP, but such combined maneuvers are more appropriate for conditions requiring large amounts of hemodynamic support, such as refractory biventricular failure and cardiogenic shock, as opposed to the more stable high-risk PCI setting. From a CPO and CBF standpoint, however, ECMO provides robust support, typically higher than other percutaneous devices.

Other drawbacks of ECMO are the rather bulky set-up and handling of the system, including risks of air embolus due to the external circuit and vascular complications, especially if a surgical cutdown is required. Smaller percutaneous ECMO systems have been developed and are gaining traction but continue to require large cannulae (Figs. 2 and 3).

Intra-aortic Balloon Pump

IABP, which was developed in the 1960s and first implanted for a patient in cardiogenic shock, works via counterpulsation synchronized to the cardiac cycle. Rather than directly pumping blood, the IABP allows the native heart to enhance forward flow through manipulation of afterload. An IABP catheter is inserted into the femoral artery and advanced under fluoroscopy until the tip is just inferior to the takeoff of the subclavian artery. The IABP inflates and deflates based on ECG triggers or pressure sensing to the appropriate time during the cardiac cycle. The IABP inflates during diastole causing both antegrade flow to the peripheral circulation and retrograde propulsion of blood flow into the great vessels and coronary arteries, increasing coronary perfusion. The IABP deflates at the initiation of systole to decrease afterload, unload the LV, decrease LV end-systolic pressure, and slightly improve stroke volume. The increase in CO is modest, however, typically approximately of 0.5 L/min to 1.0 L/min. MAP increases due to significant diastolic augmentation, which, together with the slight improvement in CO, improves CPO. The increase in MAP and CPP, as well as a reduction in afterload, improves CBF.[4] Taken together, there is a slight increase in CO, CPO, and CBF, with nominal reduction of PVA. Consistent with this, the PROTECT II trial reported that CPO was maintained during high-risk PCI to a better extent with the Impella device than with the IABP, as determined by a less significant drop in CPO from baseline with Impella 2.5 support (-0.04 ± 0.24 Watts) compared with

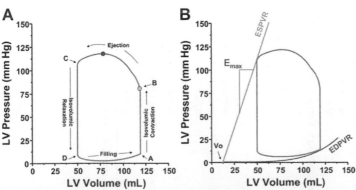

Fig. 1. (A) Pressure-volume loop. Points A thought D represent mitral valve closure (A), aortic valve opening (B), aortic valve closure (C), and mitral valve opening (D). Intervening segments are isovolumic contraction (from A to B), ejection (from B to C), isovolumic relaxation (from C to D), and ventricular filling (from D to A). (B) Relationship of pressure-volume loop to ESPVR and EDPVR, the slope of the ESPVR (E_{max}), and the volume axis intercept (Vo). (From Naidu S. Novel percutaneous cardiac assist devices, the science of and indications for hemodynamic support. Circulation 2011;123:533–43; with permission.)

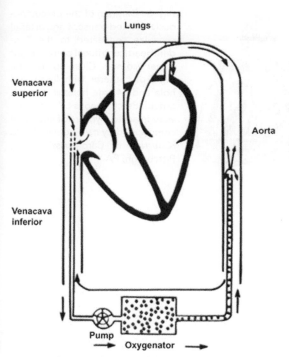

Fig. 2. Schematic drawing of the percutaneous cardio-pulmonary bypass assist device. Transfemoral venous and arterial cannulae are inserted percutaneously. Blood is pumped from the right atrium via a pump and an oxygenator to the abdominal aorta. Percutaneous LV assist devices in acute myocardial infarction complicated by cardiogenic shock. (*From* Thiele H, Smalling R, Schuler G. Percutaneous left ventricular assist devices in acute myocardial infarction complicated by cardiogenic shock. Eur Heart J 2007;28: 2057–63; with permission.)

the larger drop from baseline with the IABP (−0.14 ± 0.27 Watts) (*P* = .001).[5]

TandemHeart

TandemHeart is a form of extracorporeal bypass cardiac pump that provides a left atrial to aortic bypass circuit, powered by an external centrifugal pump. It is able to provide 3.5 L/min to 4 L/min of forward flow. Implantation of the TandemHeart requires arterial and venous femoral access, similar to ECMO but of smaller size. Via a retrograde approach through the femoral vein, a catheter is inserted and brought up to the right atrium. Transseptal puncture is performed from there into the left atrium. Once the transseptal puncture is accomplished, full anticoagulation is initiated. The transseptal puncture is then dilated up to a 2F cannula and the inflow cannula is placed into the left atrium. Two 15F catheters or one 17F catheter is

inserted into the femoral artery and advanced into the iliac artery or distal aorta. The cannulae are deaired and then connected to the centrifugal pump.

The TandemHeart decreases preload indirectly via its effect on left atrial volume, and is able to accomplish high rates of flow. The TandemHeart reduces LVEDP while simultaneously increasing CO, CPO, and MAP. As with ECMO, an increase in arterial pressure due to increased flow can increase afterload. The increase in MAP and CO results in a significant increase in CPO, whereas the indirect LV unloading can usually reduce myocardial oxygen demand despite slight increases in afterload. Accordingly, however, the reduction in myocardial oxygen demand may be inferior to a comparable flow rate with the Impella, due to the indirect versus direct unloading of the LV, because direct unloading continues to eject blood into the aorta during the isovolumic relaxation and contraction phases of the cardiac cycle.[1]

Impella 2.5, Impella CP, and Impella 5.0

The Impella, which was first approved for use in 2008, is a pump located within the shaft of a pigtail catheter (**Fig. 4**). The Impella is created in 3 forms: Impella 2.5, Impella CP, and Impella 5.0. A fourth form, the Impella RP device, is for right heart failure and is not discussed.

The Impella 2.5 is percutaneously inserted via a 13F sheath in the femoral artery; the larger CP, which can produce up to 4.0 L/min, can be placed via a 14F sheath. The Impella 5.0 version requires placement with a surgical arterial cutdown into the femoral artery, given its larger size. The internal microaxillary pump is initiated once the pigtail catheter is placed across the aortic valve, into the mid-LV cavity, creating an LV-aortic bypass that mimics normal physiology.[2,6] The Impella directly unloads the LV, markedly reducing myocardial oxygen demand to a greater extent per flow rate than the other devices, and increases CBF through both a reduction in downstream resistance and an increase in MAP and CPO. The larger devices provide more robust support of CPO and CBF, resulting in more marked reductions in myocardial oxygen demand.

DEFINITION OF HIGH-RISK PERCUTANEOUS CORONARY INTERVENTION

Historically, percutaneous mechanical circulatory support devices were used mainly for patients

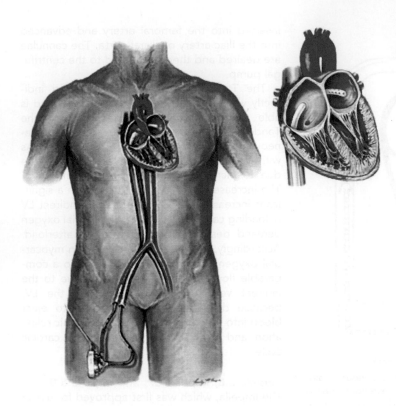

Fig. 3. Diagram of the percutaneously inserted transept and arterial cannulae connected to the TandemHeart centrifugal pump. (*Right upper corner*) Close-up of the transept catheter with large end hole and 14 side holes in the left atrium. Percutaneous LV assist devices in acute myocardial infarction complicated by cardiogenic shock. (*Courtesy of* CardiacAssist, Inc., Pittcburgh, PA.)

presenting with decompensated heart failure, cardiogenic shock, and acute coronary syndromes with hemodynamic compromise. The use of such devices has expanded over the past decade to include stable patients with complex lesions and chronically ill but hemodynamically stable patients who require PCI. The term, *high-risk PCI*, typically represents these 2 patient populations and implies a more semielective, planned PCI for improvement in cardiac function or symptoms, often in patients deemed poor candidates for surgical revascularization.

There is no consensus among cardiologists to define what is considered high-risk PCI. Multiple variables, however, are known to increase the risk of adverse outcomes in PCI and are used in decision making regarding the utility of these devices. These variables fall into 1 of 3 categories (Table 2) and should be taken into consideration prior to PCI, although the optimal mechanism to weigh each risk factor and arrive at a decision for or against cardiac support utilization remains unknown. If a patient is deemed high risk either due to hemodynamic compromise or due to an unacceptably high risk of adverse outcomes based on a combination of the noted variables, a percutaneous assist device should be considered.

Increased age has been shown in numerous studies to be a risk factor for adverse events.[7] In 1 prospective cohort study looking at outcomes in patients 80 years old or older who underwent primary PCI, in-hospital mortality was higher (17% vs 4%) with lower long-term survival rates at 3 years (cumulative survival rate 52% vs 89%).[8] Multiple validated frailty scoring systems, such as the Fried criteria, have demonstrated that increased frailty is associated with adverse long-term outcomes.[9] Short-term adverse outcomes, including complications, are also elevated in patients with frailty, because they may not tolerate ischemic PCI complications as well as more robust patients.

LV dysfunction is a marker for increased risk during PCI. A retrospective cohort study conducted on all patients who underwent elective PCI in New York State during a 1-year span (55,709 patients) evaluated the relationship between ejection fraction (EF) and hospital mortality. Patients were grouped into 5 categories based on EF (>55%, 46%–55%, 36%–45%, 26%–35%, and <26%). After multivariate adjustment, there was an increased risk for hospital mortality among EF groups of less than 26%, 26% to 35%, and 36% to 45% compared with

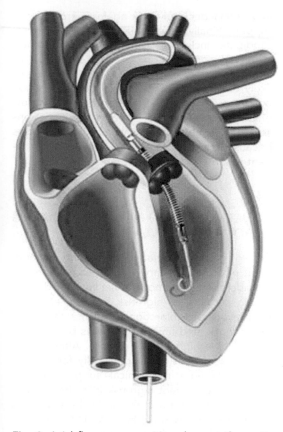

Fig. 4. Axial flow pump positioned across the aortic valve into the LV. Percutaneous LV assist devices in acute myocardial infarction complicated by cardiogenic shock. (*Courtesy of* ABIOMED, Inc., Danvers, MA.)

EF greater than 55%. As the EF decreased, the risk of hospital mortality increased, and patients with an EF less than 45% were likely to have a higher adjusted mortality rate.[10] Patients with

severe LV dysfunction (EF <25%) likely have the highest risk and have been the subject of clinical trials in this space.

Patients with chronic kidney disease have long been known to have an increased risk of the development and progression of coronary artery disease as well as mortality from cardiac causes. Chronic kidney disease requiring renal replacement therapy is an important risk factor for the development and progression of atherosclerotic coronary artery disease.[11] Patients with chronic kidney disease have poor outcomes after PCI, including increased in-hospital mortality, long-term mortality, increased rates of myocardial infarction, and increased bleeding complications, relative to patients with preserved renal function. These results were also replicated in the modern era of drug-eluting stents and antithrombotic therapy.[12-15]

Diabetes mellitus is another patient variable that increases the risk of all-cause and cardiovascular mortality. Diabetes is also a risk factor for adverse outcomes during and after PCI.[16-19] Peripheral arterial disease is also associated with increased risk for adverse outcomes for patients undergoing PCI. In the Bypass Angioplasty Revascularization Investigation trial, patients with multivessel coronary artery disease and lower extremity peripheral arterial disease randomized either to surgical or percutaneous revascularization had an adjusted relative risk of death 1.5 times greater than patients without peripheral arterial disease.[20] Despite improvement in medical therapy and coronary interventional techniques, such patients with peripheral arterial disease continue to have higher rates of myocardial infarction and mortality when undergoing PCI.[21]

Table 2
Variables known to increase the risk of adverse outcomes in percutaneous coronary intervention

Patient-Specific Variables	Lesion-Specific Variables	Clinical Setting
Increased age	Left main disease	Acute coronary syndromes
Impaired LV function	Ostial stenosis	Cardiogenic shock
Diabetes mellitus	Bifurcation disease	Acute decompensated heart failure
Chronic kidney disease	Saphenous vein graft disease	Malignant arrhythmias
Prior myocardial infarction	Heavily calcified lesions	Poor intubation candidate
Peripheral arterial disease	Chronic total occlusions	Poor surgical candidate
—	Last patent conduit	—
—	Critical 3-vessel disease	—
—	Any lesion supplying large territory	—

Patients with any lesion supplying a large area of myocardium and/or a lesion in a last remaining conduit are at high risk during PCI, because any complication may lead to catastrophic consequences from LV dysfunction and cardiogenic shock. One study looking at elective IABP use during high-risk PCI for patients with low EF characterized lesions as high risk based on the Balloon Pump–Assisted Coronary Intervention Study (BCIS-1) jeopardy score (range 0–12).[4] A score of 8 or greater indicated that the lesion was high risk. This scoring system allows broader characterization of coronary anatomy, including left main and bypass grafts and the extent of jeopardized myocardium. For example, left main stenosis greater than 50% receives a score of 8 and any diseased proximal native coronary segment is assigned a score of at least 2, with 2 additional points assigned for each major myocardial territory supplied by the segments. Protective effects of patent bypass grafts are also taken into account and represent a negative score. The scoring system has been validated by prior studies.[22–24] Aside from scoring systems, numerous studies have shown adverse in-hospital and long-term outcomes for patients undergoing PCI for left main and multivessel disease. Percutaneous revascularization on these types of lesions should be considered high risk and remain a major indication for support devices.[16,17]

Finally, the immediately preceding clinical condition of the patient may have an impact on the high-risk nature of PCI. For example, patients presenting with severe heart failure who have been recently stabilized may develop overt heart failure during PCI. Such patients, therefore, benefit from the stabilizing effect of a support device. Similarly, patients with recent malignant arrhythmias or other poorly tolerated arrhythmias are considered high risk, as is any patient with severely elevated filling pressures and/or severe pulmonary hypertension or baseline severely decreased CO or MAP.

Taken together, patients are considered high risk when a combination of all 3 variables (clinical, anatomic/lesion, and patient demographic) produces a picture of a patient who might benefit from cardiac support during PCI. In some patients, the clinical instability and LV dysfunction may make them high risk, whereas in others the lesion-specific anatomy and extent of myocardium at risk may take precedence. In most cases, baseline LV dysfunction or clinical instability is a linchpin of the concept of high risk, with anatomic lesion-specific variables and extent of myocardium in jeopardy also weighing in on a final decision for or against percutaneous support. Finally, whether a patient is a surgical candidate, including bailout surgery for emergent PCI complication, is a consideration as well as whether a patient is an airway risk or likely to fail extubation if emergent intubation becomes necessary. Such patients with low physiologic reserve or poor bailout options should be considered for support devices because such devices may avoid placing the patient in these precarious situations.

CLINICAL DATA AND GUIDELINES CONCERNING HIGH-RISK PERCUTANEOUS CORONARY INTERVENTION

Current guidelines relating to PCI and management of acute coronary syndromes recommend consideration of hemodynamic support devices in the settings of high-risk PCI, ST elevation with myocardial infarction (STEMI) with cardiogenic shock, and unstable patients being transported to a higher level of care. Although no current guidelines exist specifically for the use of percutaneous mechanical support devices during nonemergent high-risk PCI, the body of evidence supporting their use in these settings continues to grow and a Food and Drug Administration (FDA) indication was given to the Impella 2.5 device recently. In addition, an expert consensus document endorsed by multiple societies on the use of percutaneous mechanical circulatory support devices in cardiovascular care supported the use of devices for elective high-risk PCI.

Intra-aortic Balloon Pump

Initially, IABP was used as a stand-alone treatment of patients with acute myocardial infarction and cardiogenic shock. Long-term survival of these patients, however, was poor. Once it became clear coronary angiography could be performed safely with IABP, it was thought that IABP plus revascularization might improve survival. This concept has been supported, but not proved, in several uncontrolled clinical studies.[25–28] In a large National Cardiovascular Data Registry study, IABP was used in only 10.5% of 181,599 high-risk PCI patients (defined as unprotected left main, low EF, STEMI, and cardiogenic shock) but did not decrease mortality.[29] A meta-analysis of IABP use in acute myocardial infarction also found no benefit but potential harm, including higher risk of stroke.[30] Although 3 randomized trials, discussed later, did not show mortality benefit, there were some favorable results for IABP use in high-risk PCI.[4,31,32]

The Intraaortic Balloon Pump Support for Myocardial Infarction with Cardiogenic Shock II (IABP-Shock II) trial randomized 600 patients with cardiogenic shock complicating acute myocardial infarction to IABP or no IABP, with all patients planned to undergo early revascularization.[31] Mortality was similar at 30 days between the 2 groups (40% vs 41%). Secondary clinical endpoints were also similar. The 2 limitations of the trial were that the majority (83%) of IABPs were inserted after primary PCI with a 12% crossover rate of patients into the IABP arm.

The multicenter Intra-aortic Balloon Counterpulsation and infarct size in patients with acute anterior myocardial infarction without shock (CRISP AMI) trial randomized 337 patients to either IABP implantation immediately before reperfusion in patients presenting with anterior STEMI versus standard of care.[32] No reduction in infarct size was seen 3 to 5 days after PCI, as assessed by cardiac MRI, and there was no significant difference in 6-month survival.

The multicenter BCIS-1 trial randomized 301 patients at 17 centers in the United Kingdom and compared routine IABP use to provisional IABP use among patients referred for elective high-risk PCI.[4] Although major adverse cardiac endpoints at hospital discharge were similar, routine IABP use significantly reduced major procedural complications (1.3% vs 10.7%, $P<.001$) in particular procedural hypotension. Analysis at 51 months showed a 34% relative reduction in all-cause mortality with routine IABP use in patients with severe ischemic cardiomyopathy, although the trial was not powered for this endpoint.[33] Despite the limited evidence of meaningful benefit, IABP has a class IIa indication for use during STEMI complicated by cardiogenic shock in the 2013 American College of Cardiology Foundation (ACCF)/American Heart Association STEMI guidelines. IABP use without the presence of shock was not addressed except that it may be useful for mechanical complications of STEMI. A consensus statement on percutaneous mechanical circulatory support devices suggested that IABP may be helpful in patients with severely decreased LV function or decompensated heart failure undergoing noncomplex PCI.[34] It may also be helpful in patients with normal EF who are planned to undergo technically challenging or prolonged PCI. More powerful devices, however, were recommended for high-risk PCI in the setting of severe LV dysfunction or complex anatomy.

Extracorporeal Membrane Oxygenation

ECMO has little use during elective PCI. More commonly it is indicated for an inability to wean from cardiopulmonary bypass, to support patients with allograft failure post–cardiac transplant, for fulminant myocarditis, and as a bridge to more definitive VD therapy in cardiogenic shock. ECMO has also been used in patients with cardiogenic shock from acute coronary syndrome with use of other VADs concomitantly, after alternate devices have already failed, when oxygenation is inadequate, or when predominant right ventricular (RV) failure occurs. Given that ECMO typically results in more peripheral complications, requires a perfusion team, and may elevate the workload on the heart via its effect on afterload and myocardial oxygen demand, it is likely not to be used by interventional cardiologists for patients undergoing elective high-risk PCI. To date, there are no trials that have evaluated the role of ECMO in high-risk PCI. Accordingly, the role of ECMO likely is limited to patients presenting with cardiogenic shock or cardiac arrest, where the hemodynamic benefits may be of most use.[35] Even in these settings, the data for ECMO use are scarce. One systematic review of 1494 patients (from 83 studies) with cardiogenic shock, cardiac arrest, or both found that survival at discharge was slightly less than 50%,[36,37] which may not be dissimilar than the overall population presenting with cardiogenic shock. Isolated RV failure may now be treated by the dedicated Impella RP device, available as of 2015 through an FDA investigational device exemption.

TandemHeart

TandemHeart is another percutaneous mechanical circulatory support device that seems safe and feasible for high-risk PCI. No randomized trials of high-risk PCI with TandemHeart exist. In a retrospective study of 54 patients who underwent high-risk PCI using TandemHeart, procedural success rate was 97% and survival rates at 30 and 60 days were 90% and 87%, respectively.[38] None of the patients developed contrast-induced nephropathy or required hemodialysis. Major vascular complications occurred, however, in 13% of cases. Patients were considered very high risk if they had a low EF, severe left main or multivessel disease and were considered inoperable or poor surgical candidates due to comorbidities. Another small study evaluating 37 patients with cardiogenic shock or undergoing complex coronary intervention with high probability of hemodynamic collapse noted the TandemHeart was tolerated well and had a 100%

technical success rate.[39] In this study, 71% of patients in the trial survived to hospital discharge with improved functional status. One small study compared TandemHeart to IABP support in high-risk PCI.[40] The investigators randomized 33 patients within 24 hours of the onset of cardiogenic shock to 1 of the 2 devices. There was no difference in 30-day mortality or adverse events. Compared with IABP, however, the TandemHeart device resulted in increased cardiac index and decrease in pulmonary capillary wedge pressure. Use of TandemHeart for high-risk PCI has been limited, like ECMO, by large cannulae size and consequent higher complication rates, including the need for transseptal puncture.

Impella

The Impella was initially used for cardiogenic shock patients but has since been shown helpful in elective high-risk PCI. In the PROTECT I trial (A Prospective Randomized Clinical Trial of Hemodynamic Support with Impella 2.5Vs intra-Aortic Balloon pump in patients undergoing hight-risk PCI), 20 patients underwent successful high-risk PCI with the Impella 2.5, without any hemodynamic compromise.[41] The USpella registry was an observational study that included 175 patients who underwent high-risk PCI with prophylactic support of the Impella 2.5.[42] The patient population was extremely high risk: they were either deemed inoperable or had multiple patient variables that made them high risk for PCI, including chronic kidney disease, prior coronary artery bypass grafting, severe LV dysfunction, and high prevalence of New York Heart Association (NYHA) class III–IV heart failure. Overall revascularization was successful in 99% of patients, resulting in an improvement of the EF and improved functional status by 1 or more NYHA class in 51% of patients. At 30-day follow-up, the major adverse cardiac event rate was 8%, and survival was 96% and 88% at 30 days and 12 months, respectively. The PROTECT II trial, which was the largest single randomized clinical trial of high-risk PCI using mechanical circulatory support, randomized 452 symptomatic patients with complex 3-vessel or unprotected left main disease and severely depressed LV function to Impella 2.5 (n = 226) or IABP (n = 226) support during nonemergent high-risk PCI.[5] The primary endpoint of 30-day major adverse events (MAEs) was not statistically different with Impella and IABP in the intention-to-treat protocol (35% vs 40%, $P = .227$), despite the Impella providing superior hemodynamic support as represented by change in CPO during the procedure. At 90 days, a strong trend toward

decreased MAEs was observed in the Impella 2.5–supported patients compared with IABP (40.6% vs 49.3%, $P = .066$) in intention-to-treat analysis, whereas the per protocol evaluation showed a significant improvement in MAE. The limitation to this study was that it was terminated early due to projected futility. Part of the reason for this was the definition of myocardial infarction and the significant learning curve that resulted in Impella-related MAE rates that were higher in the initial patient compared with the remaining patients at each site. A subsequent analysis was performed with a less stringent definition of myocardial infarction (development of new Q waves or CK-MB 8 times the upper limit of normal).[43] Patient outcomes were compared on the composite endpoints of MAEs and major adverse cardiovascular and cerebrovascular events. At 90 days, the rates of both composite endpoints were lower in the Impella group compared with the IABP group (MAE 37% vs 49%, $P = .014$; major adverse cardiovascular and cerebrovascular events 22% vs 31%, $P = .034$).[43] This late benefit was also observed in the BCIS-1 trial (IABP support for high-risk PCI), as discussed previously. Despite multiple hypotheses as to why this is the case (ie, more stable procedural hemodynamics or more complete revascularization), future randomized trials are needed to validate these findings.

PRACTICAL IMPLICATIONS AND DEVICE SELECTION

Once a patient is deemed high risk for PCI-related complications, the operator must determine which device to use. When selecting the appropriate support device for a patient, multiple factors must be considered. For example, can a mechanical circulatory support device be inserted quickly? Is the patient stable enough to tolerate the time required for device placement? Does the patient's vascular anatomy allow for placement? What is the institution or operator familiarity with the device? Which devices are available? How much support, in the form of CPO augmentation or anti-ischemic benefit, seems required? All of these considerations and others are important when making this critical selection.

In the emergent patient, shortening the time required to unload the LV and stabilize systemic hemodynamics while reducing pulmonary congestion is of paramount importance. The earlier the device can modulate hemodynamics, the less myocardium at risk and the smaller the risk of end-organ failure as well as the risk of emergent intubation or malignant arrhythmia. Therefore, a device that can be placed percutaneously quickly in the catheterization laboratory is recommended for patients in need of emergent PCI and cardiogenic shock or impending shock. Another related factor is the ease of insertion of the device. Although this consideration may be operator dependent, it is also dependent on the equipment required for each device (ie, the centrifuge required for ECMO or the transseptal puncture for TandemHeart). Historically, due to the urgent nature of a patient in cardiogenic shock, the device of choice was the IABP. Due to its ease of insertion and the nominal time required for placement, the IABP was the device of choice for decades. Contraindications to using an IABP include aortic regurgitation, significant femoral or iliac atherosclerosis, cerebrovascular disease (due to the increased risk of stroke associated with IABP), RV failure, and aortic dissection. Relative contraindications include prosthetic graft or material in the aorta or aortic aneurysm, and tachycardia, including malignant arrhythmias or rapid atrial fibrillation, during which the effectiveness of the IABP is reduced.

The Impella 2.5 device is an option in cardiogenic shock patients undergoing PCI and provides a higher level of support compared with the IABP. The Impella is placed in the catheter laboratory percutaneously and requires a larger sheath than the IABP; therefore, femoral and iliac anatomy plays a significant role in device selection. Absolute contraindications for placement of the Impella are mechanical aortic valve, significant aortic valve stenosis with effective aortic valve area less than or equal to 1.5 cm^2, moderate to severe aortic regurgitation, and severe peripheral arterial obstructive disease. Due to the powerful hemodynamic support provided by the Impella as well as its ease of insertion, however, it is quickly becoming the device of choice for these patients. Compared with the IABP, which provides 0.5 L/min to 1.0 L/min of support, the Impella 2.5 typically provides 2.5 L/min of support; such support also provides significantly more unloading of the LV, reduction of ischemia, and enhanced coronary perfusion, all of which can improve outcomes in this setting.[44,45] In experienced centers, placement of the Impella is as rapid as placement of the IABP while providing superior support.

The Impella CP and Impella 5.0 provide better hemodynamic support than the Impella 2.5 device. The Impella CP device provides up to 4 L/min of support and can also be placed percutaneously, whereas the Impella 5.0 device requires a surgical cutdown for placement. This may present an issue if placement is needed emergently. Therefore, the Impella 5.0 is best utilized for cardiogenic shock patients, when more robust support is required.

ECMO and TandemHeart are rarely used for high-risk PCI in the current era. ECMO requires surgical expertise and large cannulae, which are associated with significant complication rates, and its use typically increases myocardial oxygen demand, which could potentially worsen ischemic complications during high-risk PCI. It is most commonly used for PCI in the setting of cardiogenic shock. In such patients, unloading of the LV with another device like the Impella may be required to reduce myocardial oxygen demand. TandemHeart requires transseptal puncture, which adds risk to an unstable high-risk PCI patient.

The 2015 Society for Cardiac Angiography and Interventions/ACCF/Heart Failure Society of America/Society for Thoracic Surgery consensus statement suggests the use of mechanical assist devices in the setting of complications of acute myocardial infarction and prophylactic use in high-risk PCI.[3] The prophylactic use for high-risk PCI was further defined as a patient population with EF less than 20% to 30% and complex coronary artery anatomy. They further recommended that when deciding between support devices it is reasonable to subdivide patients into 1 of 2 categories: normal or mildly impaired EF and severely reduced EF less than 35% or recent decompensated heart failure. The higher-risk population would benefit from Impella and/or TandemHeart, whereas the lower-risk population would benefit from either no support or IABP/Impella on standby. For example, when evaluating patients undergoing high-risk PCI of the left main or triple-vessel disease with preserved EF, it was recommended to have IABP or Impella as backup in the event of technically challenging PCI or prolonged ischemia. In patients undergoing high-risk PCI with severely reduced EF, however, it was recommended to have Impella or TandemHeart device implanted at the start of the procedure. Given the familiarity and availability of Impella as well as the presence of a large randomized trial, its utilization makes the most sense in this setting. Consistent with this, the FDA approved Impella 2.5 for use in elective and urgent high-risk PCI in 2015. It remains the only device approved for elective high-risk PCI.

SUMMARY

Despite advances in coronary technologies, some patients remain at risk for decompensated heart failure, shock, hypotension, or arrhythmias that may put a patient at risk of death or emergent intubation. Cardiac assist devices are useful in sustaining such patients through complex coronary intervention. Several devices are available for high-risk PCI, each with their own risks, benefits, complications, and ease of use. Patients deemed high risk are usually those with a confluence of patient-specific, anatomic/lesion-specific, and clinical situation-specific factors that elevate risk substantially but at minimum require significant LV dysfunction, complex anatomy, and/or significant comorbidities. In such patients, placement of an appropriate support device seems to mitigate risk and improve intermediate-term outcomes. Although several devices may be used, the most randomized controlled trial experience to date has been with the Impella 2.5 catheter, and this approach is supported by consensus statements, guidelines, and recent FDA approval. Further iterations of devices and risk scores to determine the optimal patient population are required.

REFERENCES

1. Naidu S. Novel percutaneous cardiac assist devices, the science of and indications for hemodynamic support. Circulation 2011;123:533–43.

2. Burkhoff D, Naidu S. The science behind percutaneous hemodynamic support: a review and comparison of support strategies. Catheter Cardiovasc Interv 2012;80:816–29.

3. Rihal ES, Naidu SS, Givertz MM. 2015 SCAI/ACC/HFSA/STS clinical expert consensus statement on the use of percutaneous mechanical circulatory support devices in cardiovascular care. J Am Coll Cardiol 2015;65(19):1112–4.

4. Perera D, Stables R, Thomas M, et al, for the BCIS-1 Investigators. Elective intra- aortic balloon counterpulsation during high - risk percutaneous coronary intervention, a randomized trial. JAMA 2010;304: 867–74.

5. O'Neill WW, Kleiman NS, Moses J, et al. A prospective randomized clinical trial of hemodynamic support with impella 2.5 versus intra-aortic balloon pump in patients undergoing high-risk percutaneous coronary intervention: the PROTECT II study. Circulation 2012;126:1717–27.

6. Thiele H, Smalling R, Schuler G. Percutaneous left ventricular assist devices in acute myocardial infarction complicated by cardiogenic shock. Eur Heart J 2007;28:2057–63.

7. Rynkowska-Kidawa M, Zielinska M, Chizynski K, et al. In-hospital outcomes and mortality in octogenarians after percutaneous coronary intervention. Kardiol Pol 2015;73(6):396–403.

8. Kvakkestad KM, Abdelnoor M, Claussen PA, et al. Long-term survival in octogenerians and older patients with ST-elevation myocardial infraction in the era of primary angioplasty: a prospective cohort study. Eur Heart J Acute Cardiovasc Care 2015. [Epub ahead of print].

9. Singh M, Rihal CS, Lennon RJ, et al. Influence of frailty and health status on outcomes in patients with coronary disease undergoing percutaneous revascularization. Circ Cardiovasc Qual Outcomes 2011;4:496–502.

10. Wallace TW, Berger JS, Wang A, et al. Impact of left ventricular function on hospital mortality among patients undergoing elective percutaneous coronary intervention. Am J Cardiol 2009;103:355–60.

11. Go AS, Chertow GM, Fan D, et al. Chronic kidney disease and the risks of death, cardiovascular events, and hospitalization. N Engl J Med 2004; 351:1296–305.

12. Best PJ, Lennon R, Ting HH, et al. The impact of renal insufficiency on clinical outcomes in patients undergoing percutaneous coronary interventions. J Am Coll Cardiol 2002;39:1113–9.

13. Kahn JK, Rutherford BD, McConahay DR, et al. Short- and long-term outcome of percutaneous transluminal coronary angioplasty in chronic dialysis patients. Am Heart J 1990;119:484–9.

14. Gupta R, Gurm HS, Bhatt DL, et al. Renal failure after percutaneous coronary intervention is associated with high mortality. Catheter Cardiovasc Interv 2005;64:442–8.

15. Gupta T, Paul N, Kolte D, et al. Association of chronic renal insufficiency with in-hospital outcomes after percutaneous coronary intervention. J Am Heart Assoc 2015;4:e002069.

16. Serruys PW, Morice MC, Kappetein AP, et al. Percutaneous coronary intervention versus coronary-artery bypass grafting for severe coronary artery disease. N Engl J Med 2009;360:961–72.

17. Mohr FW, Morice MC, Kappetein AP, et al. Coronary artery bypass graft surgery versus percutaneous coronary intervention in patients with three-vessel disease and left main coronary disease: 5-year follow-up of the randomized, clinical SYNTAX trial. Lancet 2013;381:629–38.

18. Farkouh ME, Domanski M, Sleeper LA, et al. Strategies for multivessel revascularization in patients with diabetes. N Engl J Med 2012;367: 2375–84.

19. Brooks MM, Alerman EL, Bates E, The BARI Investigators. The final 10-year follow-up results from the BARI randomized trial. J Am Coll Cardiol 2007;49: 1600–6.

20. Sutton-Tyrrell K, Rihal C, Sellars MA, et al. Long-term prognostic value of clinically evident noncoronary vascular disease in patients undergoing coronary revascularization in the bypass

angioplasty revascularization investigation (BARI). Am J Cardiol 1998;81:375–81.

21. Parikh SV, Saya S, Divanji P, et al. Risk of death and myocardial infarction in patients with peripheral arterial disease undergoing percutaneous coronary intervention: from the national heart, lung and blood institute dynamic registry. Am J Cardiol 2011;107:959–64.

22. Califf RM, Phillips HR III, Hindman MC, et al. Prognostic value of coronary artery jeopardy score. J Am Coll Cardiol 1985;5:1055–63.

23. Patel VG, Michael TT, Mogabgab O, et al. Clinical, angiographic, and procedural predictors of periprocedural complications during chronic total occlusion percutaneous coronary intervention. J Invasive Cardiol 2014;26:100–5.

24. Brilakis ES, Banerjee S, Karmpaliotis D, et al. Procedural outcomes of chronic total occlusion percutaneous coronary intervention: a report from the national cardiovascular data registry. JACC Cardiovasc Interv 2015;8:245–53.

25. Willerson JT, Curry GC, Watson JT, et al. Intraaortic balloon counterpulsation in patients in cardiogenic shock, medically refractory left ventricular failure and/or recurrent ventricular tachycardia. Am J Med 1975;58:183–91.

26. Baron DW, O'Rourke MR. Long-term results of arterial counterpulsation in acute severe cardiac failure complicating myocardial infarction. Br Heart J 1976; 38:285–8.

27. McEnany MT, Kay HR, Buckley MJ, et al. Clinical experience with intra-aortic balloon pump support in 728 patients. Circulation 1978;58:124–32.

28. DeWood MA, Notshe RN, Hensley GR, et al. Intraaortic balloon counterpulsation with and without reperfusion for myocardial infarction shock. Circulation 1980;61:1105–12.

29. Curtis JP, Rathore SS, Wang Y, et al. Use and effectiveness of intra-aortic balloon pumps among patients undergoing high risk percutaneous coronary intervention: insights from the national cardiovascular data registry. Circ Cardiovasc Qual Outcomes 2012;5:21–30.

30. Siauw KD, Engstrom AE, Vis MM, et al. A systemic review and meta-analysis or intra-aortic balloon pump therapy in ST-elevation myocardial infarction: should we change the guidelines? Eur Heart J 2009;30:459–68.

31. Thiele H, Schuler G, Neumann FJ, et al. Intra-aortic balloon counterpulsation in acute myocardial infarction complicated by cardiogenic shock: design and rationale of the intra-aortic balloon pump in cardiogenic shock II (IABP-SHOCK II) trial. Am Heart J 2012;163:938–45.

32. Patel MR, Smalling RW, Thiele H, et al. Intra-aortic balloon counterpulsation and infarct size in patients with acute anterior myocardial infarction

without shock: the crisp AMI randomized trial. JAMA 2011;306:1329–37.

33. Perera D, Stables R, Clayton T, et al. Long-term mortality data from the balloon pump-assisted coronary intervention study (BCIS-1): a randomized, controlled trial of elective balloon counterpulsation during high-risk percutaneous coronary intervention. Circulation 2013;127:207–12.

34. Rihal CS, Naidu SS, Givertz MM, et al. 2015 SCAI/ ACC/HFSA/STS clinical expert consensus statement on the use of percutaneous mechanical circulatory support devices in cardiovascular care. J Am Coll Cardiol 2015;65:e7–26.

35. Haines NM, Rycus PT, Zwischenberger JB, et al. Extracorporeal life support registry report 2008: neonatal and pediatric cardiac cases. ASAIO J 2009;55:111–6.

36. Nichol G, Karmy-Jones R, Salerno C, et al. Systemic review of percutaneous cardiopulmonary bypass for cardiac arrest or cardiogenic shock states. Resuscitation 2006;70:381–94.

37. Takayama H, Truby L, Koekort M, et al. Clinical outcome of mechanical circulatory support for refractory cardiogenic shock in the current era. J Heart Lung Transplant 2013;32:106–11.

38. Alli OO, Singh M, Holmes DR Jr, et al. Percutaneous left ventricular assist device with tandemheart for high-risk percutaneous coronary intervention: the mayo clinic experience. Catheter Cardiovasc Interv 2012;80:728–34.

39. Thomas JL, Al-Ameri H, Economides C, et al. Use of percutaneous left ventricular assist device for high-risk cardiac interventions and cardiogenic shock. J Invasive Cardiol 2010;22:360–4.

40. Burkhoff D, Cohen H, Brunckhorst C, et al. A randomized multicenter clinical study to evaluate the safety and efficacy of the TandemHeart percutaneous ventricular assist device versus conventional therapy with intra-aortic balloon pumping for the treatment of cardiogenic shock. Am Heart J 2006;152:469.e1–8.

41. Dixon SR, Henriques JPS, Mauri L, et al. A prospective feasibility trial investigating the use of the impella 2.5 system in patients undergoing high-risk percutaneous coronary intervention (the protect I trial). JACC Cardiovasc Interv 2009;2:91–6.

42. Maini B, Naidu SS, Mulukutla S, et al. Real-world use of the impella 2.5 circulatory support system in complex high-risk percutaneous coronary intervention: USpella registry. Catheter Cardiovasc Interv 2012;80:717–25.

43. Dangas GD, Kini AS, Sharma SK, et al. Impact of hemodynamic support with impella 2.5 versus intra-aortic balloon pump on prognostically important clinical outcomes in patients undergoing highrisk percutaneous coronary intervention (from the

protect II randomized trial). Am J Cardiol 2014;113: 222–8.

44. Jensen LO, Kaltoft A, Thayssen P, et al. Outcome in high risk patients with unprotected left main coronary artery stenosis treated with percutaneous coronary intervention. Catheter Cardiovasc Interv 2010;75:101–8.

45. Anderson HV, Shaw RE, Brindis RG, et al. A contemporary overview of percutaneous coronary interventions. The American College of Cardiology - National Cardiovascular Data Registry (ACC-NCDR). J Am Coll Cardiol 2002;39: 1096–103.

Management of Complications

Peter P. Monteleone, MD, MS[a], Robert W. Yeh, MD, MSc, MBA[b],*

KEYWORDS

- Complications • Vasovagal • Coronary dissection • Coronary perforation • Stent thrombosis
- No reflow • Stent loss • Embolization

KEY POINTS

- As the complexity of percutaneous coronary intervention (PCI) cases has grown, so too has the opportunity for procedural complications.
- The estimated risk associated with diagnostic coronary angiography of death, myocardial infarction (MI), or stroke in patients who are stable at the time of presentation to a catheterization laboratory is less than 0.1% for each.
- Vascular complications, allergic complications, renal injury, and radiation injury are all complications to be remembered during performance of cardiac catheterization procedures.
- Meticulous and focused technique, applied consistently, is mandatory to prevent the intracoronary complications of PCI.
- Operators must be constantly vigilant for intracoronary complications and prepared to initiate treatment of them when they occur immediately and expertly.

INTRODUCTION

Over the past 4 decades, PCI has made incredible progress in the management of obstructive coronary artery disease. From the first percutaneous balloon angioplasty by Gruntzig in 1977, through the first scaffolding coronary stent placed by Puel and Sigwart in 1986 to prevent vessel closure, through the commercialization of drug-eluting stent (DES) technologies in 2002 to slow restenosis, the rapid growth of technology has progressively improved the ability to combat the complications of PCI.[1] The use of dual antiplatelet therapy, anticoagulation strategies, improved guiding catheters, atherectomy devices, novel balloons, improved stent materials, embolic protection devices, percutaneous hemodynamic support devices, and untold other technologies has enhanced interventionalists' ability to successfully open obstructive coronary lesions while minimizing the incidence of periprocedural complications.[2]

PERCUTANEOUS CORONARY INTERVENTION AND FOUNDATIONAL ELEMENTS OF INFORMED CONSENT

The many distinct complications of PCI run the gamut from the general (eg, death, stroke, and periprocedural MI) to the exceedingly specific (eg, balloon rupture and stent embolization). To discuss the specific incidence and characteristics of every possible complication that could occur during preprocedural consent is time prohibitive. More importantly, providing such an abundance of information likely would cloud a preprocedure patient's ability to understand the fundamental elements of the catheterization procedure and the major points of the associated procedural risk. Operators thus develop

Disclosure Statement: Dr R.W. Yeh reports the following disclosures: Personal Fees and Consulting: Abbott Vascular, Boston Scientific, Gilead Sciences. Expert Witness Testimony: Merck.
[a] Division of Cardiology, Department of Medicine, Massachusetts General Hospital, Harvard Medical School, 55 Fruit Street, Boston, MA 02114, USA; [b] Division of Cardiology, Smith Center for Outcomes Research in Cardiology, Beth Israel Deaconess Medical Center, Harvard Medical School, 185 Pilgrim Road, Baker 4, Boston, MA 02215, USA
* Corresponding author.
E-mail address: ryeh@bidmc.harvard.edu

their own consent process, with unique discussion points and demonstrative techniques by which to ensure that their patients are well informed about the processes and the risks of PCI.[3] Regardless of interoperator consent variability, however, there are certain fundamental risks and statistics that ideally should be included in any informed consent process prior to performance of coronary angiography and intervention.

General Risks of Diagnostic Coronary Angiography

Diagnostic coronary angiography carries its own general risks, and, in that many coronary procedures are performed as angiography with the possibility of performing ad hoc PCI, it is important to prespecify to patients the potential risks of both coronary angiography and PCI.

Death secondary to coronary angiography is rare. A registry of 200,000 patients reported that the procedural mortality of diagnostic coronary angiography had fallen to 0.1%.[4] Advanced age, advanced heart failure, severe left main disease, valvular heart disease, and chronic kidney disease have been identified as risk factors for procedural mortality.[4,5] The risk of periprocedural MI is less than 0.1%.[4,6] The risk of stroke is also approximately 0.1%.[7]

Although every patient, and thus every case, is different, a statistic that is frequently cited during the informed consent process is that the risks associated with diagnostic coronary angiography of death, MI, or stroke in patients who are stable at the time of presentation to a catheterization laboratory are less than 0.1% for each.[8,9]

General Risks of Percutaneous Coronary Intervention

The risk of short-term mortality immediately due to PCI is widely variable secondary to underlying patient risk factors as well as the degree of PCI complexity. The American College of Cardiology National Cardiovascular Data Registry (NCDR), which included more than 100,000 PCIs performed between 1998 and 2000, with stent placement in 77%, reported a risk of death secondary to PCI of 1.4%, ranging within individual participating hospitals from a low of 0% to a high of 4%.[10] A 2013 analysis of the Cleveland Clinic's institutional PCI registry of 4078 PCI patients reported a 2% risk of death within 30 days, with 42% of these deaths deemed secondary to PCI-related complications.[11]

The risk of periprocedural MI is even more difficult to report because every measurement

of periprocedural MI incidence has changed with the improving technology that has both reduced the risk of complications and simultaneously allowed operators to tackle more complex lesions. Perhaps even more importantly, the measured frequency of periprocedural MI has changed with changing definitions of periprocedural MI itself, as well as with the increasing sensitivity of biochemical markers of MI.[12] This effect of the changing definition of postprocedural MI becomes clear when up to 43% of patients who go into a PCI with a normal troponin level have some elevation of troponin at the completion of the case.[13] The 2011 American College of Cardiology/American Heart Association guidelines for PCI describe the 2007 universal definition of MI as occurring when cardiac biomarkers post-PCI climb to above the 99th percentile upper reference limit of normal and thus indicate myocardial necrosis. These guidelines also report, however, that the increase of biomarkers greater than 3 times the 99th percentile upper reference limit defines PCI-related MI.[2] According to this definition, approximately 15% of patients undergoing PCI experience a periprocedural MI.[14] In an attempt to define a group at risk for a clinically negative outcome and to develop a definition of periprocedural MI applicable to patients with elevated baseline troponin levels, the 2012 Third Universal Definition of Myocardial Infarction was formulated by a joint European Society of Cardiology/American College of Cardiology Foundation/American Heart Association/World Health Federation task force. This definition somewhat arbitrarily defines MI associated with PCI as elevation of troponin values greater than 5 times the 99th percentile upper reference limit in patients with normal baseline values or a rise of troponin values greater than 20% if the baseline values are elevated and are stable or falling. Patients must also experience symptoms suggestive of myocardial ischemia, new ischemic electrocardiographic changes, new left bundle branch block, angiographic loss of patency of a major coronary artery or a side branch, persistent diminished flow or embolization, or imaging demonstration of new loss of viable myocardium or new regional wall motion abnormality. The incidence of periprocedural PCI meeting this definition is currently poorly delineated.[15]

An NCDR report describes a 0.4% risk of conversion to emergency coronary artery bypass surgery.[16] The incidence of PCI-related stroke, defined as development of a central neurologic deficit persisting greater than 72 hours with its onset starting anytime from the time of PCI until the time of discharge, in a recent NCDR analysis was 0.22%.[17] The risk of PCI-associated vascular complications varies greatly with reports, ranging from 2% to 6%.[2]

NONCORONARY COMPLICATIONS
Vascular Access Complications
Vascular complications associated with PCI are most commonly attributed to femoral arterial access and include but are not limited to local bleeding/hematoma, retroperitoneal hematoma, pseudoaneurysm formation, arteriovenous fistula, ileofemoral arterial dissection, thromboembolic arterial occlusion, and infection. Although specific description of all vascular complications is beyond the scope of this article, certain fundamental elements of vascular access technique are worth mentioning as a means of avoiding and treating many if not all of these complications.

Utilization of radial access is perhaps the best defense against development of many of the vascular complications that have plagued femoral arterial access. Radial access itself carries a distinct complication list. When femoral access is required, fluoroscopic with or without ultrasound guidance as well as micropuncture techniques can be considered a means of ensuring that the arterial puncture overlies the middle to lower third of the femoral head. This allows for compression of the arteriotomy site against the femoral head after sheath removal and also ensures anatomically that bleeding into the arteriotomy area is constrained within the fixed compartment of the leg below the inguinal ligament. Careful and protocolized monitoring of anticoagulation strategies used both before and during PCI is absolutely mandatory, as are clear algorithms to ensure the removal of arterial sheaths as soon as is safely possible and with the use of excellent technique. Vascular closure devices lead to early sheath removal and patient satisfaction and may facilitate hemostasis.

Vasovagal Reactions
Vasovagal reactions are important occurrences both during coronary catheterization and during the postprocedural period. Vasovagal reactions can be marked by bradycardia, hypotension, diaphoresis, and nausea and can occur in up to 3% of patients undergoing cardiac catheterization.[4] Events are the result of stimulation of the parasympathetic nervous system with physical manifestations activated by the vagus nerve. When the vagus nerve is stimulated, outgoing impulses travel from the brainstem via the vagal nerve to the heart. The heart is slowed via action on the sinus node. Vasodilatation is mediated via cardiac baroreceptor and arterial baroreceptor activation. Other organs are also affected, resulting in nausea, pallor, diaphoresis, yawning, and so forth. These events can be associated with pulse palpation, manual compression, needle vascular access, coronary injection, or any episode of discomfort/pain.

Atropine can be given to block the vagally induced effects on heart rate and blood pressure. Doses of 0.6 mg to 1.2 mg intravenously (IV) can be given to rapidly reverse symptoms within minutes. IV saline bolus infusion can also be concurrently provided. Vasopressor medications, including epinephrine, are reserved for refractory hypotension.

Other Noncoronary Complications
The risk of contrast-induced nephropathy can be reduced by adequate hydration with IV fluid prior to coronary angiography. Allergic reactions, including anaphylaxis, can occur after exposure to contrast media. Its symptoms and effects can be easily mistaken for other intracoronary complications. Early diagnosis and treatment are imperative to minimize the risk of hemodynamic collapse and respiratory failure. Radiation injury can carry both deterministic and stochastic risks that may plague patients from days after to decades after their procedures.

COMPLICATIONS OF PERCUTANEOUS CORONARY INTERVENTION
Coronary Dissection
Coronary dissection is an uncommon yet potentially devastating complication of PCI. Iatrogenic dissection during catheterization can be caused by the catheter, guide wire, contrast injection, or any device inserted into a coronary artery. Dissection can progress antegrade into the coronary vessel or can also track retrograde and even back into the aorta, leading to aortic dissection. The natural history of dissections can vary.[18] Small dissections can lead to minimal injury with maintenance of normal Thrombolysis in Myocardial Infarction (TIMI)-3 flow into the distal coronary bed beyond the dissection, resulting in no damage to heart muscle. This situation can often heal without any intervention.[19] In other cases, dissection can lead to acute closure of the dissected coronary vessel with resultant myocardial malperfusion, injury, and MI.[20] Retrograde dissection can extend back to involve the aorta, and the resultant ascending aortic dissection can either be clinically insignificant or emergently life threatening.[21]

Excellent angiographic technique, including optimization of guiding catheter selection, is of the utmost importance to avoid dissection. Of extreme importance is awareness that injection (contrast or saline) can continuously extend previously created coronary dissection planes. Thus, operators must weigh the risks and benefits of performing repeated injections to delineate a coronary dissection because they can propagate the dissection and increase the size of the false channel.

The patency of the vessel distal to the dissection flap and the size of the myocardial territory at risk determines the optimum treatment strategy for coronary dissection. If flow distal to the dissection is compromised, as is the case with acute closure of a coronary artery, urgent PCI or coronary artery bypass grafting is indicated to prevent MI. Revascularization should be strongly considered if flow to the distal arterial bed is compromised by the dissection, especially in the presence of clinical ischemia, including chest pain, ECG changes, dysrhythmia, or hemodynamic instability. A soft-tipped coronary wire should be used for attempted passage into the true lumen of the coronary. Minimal contrast injections should be performed to avoid dissection propagation. To confirm that an over-the-wire coronary balloon has passed back into the true coronary lumen, injections can be performed through the distal over-the-wire balloon port. Passing a coronary wire beyond the site of a coronary dissection that has resulted in complete closure of the vessel is particularly challenging because the coronary wire is likely to pass into and extend the dissection flap rather than find the true lumen. In this situation, dissection reentry techniques can be considered. Many of the advanced techniques for navigating dissection planes that have been utilized in chronic total occlusion PCI can be applicable to this emergent scenario.

If the vessel remains patent with no obstruction to flow, the optimal clinical management of the dissection is less clear. Although conservative management has been used successfully in this situation, the use of an intra-aortic balloon pump is controversial. Increased coronary perfusion pressure provided by the intra-aortic balloon pump may help maintain vessel patency, whereas increased coronary perfusion can simply extend the dissection and possibly close down the vessel entirely.

If retrograde dissection propagates back into the aorta, emergent management may be necessary. Contrast injections into the dissection should be limited to avoid further propagation.

It should be determined if the dissection extends only into the coronary cusp or if it continues to extend beyond the cusp into the aortic wall. Small dissection can be managed conservatively with close monitoring for propagation and beta-blockade for blood pressure control to decrease shear wall stress in the aorta. Advanced imaging (CT angiography of the aorta or transesophageal echocardiogram) should be strongly considered to delineate the extent of the dissection.

If the dissection propagates retrograde into the aorta and compromises coronary perfusion, emergent PCI of the ostial left main or ostial right coronary artery may be utilized to tack up the entrance flap of the dissection, thus prohibiting further propagation. Emergent surgical consultation should be considered for these cases and emergent aortic surgery may be necessary in extreme cases.

Coronary Artery Perforation

Coronary artery perforation can be caused by distal wire migration, angioplasty balloon rupture, stent oversizing, high-pressure postdilatation, and multiple other causes and results in outcomes, ranging from microperforation to frank rupture with rapid filling of the pericardial space resulting in cardiac tamponade. As interventional coronary techniques continue to progress to include more aggressive equipment and to tackle more complex lesions, coronary artery perforation will remain a potential complication during PCI.

Advanced patient age, female gender and utilization of atherectomy devices are associated with an increased frequency of coronary artery perforation. Distal guide wire perforation remains, however, the most common cause. A series of more than 10,000 PCIs during the stent era reported the incidence of coronary perforation as 0.84%.[22] Ellis and colleagues proposed an angiographic classification system for coronary perforation in 1994.[23]

- Class I = extraluminal crater without extravasation
- Class II = pericardial or myocardial blushing
- Class III = perforation greater than or equal to 1-mm diameter with contrast streaming and cavity spilling

Class III perforation can often result in abrupt onset of cardiac tamponade requiring emergent pericardiocentesis. Case series report morality from coronary perforations up to 10%.[24] Class III perforations are causative for most if not all of this mortality.[23]

Excellent and focused technique is the key to the prevention of coronary artery perforation. Avoiding distal wire migration especially when utilizing hydrophilic wires can reduce the majority of wire perforations, as can careful vessel preparation and avoiding overaggressive balloon and stent sizing to reduce the risk of other causes of perforation.

The key to the successful management of coronary artery perforation is early diagnosis and prompt treatment. The first step is often balloon occlusion of the perforated vessel to prevent active continued extravasation into the pericardium. This may lead, however, to ischemia of the myocardial territory fed by the perforated vessel, resulting in electrical or hemodynamic instability.

Anticoagulation should, in many cases, be discontinued and/or reversed. Protamine sulfate can be administered to achieve an activated clotting time of less than 150 seconds. The often-stated typical dose of protamine is 10 mg for 1000 units of heparin provided. If enoxaparin is in place for the procedure, 1 mg protamine can be given for 1 mg enoxaparin if it is required less than 8 hours from the last use of enoxaparin. The maximum dose of protamine is 50 mg. Bivalirudin is a direct selective thrombin inhibitor that interacts with both the active site and exosite of thrombin, producing a transient inhibition of thrombin function. Although hemodialysis can remove 25% of bivalrudin's function and hemofiltration can remove 43% to 65% of bivalrudin's activity, these reversal modalities are not available emergently in a catheterization laboratory. Reversal of bivalirudin can be attempted with use of recombinant activated factor VII, which has been used at a dose of 90 µg/kg IV. A second dose can be given if the bleeding recurs. Blood products, such as fibrinogen, fresh frozen plasma, and cryoprecipitate, have been utilized for reversal of bivalirudin and should be considered.

If rapid accumulation of a pericardial effusion and resultant pericardial tamponade occurs, emergent pericardiocentesis is indicated. Large volumes of blood can be removed in this situation from the pericardial space and can potentially be reinfused through a femoral venous sheath to avoid rapid exsanguination. After stability is achieved, pericardial drain placement at the time of pericardiocentesis is common. If unsuccessful, emergent pericardial window may be needed to prevent hemodynamic collapse.

Coil embolization of perforated coronary side branches can be performed. The Jostent coronary stent graft (Jomed), which is a covered stent composed of 2 stents sandwiching polytetrafluoroethylene graft material to create a covered stent, can be used to exclude perforation. These stents can be associated with subacute stent thrombosis in up to 6% of cases in the months after stent placement.[25] Restenosis can occur in up to one-third of Jostent placements.[25] The current generation of Jostent can be inserted through a 6F guide catheter.

Stent Thrombosis

Stent thrombosis describes the formation of thrombus and subsequent occlusion of a coronary stent. It is categorized as definite, probable, or possible based on the diagnostic testing used and the degree of certainty that it has occurred. Stent thrombosis presents as an acute MI in more than 50% of patients and carries a mortality rate of 20% to 40%.[26] It is further categorized as occurring early (in the first 30 days of stent implantation), late (between 1 month and 1 year after implantation), and very late (occurring beyond 1 year after implantation).[27] The rate of stent thrombosis has been compared in various studies and trials between bare metal stents (BMSs) and DESs of multiple generations. Various studies have reported rates of stent thrombosis between DESs and BMSs that were no different at 1 year. Famously, the incidence of very late stent thrombosis was reported as increased with first-generation DESs.[28] Other studies, however, including a large multicenter randomized controlled trial, found no difference between BMSs and DESs in very late stent thrombosis with sirolimus-eluting stents.[29] Predictors for occurrence of stent thrombosis include longer total stent length, smaller minimum luminal diameter of stent, persistent coronary dissection, stent underexpansion or undersizing, and occurrence during PCI for an acute coronary syndrome.[30,31] For late stent thrombosis, incomplete neointimal coverage of the placed stent may play a significant role.[32] The latest generation of DESs has overall low rates of stent thrombosis.[33]

Optimal stent size selection and assurance of complete deployment and expansion are extremely important to prevention of stent thrombosis. Strict patient adherence to combined dual antiplatelet therapy is recommended, and its premature cessation is the strongest independent predictor for developing stent thrombosis.[34]

Prompt reperfusion is the primary goal of therapy. In addition to appropriate anticoagulation and antiplatelet therapy, endovascular imaging, including intravascular ultrasound or optical coherence tomography, to seek causative etiologies of thrombosis, including edge dissection, underexpansion, and geographic miss, should be strongly considered. If stent underexpansion is identified, additional postdilatation should be performed. If residual dissection or geographic miss of the primary lesion is identified, further stenting should be pursued.

No-Reflow

No-reflow describes a persistent decrease in myocardial blood flow present despite a fully patent epicardial coronary artery. This most commonly occurs in patients who undergo primary PCI for ST-segment elevation MI (STEMI), saphenous vein graft intervention, and atherectomy procedures. The underlying etiology of no-reflow is complex and often multifactorial. Mechanical obstruction of the distal microvasculature secondary to microembolization to the coronary capillary network is a major proposed cause. Direct ischemic injury to the distal tissues may also play a role in that ischemic myocytes are edematous and can protrude into the intima and decrease flow. Furthermore, with the opening of an occluded artery, rapid tissue reperfusion can induce the release of inflammatory cytokines as well as potent vasoconstricting factors into the distal capillary bed, further worsening microvascular inflammation, edema, and constriction.

The preventative use of embolic protection devices during saphenous vein graft intervention has resulted in significant improvements in post-PCI flow.[35] Aspiration thrombectomy increased in popularity for the treatment of patients with STEMI after the Thrombus Aspiration During Percutaneous Coronary Intervention in Acute Myocardial Infarction Study (TAPAS) demonstrated improved reperfusion, decreased mortality, and decreased adverse events at 30 days and at 1 year.[36] More recent randomized controlled trials have tempered this optimism about the benefits of this strategy and have led to the belief that the targeted use of this treatment to more individualized scenarios is appropriate.[37,38]

When no-reflow phenomenon occurs, the primary mechanism of treatment is with intracoronary pharmacologic intervention. Intracoronary adenosine, nitroprusside, verapamil, and nicardipine have all been used in patients with no-reflow to improve TIMI flow grade as well as myocardial blush grade. These agents should be administered through a microcatheter to enhance delivery to the distal coronary bed rather than though the guiding catheter. All were equally effective when studied in decreasing the clinical composite endpoint of heart failure, cardiogenic shock, or death.[39] The 2011 PCI guidelines thus recommend utilization of these medications in this setting.[2] High doses of intracoronary adenosine decreased the incidence of the no-reflow phenomenon when given in advance of PCI.[40]

Embolization

Embolization of air, thrombus, or atherosclerotic debris can all occur during coronary angiography or PCI and result in various degrees of morbidity or mortality depending on the burden of embolization and the amount of myocardial tissue injured in the process. Air embolization can occur as the simple result of imperfect manifold or catheter manipulation and result in air lock, in which a column of air injected within the coronary artery prevents passage of blood to the coronary capillary network. Meticulous preparation of the manifold and vigilance for entrapped air are vital to prevent this occurrence. Supplemental oxygen can facilitate resolution of air embolism. Rapid infusion of normal saline into the coronary can help displace the air. Similarly, passage of a 0.014 inch coronary wire into the air embolus can also help reduce the surface tension of the air embolus within the blood and thus help break up the air embolus, expose more of it to the blood interface, and improve its absorption. Hypotension should be aggressively treated with vasopressors, including epinephrine or phenylephrine. Intra-aortic balloon pump should be considered in extreme, refractory cases of hypotension. Bradycardia can be treated with atropine. Aspiration thrombectomy can be performed after passage of a coronary wire into the affected vessel in hopes of removing the embolized thrombus or air.

Stent Loss

Stent loss can occur when an undeployed or partially deployed stent unintentionally comes off of the intracoronary balloon on which it is mounted, potentially leading to a catastrophic scenario. It most commonly occurs when a stent that cannot be advanced to its intended location is withdrawn back into a guiding catheter that is not coaxial to the stent balloon and the stent is effectively stripped off of its deployment balloon. Similarly, when stent passage is attempted across a previously placed stent, the stent can easily be stripped off the balloon by the initial stent. Any failed attempt at passage of a stent through tortuous or complex lesions can result in the stent becoming stuck within the coronary artery, and removal of the stent balloon catheter can effectively strip the undeployed stent off of its balloon. Careful inspection of the stent balloon that is withdrawn after every failed attempt at stent passage is imperative to ensure that the stent has not been stripped off and left undeployed within the coronary or any other vascular bed.

Optimal guiding catheter selection and utilization to ensure appropriate coaxial alignment are important to avoid this complication. Furthermore, adequate lesion preparation with predilatation angioplasty and atherectomy, when clinically indicated, can help prevent stents from being stripped off of stent balloons by complex or tortuous unprepared coronary disease.

When a stent is lost within the coronary circulation, 3 basic strategies exist for rescue treatment. If the stent remains on the coronary delivery guide wire, a small angioplasty balloon (1.25 mm or 1.5 mm) can sometimes be successfully passed into or distal to the stent and then inflated, resulting in the capture of the stent so that it can be retrieved into the guiding catheter and removed. If the stent does not fit into the guiding catheter, the lost stent can be brought to the tip of the guiding catheter and the entire ensemble can be removed as a unit. Through a similar technique, the stent can be captured on a small balloon inflated within it, followed by serial inflations with larger balloons to expand and fully deploy the stent at its current location if the stent was lost in a position acceptable for deployment. If the delivery guide wire remains through the undeployed stent but a small balloon cannot be passed through it, a second coronary guide wire can be advanced into the same coronary artery and twisted around the first guide wire. The tangling of wires may lead to capture of the stent, and the wires can then be carefully removed taking the undeployed stent with them. Gooseneck-type or other intracoronary snares can also be used to retrieve a lost stent. If a wire can be passed through the struts of the undeployed lost stent, this wire can also then be snared with all of the equipment being removed together as a unit.

If the lost stent cannot be retrieved or deployed, another stent can be deployed to cover and crush the lost stent against the coronary wall. If the stent can be removed from the coronary circulation but cannot be removed through the access sheath, the stent can potentially be deployed (and overexpanded) or crushed in the ileofemoral tree to remove the risk of intracoronary complications. If a lost partially deployed stent or other device does not fit through and thus cannot be retrieved through the sheath in which it is placed, a larger-bore femoral arterial sheath can be placed in the contralateral femoral site so that a snare can capture the device, externalizing it and thus retrieving it.

SUMMARY

PCI is a safe and effective treatment of severe coronary artery disease. As indications for PCI continue to expand, including more complex lesions, the potential for life-threatening complications increases. Constant and meticulous attention to technique and detail, both basic and advanced, within a catheterization laboratory can minimize the risk of complications. The physical and mental fatigue that can occur during prolonged cases is a real phenomenon, and, when an operator or a team loses focus for even a single second, patients can be hurt or killed. As PCI continues to advance and to grow, so will its potential risks and so must its current and future operators.

REFERENCES

1. Bennett J, Dubois C. Percutaneous coronary intervention, a historical perspective looking to the future. J Thorac Dis 2013;5(3):367–70.
2. Levine GN, Bates ER, Blankenship JC, et al. 2011 ACCF/AHA/SCAI guideline for percutaneous coronary intervention. A report of the american college of cardiology foundation/american heart association task force on practice guidelines and the society for cardiovascular angiography and interventions. J Am Coll Cardiol 2011;58(24): e44–122.
3. Arnold SV, Decker C, Ahmad H, et al. Converting the informed consent from a perfunctory process to an evidence-based foundation for patient decision making. Circ Cardiovasc Qual Outcomes 2008;1(1):21–8.
4. Johnson LW, Lozner EC, Johnson S, et al. Coronary arteriography 1984-1987: a report of the registry of the society for cardiac angiography and interventions. I. results and complications. Cathet Cardiovasc Diagn 1989;17(1):5–10.
5. Laskey W, Boyle J, Johnson LW. Multivariable model for prediction of risk of significant complication during diagnostic cardiac catheterization. The registry committee of the society for cardiac angiography & interventions. Cathet Cardiovasc Diagn 1993;30(3):185–90.
6. Noto TJ Jr, Johnson LW, Krone R, et al. Cardiac catheterization 1990: a report of the registry of the

society for cardiac angiography and interventions (SCA&I). Cathet Cardiovasc Diagn 1991;24(2):75–83.

7. Korn-Lubetzki I, Farkash R, Pachino RM, et al. Incidence and risk factors of cerebrovascular events following cardiac catheterization. J Am Heart Assoc 2013;2(6):e000413.

8. Bashore TM, Balter S, Barac A, et al. 2012 American college of cardiology foundation/society for cardiovascular angiography and interventions expert consensus document on cardiac catheterization laboratory standards update: a report of the american college of cardiology foundation task force on expert consensus documents developed in collaboration with the society of thoracic surgeons and society for vascular medicine. J Am Coll Cardiol 2012;59(24):2221–305.

9. Dehmer GJ, Weaver D, Roe MT, et al. A contemporary view of diagnostic cardiac catheterization and percutaneous coronary intervention in the united states: A report from the CathPCI registry of the national cardiovascular data registry, 2010 through june 2011. J Am Coll Cardiol 2012;60(20):2017–31.

10. Anderson HV, Shaw RE, Brindis RG, et al. A contemporary overview of percutaneous coronary interventions. The American college of cardiology-national cardiovascular data registry (ACC-NCDR). J Am Coll Cardiol 2002;39(7):1096–103.

11. Aggarwal B, Ellis SG, Lincoff AM, et al. Cause of death within 30 days of percutaneous coronary intervention in an era of mandatory outcome reporting. J Am Coll Cardiol 2013;62(5):409–15.

12. Sherwood MW, Kristin Newby L. High-sensitivity troponin assays: evidence, indications, and reasonable use. J Am Heart Assoc 2014;3(1):e000403.

13. Prasad A, Rihal CS, Lennon RJ, et al. Significance of periprocedural myonecrosis on outcomes after percutaneous coronary intervention: an analysis of preintervention and postintervention troponin T levels in 5487 patients. Circ Cardiovasc Interv 2008;1(1):10–9.

14. Alcock RF, Roy P, Adorini K, et al. Incidence and determinants of myocardial infarction following percutaneous coronary interventions according to the revised joint task force definition of troponin T elevation. Int J Cardiol 2010;140(1):66–72.

15. Thygesen K, Alpert JS, Jaffe AS, et al. Third universal definition of myocardial infarction. Circulation 2012;126(16):2020–35.

16. Kutcher MA, Klein LW, Ou FS, et al. Percutaneous coronary interventions in facilities without cardiac surgery on site: a report from the national cardiovascular data registry (NCDR). J Am Coll Cardiol 2009;54(1):16–24.

17. Aggarwal A, Dai D, Rumsfeld JS, et al, American College of Cardiology National Cardiovascular Data Registry. Incidence and predictors of stroke associated with percutaneous coronary intervention. Am J Cardiol 2009;104(3):349–53.

18. Boyle AJ, Chan M, Dib J, et al. Catheter-induced coronary artery dissection: risk factors, prevention and management. J Invasive Cardiol 2006;18(10):500–3.

19. Nikolsky E, Boulos M, Amikam S. Spontaneous healing of long, catheter-induced right coronary artery dissection. Int J Cardiovasc Intervent 2003;5(4):211.

20. Awadalla H, Sabet S, El Sebaie A, et al. Catheter-induced left main dissection incidence, predisposition and therapeutic strategies experience from two sides of the hemisphere. J Invasive Cardiol 2005;17(4):233–6.

21. Goldstein JA, Casserly IP, Katsiyiannis WT, et al. Aortocoronary dissection complicating a percutaneous coronary intervention. J Invasive Cardiol 2003;15(2):89–92.

22. Stankovic G, Orlic D, Corvaja N, et al. Incidence, predictors, in-hospital, and late outcomes of coronary artery perforations. Am J Cardiol 2004;93(2):213–6.

23. Ellis SG, Ajluni S, Arnold AZ, et al. Increased coronary perforation in the new device era. Incidence, classification, management, and outcome. Circulation 1994;90(6):2725–30.

24. Gruberg L, Pinnow E, Flood R, et al. Incidence, management, and outcome of coronary artery perforation during percutaneous coronary intervention. Am J Cardiol 2000;86(6):680–2. A8.

25. Gercken U, Lansky AJ, Buellesfeld L, et al. Results of the jostent coronary stent graft implantation in various clinical settings: procedural and follow-up results. Catheter Cardiovasc Interv 2002;56(3):353–60.

26. Holmes DR Jr, Kereiakes DJ, Garg S, et al. Stent thrombosis. J Am Coll Cardiol 2010;56(17):1357–65.

27. Cutlip DE, Windecker S, Mehran R, et al. Clinical end points in coronary stent trials: a case for standardized definitions. Circulation 2007;115(17):2344–51.

28. Roukoz H, Bavry AA, Sarkees ML, et al. Comprehensive meta-analysis on drug-eluting stents versus bare-metal stents during extended follow-up. Am J Med 2009;122(6):581.e1–10.

29. Weisz G, Leon MB, Holmes DR Jr, et al. Five-year follow-up after sirolimus-eluting stent implantation results of the SIRIUS (sirolimus-eluting stent in de-novo native coronary lesions) trial. J Am Coll Cardiol 2009;53(17):1488–97.

30. Cutlip DE, Baim DS, Ho KK, et al. Stent thrombosis in the modern era: a pooled analysis of multicenter coronary stent clinical trials. Circulation 2001;103(15):1967–71.

31. Kukreja N, Onuma Y, Garcia-Garcia HM, et al. The risk of stent thrombosis in patients with acute

coronary syndromes treated with bare-metal and drug-eluting stents. JACC Cardiovasc Interv 2009; 2(6):534–41.

32. Hasegawa K, Tamai H, Kyo E, et al. Histopathological findings of new in-stent lesions developed beyond five years. Catheter Cardiovasc Interv 2006;68(4):554–8.

33. Palmerini T, Biondi-Zoccai G, Della Riva D, et al. Stent thrombosis with drug-eluting and bare-metal stents: evidence from a comprehensive network meta-analysis. Lancet 2012;379(9824): 1393–402.

34. Spertus JA, Kettelkamp R, Vance C, et al. Prevalence, predictors, and outcomes of premature discontinuation of thienopyridine therapy after drug-eluting stent placement: results from the PREMIER registry. Circulation 2006;113(24):2803–9.

35. Sturm E, Goldberg D, Goldberg S. Embolic protection devices in saphenous vein graft and native vessel percutaneous intervention: a review. Curr Cardiol Rev 2012;8(3):192–9.

36. Vlaar PJ, Svilaas T, van der Horst IC, et al. Cardiac death and reinfarction after 1 year in the thrombus aspiration during percutaneous coronary intervention in acute myocardial infarction study (TAPAS): a 1-year follow-up study. Lancet 2008; 371(9628):1915–20.

37. Jolly SS, Cairns JA, Yusuf S, et al. Randomized trial of primary PCI with or without routine manual thrombectomy. N Engl J Med 2015;372(15):1389–98.

38. Frobert O, Lagerqvist B, Gudnason T, et al. Thrombus aspiration in ST-elevation myocardial infarction in scandinavia (TASTE trial). A multicenter, prospective, randomized, controlled clinical registry trial based on the swedish angiography and angioplasty registry (SCAAR) platform. Study design and rationale. Am Heart J 2010;160(6): 1042–8.

39. Rezkalla SH, Dharmashankar KC, Abdalrahman IB, et al. No-reflow phenomenon following percutaneous coronary intervention for acute myocardial infarction: incidence, outcome, and effect of pharmacologic therapy. J Interv Cardiol 2010;23(5): 429–36.

40. Marzilli M, Orsini E, Marraccini P, et al. Beneficial effects of intracoronary adenosine as an adjunct to primary angioplasty in acute myocardial infarction. Circulation 2000;101(18):2154–9.

In-stent Restenosis

Michael S. Lee, MD[a,*], Gaurav Banka, MD[b]

KEYWORDS

- Percutaneous coronary intervention • In-stent restenosis • Neointimal hyperplasia
- Target vessel revascularization • Target lesion revascularization

KEY POINTS

- In-stent restenosis (ISR) typically presents as recurrent angina, but can also present as a myocardial infarction in some patients. ISR typically presents 6 to 12 months after percutaneous coronary intervention.
- Patient characteristics associated with ISR include age, female gender, diabetes, chronic kidney disease, and multivessel coronary artery disease. Lesion characteristics associated with ISR include smaller reference artery diameter, ostial lesion, and initial plaque burden.
- Anatomic assessment of ISR with intravascular imaging provides insight into the cause of ISR and true vessel sizing for appropriate stent size. Hemodynamic assessment with fractional flow reserve (FFR) is valuable to evaluate for functional ischemia because there is a poor correlation with estimated percent diameter stenosis and FFR in patients with diffuse restenosis.
- Treatment of ISR with drug-eluting stents has been shown to be superior to balloon angioplasty alone.
- Brachytherapy, excimer laser angioplasty, and routine angiographic surveillance are not recommended treatment and diagnostic options.

INTRODUCTION

In-stent restenosis (ISR) is the gradual renarrowing of a stented coronary artery lesion from arterial damage with subsequent neointimal tissue proliferation.[1] Binary angiographic restenosis is defined as greater than 50% luminal narrowing at follow-up angiography (Figs. 1 and 2). Clinical restenosis is defined as greater than 50% diameter stenosis and one of the following: positive history of recurrent angina, objective signs of ischemia (eg, electrocardiogram [ECG] changes), fractional flow reserve (FFR) less than 0.80, intravascular ultrasonography (IVUS) minimum cross-sectional area less than 4 mm^2 (<6 mm^2 for left main), or restenosis (>70% reduction in lumen diameter) even in the absence of clinical symptoms or signs (Box 1). Clinical restenosis is a requirement for target lesion revascularization (TLR). The Mehran system is a morphologic classification of ISR lesions: Pattern I includes focal (≤10 mm in length) lesions, pattern II is ISR greater than 10 mm within the stent, pattern III includes ISR greater than 10 mm extending outside the stent, and pattern IV is totally occluded ISR. This classification system can predict the need for repeat revascularization after intervention (19%, 35%, 50%, and 98%, respectively).[2]

CLINICAL PRESENTATION

The mean time from percutaneous coronary intervention (PCI) with drug-eluting stents (DESs) to ISR was 12 months.[3] In bare-metal stents (BMSs), ISR was reported an average of 6 months post-PCI.[4] ISR typically presents as recurrent angina 25% to 50% of the time, but also presents as myocardial infarction (MI) in approximately 3.5% to 20% of patients.[1,3,5,6] In

[a] Cardiology Division, Department of Medicine, UCLA Medical Center, 100 Medical Plaza Suite 630, Los Angeles, CA 90095, USA; [b] UCLA Medical Center, Los Angeles, CA, USA
* Corresponding author.
E-mail address: mslee@mednet.ucla.edu

Intervent Cardiol Clin 5 (2016) 211–220
http://dx.doi.org/10.1016/j.iccl.2015.12.006
2211-7458/16/$ – see front matter © 2016 Elsevier Inc. All rights reserved.

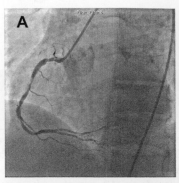
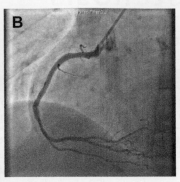
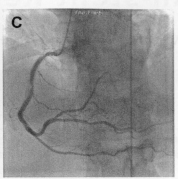

Fig. 1. (A) A 40-year-old man with history of lupus, end-stage renal disease secondary to lupus nephritis, and hypertension presented with stable angina. He was found to have a proximal right coronary artery (RCA) 45% lesion followed by a long eccentric 90% RCA lesion. (B) Percutaneous coronary intervention (PCI) of the proximal RCA with a 3.5 × 15 mm Xience Xpedition drug eluting stent and PCI of the mid RCA with a 3.0 × 38 mm Promus Premier drug eluting stent. (C) The patient presented 1 year later with chest pain and repeat angiogram showed severe ISR of the RCA stents. The patient also had coronary artery disease in the left anterior descending artery and was referred for coronary artery bypass surgery.

contrast, stent thrombosis is an abrupt thrombotic occlusion that presents as either MI or sudden cardiac death.[7]

It is also possible for neointimal hyperplasia plus focal thrombosis to be present inside the stent. Factors that are more suggestive of ISR, as opposed to thrombosis, are longer time from implantation, absence of angiographic factors such as thrombus, length of stent, IVUS findings showing neointimal hyperplasia, and findings during catheterization such as balloon slippage associated with hard neointimal tissue from ISR, in contrast with soft thrombi.[1]

INCIDENCE

Rates of ISR with DESs range from 3% to 20%. In the j-Cypher registry of 12,812 patients who received sirolimus-eluting stents (SESs), the TLR rate was 7.3% at 1 year, after which the rate was ~2.2% per year, and 15.9% at 5 years. The stent thrombosis rate was 0.3% at 30 days, 0.6% at 1 year, and 1.6% at 5 years (very late stent thrombosis continued to occur up 5 years after implantation).[8] In the Endeavor IV trial, 1548 patients were randomized to zotarolimus-eluting stent (ZES) or paclitaxel-eluting stent (PES).[9] At 3 years, rates of ischemia-driven TLR were similar. However, the rate of very late stent thrombosis (1–3 years) was significantly lower in ZES patients (0.1% vs 1.6%; hazard ratio [HR], 0.09; confidence interval [CI], 0.01–0.71; P = .004). In the Sirolimus-Eluting Versus Paclitaxel-Eluting Stents for Coronary Revascularization (SIRTAX) LATE study study, 1012 patients were randomly assigned to SES or PES. Of 444 patients who had repeat angiography, 5-year

rates of TLR were 13.1% and 15.1% respectively (P = .29).[10]

The use of DESs has significantly reduced the rate of restenosis and TLR compared with BMSs. A meta-analysis of 38 randomized controlled trials with more than 18,000 patients showed that there was significant reduction in TLR with both SESs and PESs compared with BMSs.[11] SESs were associated with the lowest risk of MI (HR 0.81, 95% CI 0.66-0.97, P = .030 vs BMS; HR 0.83, 95% CI 0.71–1.00, P = .045 vs PES). The reduction in TLR seen with DES compared with BMS was more pronounced with SES than with PES (HR 0.70; 95% CI, 0.56–0.84; P = .0021). Although there was no significant difference in definite stent thrombosis from 0 to 4 years, the risk of late stent thrombosis (>30 days) was increased for PESs.

There is also late catch-up in neointimal hyperplasia in DESs, shown in both first-generation and second-generation stents.[12] BMSs show a late decrease in neointimal hyperplasia. Nevertheless, the overall neointimal hyperplasia is still significantly less in DESs than in BMSs.[12–14]

PREDICTORS OF IN-STENT RESTENOSIS

The predictors of ISR include patient, lesion, and procedural characteristics (Table 1). Patient characteristics associated with ISR include age, female gender, diabetes, chronic kidney disease, and multivessel coronary artery disease.[1,15,16] Lesion characteristics associated with ISR include smaller reference artery diameter, ostial lesion, initial plaque burden, and residual plaque after implantation. In contrast with BMSs, DESs tend

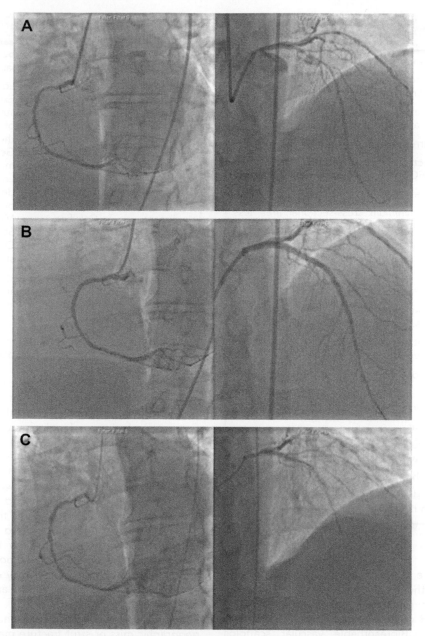

Fig. 2. (A) A 57-year-old man with end-stage renal disease on hemodialysis who presented for kidney transplant evaluation. Preoperative stress test was positive and the patient underwent coronary angiogram, which showed diffuse 80% to 90% stenosis of the left anterior descending (LAD) artery and heavy calcification with proximal 70% stenosis of the RCA. (B) The patient refused coronary artery bypass surgery (CABG) and underwent staged PCI of the LAD and then RCA. Rotational atherectomy was performed and 3.0 × 24 mm and 2.75 × 38 mm Xience Xpedition everolimus-eluting stents (EES) were placed in the proximal and mid-LAD. Three weeks later, several runs of rotational atherectomy of the proximal to mid-RCA were performed. The proximal to mid-RCA was stented with a 3.0 × 38 mm Xience Xpedition EES. (C) Repeat stress test 6 months later was positive for ischemia. Repeat angiogram showed severe ISR of proximal and mid-LAD stents and mid-RCA stent. The patient underwent CABG.

to have a more focal pattern of ISR, except in diabetics, and the ISR tends to be more confined to the stent edges.[17,18] Focal ISR has been associated with a lower rate of ISR recurrence than nonfocal ISR.[19]

Patients undergoing PCI for ISR have higher risk of clinical events than patients with ISR not undergoing PCI in registry data analysis, but also tend to have more baseline comorbidities/complex disease.[20] The two layers of stent

Box 1
Characteristics of ISR

ISR definitions

- Binary angiographic restenosis: greater than 50% luminal narrowing.
- Clinical restenosis: greater than 50% diameter stenosis and one of the following:
  1. Recurrent angina
  2. Objective signs of ischemia or exercise (eg, ECG changes)
  3. FFR less than 0.80
  4. IVUS minimum cross-sectional area less than 4 mm^2 (<6 mm^2 for left main)
  5. Restenosis greater than 70% reduction in lumen diameter even in the absence of clinical symptoms or signs

Clinical presentation

- Mean time to presentation: bare-metal stents 6 months. Drug-eluting stents 12 months.
- Recurrent angina 25% to 50% of the time. Acute myocardial infarction in 3% to 20%.

Factors more suggestive of ISR than stent thrombosis

- Longer time from stent implantation.
- Long stent.
- Intravascular ultrasonography showing neointimal hyperplasia.
- Lack of thrombus visualization on angiogram.
- Balloon slippage associated with hard intimal tissue in ISR. Thrombi more soft.

Table 1
Predictors of ISR

Patient Characteristics	Lesions Characteristics	Procedural Characteristics
• Female gender • Diabetes • Multivessel coronary artery disease • Age • Chronic kidney disease	• Small arteries • Ostial lesions • High initial plaque burden • Residual plaque after implantation • ISR • Calcified lesions	• Longer stent • Excessive straightening of vessel by the stent • Geographic miss • Low deployment pressures • Malapposition • Strut fracture • Overlapping stents

Adapted from Dangas GD, Claessen BE, Caixeta A, et al. In-stent restenosis in the drug-eluting stent era. J Am Coll Cardiol 2010;56:1897–907; with permission.

may be the cause of the higher rates of ISR. However, the higher target lesion failure rate of PCI for patients with ISR versus patients without ISR cease to exist with case-controlled matching.[21] Bioresorbable vascular scaffolds and drug-coated balloons (DCBs) may be potential future treatments of ISR because they would avoid multiple stent layers.

Procedural characteristics associated with higher rates of ISR include longer stented stenosis and stent length. Each 10 mm of excess stent length independently increases percent diameter stenosis by 4% and increases TLR at 9 months (odds ratio [OR], 1.12; 95% CI, 1.02–1.24).[22–25] Other important factors are stent/lesion ratio, use of coil stents, excessive straightening effect of the stent on the vessel, and post-procedural percent diameter stenosis and vessel size (large luminal areas allow for greater extent of hyperplasia before restenosis occurs). Stent fracture can trigger focal ISR or thrombosis,[1,26–28] which can result in a reduction in drug delivery at the breakage point of the stent. This outcome occurs more frequently in the right coronary artery, overlapping stents, longer stents, SESs (because of the ridged closed cell structure), or excessively tortuous, angulated vessels. In malapposition, stent struts are not completely apposed to the vessel wall, which allows blood between the stent and the arterial wall and may contribute to ISR and thrombosis.[1] Nonuniform drug delivery can also predispose to ISR and can be influenced by local blood flow alterations, strut overlap, and polymer damage.[1,29] Difficult stent delivery may cause alterations to the stent composition and prevent optimal drug distribution.

DESs decrease neointimal growth. As a result, geographic miss or strut fracture may be larger factors of ISR in DESs compared with BMSs.[30] Geographic miss occurs when the stent does not fully cover the injured or diseased segment of the artery (axial miss) or the ratio of balloon to artery size is less than 0.9 or greater than 1.3 (longitudinal miss). Geographic miss is associated with increased risk of TLR and MI at 1 year.[1,31] Underexpansion is a major risk factor for ISR and can be caused by undersizing the stent, use of low deployment pressures, or presence of heavily calcified lesions. However, oversized stents can also lead to extensive trauma to the vessel wall and increased proliferative reaction.[1,32]

ANATOMIC AND HEMODYNAMIC ASSESSMENT

Routine Surveillance

Routine angiographic surveillance is not recommended because it has been shown to increase the rates of oculostenotic revascularization. One study compared long-term outcomes of patients assigned to routine angiographic follow-up in 3 large-scale TAXUS trials versus those assigned to clinic follow-up alone.[33] The rate of TLR at 5 years was significantly higher in the angiographic cohort compared with the clinic follow-up only cohort (18% vs 11%; P<.001), which was caused by treatment of more intermediate lesions (40%–70% stenosis). However, there was no reduction in rates of cardiac death or MI (8.9% vs 8.8%; P = .93).

Intravascular Ultrasonography

Intravascular ultrasonography is an important imaging modality to identify the cause of ISR. It can help differentiate between device underexpansion, neointimal hyperplasia, stent fracture, or edge restenosis. In addition, it can provide insights into optimal vessel sizing for choosing the appropriate stent size. However, IVUS provides limited axial resolution (150 μm).

Optical coherence tomography

Optical coherence tomography (OCT) can provide better axial resolution (15 μm), allowing better resolution of the lumen, neointimal tissue, and stent struts. However, tissue penetration is worse with OCT, leading to poor visualization of the residual plaque behind the stent.[30]

Fractional Flow Reserve

Studies have found a discrepancy between functional ischemia measured through FFR and angiographic estimates of stenosis.[34] One study showed that FFR and percent diameter stenosis have a negative correlation (−0.61; P<.001).[35] However, in lesions with diffuse restenosis there was not a statically significant correlation. Thus, FFR may be a valuable tool in patients with diffuse restenosis to confirm functional ischemia.

TREATMENT

Balloon Angioplasty

Balloon angioplasty is used to treat ISR by displacing tissue from the lumen to the outer portion of the vessel wall as well as further expanding the stent. During balloon inflation, slippage or watermelon seeding can occur, leading to edge-related complications. Cutting or scoring balloons can help minimize this, but also have limitations in delivery through stented

regions or distal areas.[1] Lateral blades or atherotomes anchor the balloon in the lesion and minimize slippage.[30] The Restenosis Cutting balloon Evaluation trial (RESCUT) randomized 428 patients with ISR to conventional balloon angioplasty versus cutting balloon angioplasty.[36] There was less balloon slippage in the cutting balloon group (6.5% vs 25%; P<.01). Fewer balloons were used in the cutting balloon group (82% of cutting balloon cases vs 75% of balloon angioplasty cases required just one balloon; P = .03) and the cutting balloon group had a trend toward a lower need for additional stenting (3.9% vs 9.0%; P = .07). At 7 months, there was no difference in binary restenosis rate and clinic events between the two groups. Scoring balloons add the advantage of being more flexible and having increased deliverability compared with conventional balloons.[30] Balloon angioplasty should target the lesion, not the entire stented segment, while trying to avoid watermelon seeding. A buddy-wire technique can be used to stabilize the balloon.[37] Progressive balloon dilations and small/short balloons can also prevent side effects from balloon slippage. If a dog-bone effect occurs, shift to aggressive dilations with noncompliant balloons.[30]

Treatment with Drug-eluting Stents

Balloon angioplasty alone carries a high risk of recurrent stenosis, especially in diffuse and/or severe ISR.[5,38,39] When ISR requires intervention, a DES is typically placed. In The Intracoronary Stenting or Angioplasty for Restenosis Reduction - Drug-Eluting Stents for In-Stent Restenosis (ISAR-DESIRE) trial, 300 patients with restenosis of at least 50% after implantation of any limuseluting stent were randomized to SES, PES, and balloon angioplasty. At 6-month follow-up, the binary angiographic restenosis rate was 14% in the SES group (P<.001 vs angioplasty), 19% in PES group (P = .001 vs angioplasty), and 44% in the balloon angioplasty group.[40] The Restenosis Intrastent: Balloon Angioplasty versus Elective Sirolimus-Eluting Stenting (RIB-II trial) randomized patients with ISR to balloon angioplasty or SES. The trial showed improved outcomes at 4 years with SES compared with balloon angioplasty. Event-free survival was 76% in the SES cohort versus 65% in the balloon angioplasty cohort (P = .019).[41]

There is no clear evidence on which type of DES should be used to treat ISR of a DES. Some clinicians argue that using a different type of DES helps to overcome drug resistance, but no strong data support this. In the

ISAR-DESIRE 2 trial, patients with ISR in SESs were randomized to PES or SES with no significant differences in outcome.[42] In the RIBS-III trial, a prospective registry also showed that the results of a hetero-DES and homo-DES strategy were similar.[43] BMSs are not typically used because studies have shown that they are not superior to balloon angioplasty alone.[44,45]

As a result, the 2005 and 2009 update of the American College of Cardiology/American Heart Association/Society for Cardiovascular Angiography and Interventions guideline update for PCI and the 2005 European Society of Cardiology Task Force recommend DES for ISR whether the initial stent was BMS or DES.[46–48]

Brachytherapy
Brachytherapy inhibits neointimal formation within the stent, but not the stent edges, by delivering radiation to the areas of ISR. The randomized trials Paclitaxel-eluting Stents versus Brachytherapy for In-stent Restenosis (TAXUS V ISR) and Sirolimus-eluting Stents versus Vascular brachytherapy (SISR) trial showed significantly better outcomes for DES compared with brachytherapy.[49,50] Brachytherapy is only available at a few centers and can be used if DES has failed as an initial treatment for ISR.

Drug-coated Balloon Angioplasty
Repeat stenting for ISR raises concerns for creating multiple stent layers. Drug-coated balloon angioplasty is at least noninferior to DES for treating ISR. Unverdorben and colleagues[51] randomized patients with BMS ISR to paclitaxel-coated balloon versus PES. At 36 months, the lesion-related rates of major adverse cardiac events were not significantly different (9.1% vs 18.5%; $P = .14$). Similarly, the rate of TLR was not significantly different (6.2% versus 15.4%; $P = .10$). In the RIBS-V trial, 189 patients with BMS ISR were randomized to DCB or everolimus-eluting stent (EES).[52] The EES group had significantly larger minimal lumen diameter (2.36 mm vs 2.01 mm; $P<.001$) and a lower percentage of diameter stenosis (13% vs 25%; $P<.001$) when angiography was performed at a median of 249 days. The EES group also showed a trend toward better outcomes in late loss (0.04 mm vs 0.14 mm; $P = .14$), binary restenosis rate (4.7% vs 9.5%; $P = .22$), and need for target vessel revascularization (2% vs 6%; HR, 0.32; 95% CI, 0.07–1.59; $P = .17$). The ISAR-DESIRE 3 trial randomized 402 patients with ISR in DES to paclitaxel-eluting balloon (PEB) versus PES versus balloon angioplasty.[53,54] At a median follow-up of

3 years, the risk of TLR was similar with PEB versus PES ([HR, 1.46; 95% CI, 0.91–2.33; $P = .11$) and lower with PEB versus balloon angioplasty (HR, 0.51; 95% CI, 0.34–0.74; $P<.001$). The risk of death/MI was lower, but not statistically significant, with PEB versus PES (HR, 0.55; 95% CI, 0.28–1.07; $P = .08$). This finding was driven by a lower risk of death (HR, 0.38; 95% CI, 0.17–0.87; $P = .02$). The risk of death/MI was similar with PEB versus balloon angioplasty (HR, 0.96; 95% CI, 0.46–2.0; $P = .91$).

A meta-analysis of randomized controlled trials comparing DCB, DES, and balloon angioplasty for the treatment of ISR reported that treatment with DCB had a trend toward better outcomes than with DES.[55] This analysis included 2059 patients from 11 RCTs. The risk of TLR was lower in patients treated with DEB (OR, 0.22; 95% CI, 0.10–0.42) or DES (OR, 0.24; 95% CI, 0.11–0.47) than in those treated with balloon angioplasty. In a comparison of DEB and DES, the risk of TLR (OR, 0.92; 95% CI, 0.43–1.90) was similar. The risk of major adverse cardiac events, which was mainly driven by TLR, was also significantly lower in the DEB and DES groups (OR, 0.28; 95% CI, 0.14–0.53) than in the balloon angioplasty group, but it was similar between the DEB and DES groups (OR, 0.84; 95% CI, 0.45–1.50). For MI, both DES and DEB were superior to balloon angioplasty. For TLR, the probability of being ranked as the best treatment was 59.9% (DEB), 40.1% (DES), and 0.1% (balloon angioplasty). For MI, the probability of being ranked as the best treatment was 63.0% (DEB), 35.3% (balloon angioplasty), and 1.7% (DES). The United States Food and Drug Administration has approved DCB for use in peripheral arterial disease but not yet for coronary artery disease. The ongoing RIBS-IV trial and ISAR DESIRE-4 trial will help provide additional data.

Excimer Laser Angioplasty
Excimer laser angioplasty (ELA) produces monochromatic light energy, which generates heat and shock waves that disrupt plaque. Mehran and colleagues[56] compared results of ELA versus rotational atherectomy (RA), both followed by Percutaneous transluminal coronary angioplasty (PTCA). 119 patients with 158 ISR lesions were treated with ELA plus PTCA and 130 patients with 161 ISR lesions were treated with RA plus PTCA. Volumetric IVUS analysis showed a greater reduction in intimal hyperplasia volume after RA than after ELA (43 vs 19 mm^3; $P<.001$). However, the 1-year TLR rates were similar: 26% with ELA plus PTCA versus 28% with RA plus PTCA

(*P* = nonsignificant). Dahm and Kuon[57] followed 39 patients with diffuse ISR treated with ELA followed by PTCA. Diameter stenosis decreased from 84% to 23% after ELA (*P* = .001), 9% after PTCA (*P* = .001), and was 31% at follow-up (*P*<.01). Minimal lumen diameter increased from 0.7 mm to 2.2 mm after ELA (*P* = .001), to 2.7 mm after PTCA (*P* = .001), to 1.7 mm at follow-up (*P* = .005).

However, ELA has been associated with serious complications. In a series of 3000 consecutive patients treated with ELA, complications included in-hospital bypass surgery (3.8%), Q wave MI (2.1%), and death (0.5%).[58] Coronary artery perforation occurred in 1.2% of patients, but decreased to 0.4% in the last 1000 patients (0.3% of lesions).[58] In the Laser Angioplasty versus Angioplasty (LAVA) trial, 215 patients with 244 lesions were prospectively randomized at 14 clinical centers to laser-facilitated PTCA versus PTCA alone.[59] There was no difference in postprocedural diameter stenosis after laser treatment compared with PTCA (18.3% vs 19.5%; *P* = .50). However, use of the laser versus angioplasty alone did result in more major and minor procedural complications (18.0% vs 3.1%; *P* = .0004), MI (4.3% vs 0%; *P* = .04), and total in-hospital major adverse events (10.3% vs 4.1%; *P* = .08). At a mean follow-up time of 11 months, there was no difference in event-free survival in patients assigned to laser treatment versus PTCA alone. In the Excimer Laser, Rotational Atherectomy, and Balloon Angioplasty Comparison (ERBAC) study, 685 patients with symptomatic coronary disease warranting elective PCI for a complex lesion were randomly assigned to balloon angioplasty (n = 222), ELA (n = 232), or RA (n = 231).[60] The patients who underwent ELA had a lower rate of procedural success than those who underwent RA or conventional balloon angioplasty (77% vs 89% and 80%; *P* = .0019). However, there was no difference in major in-hospital complications (4.3% vs 3.2% vs 3.1%; *P* = .71). At 6 months, revascularization of the original target lesion was performed more frequently in the RA group (42.4%) and the ELA group (46.0%) than in the angioplasty group (31.9%; *P* = .013). ELA is not currently a well-accepted treatment for ISR, but the ultimate role of this therapy is still unclear.

SUMMARY

ISR is a common clinical problem encountered by patients after PCI. ISR typically presents as recurrent angina, but presents as MI in some patients. A variety of patient, lesion, and procedural characteristics are associated with ISR. The incidence of ISR has dramatically decreased since the use of DESs. Treatment options for ISR include DES and DCB. Further studies are required to identify the optimal treatment strategy for patients with ISR.

REFERENCES

1. Dangas GD, Claessen BE, Caixeta A, et al. In-stent restenosis in the drug-eluting stent era. J Am Coll Cardiol 2010;56:1897–907.
2. Mehran R, Dangas G, Abizaid AS, et al. Angiographic patterns of in-stent restenosis: classification and implications for long-term outcome. Circulation 1999;100:1872–8.
3. Lee MS, Pessegueiro A, Zimmer R, et al. Clinical presentation of patients with in-stent restenosis in the drug-eluting stent era. J Invasive Cardiol 2008;20:401–3.
4. Nayak AK, Kawamura A, Nesto RW, et al. Myocardial infarction as a presentation of clinical in-stent restenosis. Circ J 2006;70:1026–9.
5. Bossi I, Klersy C, Black AJ, et al. In-stent restenosis: long-term outcome and predictors of subsequent target lesion revascularization after repeat balloon angioplasty. J Am Coll Cardiol 2000;35: 1569–76.
6. Chen MS, John JM, Chew DP, et al. Bare metal stent restenosis is not a benign clinical entity. Am Heart J 2006;151:1260–4.
7. Stone GW, Ellis SG, Colombo A, et al. Offsetting impact of thrombosis and restenosis on the occurrence of death and myocardial infarction after paclitaxel-eluting and bare metal stent implantation. Circulation 2007;115:2842–7.
8. Kimura T, Morimoto T, Nakagawa Y, et al. Very late stent thrombosis and late target lesion revascularization after sirolimus-eluting stent implantation: five-year outcome of the j-Cypher registry. Circulation 2012;125:584–91.
9. Leon MB, Nikolsky E, Cutlip DE, et al. Improved late clinical safety with zotarolimus-eluting stents compared with paclitaxel-eluting stents in patients with de novo coronary lesions: 3-year follow-up from the ENDEAVOR IV (Randomized Comparison of Zotarolimus- and Paclitaxel-Eluting Stents in Patients with Coronary Artery Disease) trial. JACC Cardiovasc Interv 2010;3:1043–50.
10. Raber L, Wohlwend L, Wigger M, et al. Five-year clinical and angiographic outcomes of a randomized comparison of sirolimus-eluting and paclitaxel-eluting stents: results of the Sirolimus-Eluting Versus Paclitaxel-Eluting Stents for Coronary Revascularization LATE trial. Circulation 2011; 123:2819–28, 6 p following 2828.

11. Stettler C, Wandel S, Allemann S, et al. Outcomes associated with drug-eluting and bare-metal stents: a collaborative network meta-analysis. Lancet 2007;370:937–48.

12. Aoki J, Colombo A, Dudek D, et al. Persistent remodeling and neointimal suppression 2 years after polymer-based, paclitaxel-eluting stent implantation: insights from serial intravascular ultrasound analysis in the TAXUS II study. Circulation 2005; 112:3876–83.

13. Claessen BE, Beijk MA, Legrand V, et al. Two-year clinical, angiographic, and intravascular ultrasound follow-up of the XIENCE V everolimus-eluting stent in the treatment of patients with de novo native coronary artery lesions: the SPIRIT II trial. Circ Cardiovasc Interv 2009;2:339–47.

14. Aoki J, Abizaid AC, Serruys PW, et al. Evaluation of four-year coronary artery response after sirolimus-eluting stent implantation using serial quantitative intravascular ultrasound and computer-assisted grayscale value analysis for plaque composition in event-free patients. J Am Coll Cardiol 2005;46: 1670–6.

15. Kastrati A, Schomig A, Elezi S, et al. Predictive factors of restenosis after coronary stent placement. J Am Coll Cardiol 1997;30:1428–36.

16. Ivens K, Gradaus F, Heering P, et al. Myocardial revascularization in patients with end-stage renal disease: comparison of percutaneous transluminal coronary angioplasty and coronary artery bypass grafting. Int Urol Nephrol 2001;32:717–23.

17. Rathore S, Kinoshita Y, Terashima M, et al. A comparison of clinical presentations, angiographic patterns and outcomes of in-stent restenosis between bare metal stents and drug eluting stents. EuroIntervention 2010;5:841–6.

18. Stone GW, Ellis SG, Cox DA, et al. A polymer-based, paclitaxel-eluting stent in patients with coronary artery disease. N Engl J Med 2004;350: 221–31.

19. Cosgrave J, Melzi G, Biondi-Zoccai GG, et al. Drug-eluting stent restenosis the pattern predicts the outcome. J Am Coll Cardiol 2006;47:2399–404.

20. Lee MS, Yang T, Lasala JM, et al. Two-year clinical outcomes of paclitaxel-eluting stents for in-stent restenosis in patients from the arrive programme. EuroIntervention 2011;7:314–22.

21. Lee MS, Yang T, Mahmud E, et al. Clinical outcomes in the percutaneous coronary intervention of in-stent restenosis with everolimus-eluting stents. J Invasive Cardiol 2014;26:420–6.

22. Kobayashi Y, De Gregorio J, Kobayashi N, et al. Stented segment length as an independent predictor of restenosis. J Am Coll Cardiol 1999;34:651–9.

23. Goldberg SL, Loussararian A, De Gregorio J, et al. Predictors of diffuse and aggressive intra-stent restenosis. J Am Coll Cardiol 2001;37:1019–25.

24. Serruys PW, Kay IP, Disco C, et al. Periprocedural quantitative coronary angiography after Palmaz-Schatz stent implantation predicts the restenosis rate at six months: results of a meta-analysis of the Belgian Netherlands stent study (BENESTENT) I, BENESTENT II pilot, BENESTENT II and MUSIC trials. Multicenter ultrasound stent in coronaries. J Am Coll Cardiol 1999;34:1067–74.

25. Mauri L, O'Malley AJ, Cutlip DE, et al. Effects of stent length and lesion length on coronary restenosis. Am J Cardiol 2004;93:1340–6. A5.

26. Lee MS, Jurewitz D, Aragon J, et al. Stent fracture associated with drug-eluting stents: clinical characteristics and implications. Catheter Cardiovasc Interv 2007;69:387–94.

27. Umeda H, Gochi T, Iwase M, et al. Frequency, predictors and outcome of stent fracture after sirolimus-eluting stent implantation. Int J Cardiol 2009;133(3):321–6.

28. Aoki J, Nakazawa G, Tanabe K, et al. Incidence and clinical impact of coronary stent fracture after sirolimus-eluting stent implantation. Catheter Cardiovasc Interv 2007;69:380–6.

29. Balakrishnan B, Tzafriri AR, Seifert P, et al. Implications for single and overlapping drug-eluting stents. Circulation 2005;111:2958–65.

30. Alfonso F, Byrne RA, Rivero F, et al. Current treatment of in-stent restenosis. J Am Coll Cardiol 2014;63:2659–73.

31. Costa MA, Angiolillo DJ, Tannenbaum M, et al. Impact of stent deployment procedural factors on long-term effectiveness and safety of sirolimus-eluting stents (final results of the multicenter prospective STLLR trial). Am J Cardiol 2008;101:1704–11.

32. Fujii K, Mintz GS, Kobayashi Y, et al. Contribution of stent underexpansion to recurrence after sirolimus-eluting stent implantation for in-stent restenosis. Circulation 2004;109:1085–8.

33. Uchida T, Popma J, Stone GW, et al. The clinical impact of routine angiographic follow-up in randomized trials of drug-eluting stents: a critical assessment of "oculostenotic" reintervention in patients with intermediate lesions. JACC Cardiovasc Interv 2010;3:403–11.

34. Meijboom WB, Van Mieghem CA, van Pelt N, et al. Comprehensive assessment of coronary artery stenoses: computed tomography coronary angiography versus conventional coronary angiography and correlation with fractional flow reserve in patients with stable angina. J Am Coll Cardiol 2008; 52:636–43.

35. Nam CW, Rha SW, Koo BK, et al. Usefulness of coronary pressure measurement for functional evaluation of drug-eluting stent restenosis. Am J Cardiol 2011;107:1783–6.

36. Albiero R, Silber S, Di Mario C, et al. Cutting balloon versus conventional balloon angioplasty for the treatment of in-stent restenosis: results of the restenosis cutting balloon evaluation trial (RESCUT). J Am Coll Cardiol 2004;43:943–9.

37. Alfonso F, Perez-Vizcayno MJ, Cruz A, et al. Treatment of patients with in-stent restenosis. EuroIntervention 2009;5(Suppl D):D70–8.

38. Bauters C, Banos JL, Van Belle E, et al. Six-month angiographic outcome after successful repeat percutaneous intervention for in-stent restenosis. Circulation 1998;97:318–21.

39. Eltchaninoff H, Koning R, Tron C, et al. Balloon angioplasty for the treatment of coronary in-stent restenosis: immediate results and 6-month angiographic recurrent restenosis rate. J Am Coll Cardiol 1998;32:980–4.

40. Kastrati A, Mehilli J, von Beckerath N, et al. Sirolimus-eluting stent or paclitaxel-eluting stent vs balloon angioplasty for prevention of recurrences in patients with coronary in-stent restenosis: a randomized controlled trial. JAMA 2005;293:165–71.

41. Alfonso F, Perez-Vizcayno MJ, Hernandez R, et al. A randomized comparison of sirolimus-eluting stent with balloon angioplasty in patients with in-stent restenosis: results of the Restenosis Intrastent: Balloon Angioplasty Versus Elective Sirolimus-Eluting Stenting (RIBS-II) trial. J Am Coll Cardiol 2006;47:2152–60.

42. Garg S, Smith K, Torguson R, et al. Treatment of drug-eluting stent restenosis with the same versus different drug-eluting stent. Catheter Cardiovasc Interv 2007;70:9–14.

43. Alfonso F, Perez-Vizcayno MJ, Dutary J, et al. Implantation of a drug-eluting stent with a different drug (switch strategy) in patients with drug-eluting stent restenosis. results from a prospective multicenter study (RIBS III [restenosis intra-stent: balloon angioplasty versus drug-eluting stent]). JACC Cardiovasc Interv 2012;5:728–37.

44. Alfonso F, Auge JM, Zueco J, et al. Long-term results (three to five years) of the Restenosis Intrastent: Balloon Angioplasty Versus Elective Stenting (RIBS) randomized study. J Am Coll Cardiol 2005;46:756–60.

45. Mehran R, Dangas G, Abizaid A, et al. Treatment of focal in-stent restenosis with balloon angioplasty alone versus stenting: short- and long-term results. Am Heart J 2001;141:610–4.

46. Smith SC Jr, Feldman TE, Hirshfeld JW Jr, et al. ACC/AHA/SCAI 2005 guideline update for percutaneous coronary intervention: a report of the American College of Cardiology/American Heart Association Task Force on Practice Guidelines (ACC/AHA/SCAI Writing Committee to Update the 2001 Guidelines for Percutaneous Coronary Intervention). J Am Coll Cardiol 2006;47:e1–121.

47. Silber S, Albertsson P, Aviles FF, et al. Guidelines for percutaneous coronary interventions. The Task Force for Percutaneous Coronary Interventions of the European Society of Cardiology. Eur Heart J 2005;26:804–47.

48. Kushner FG, Hand M, Smith SC Jr, et al. 2009 Focused updates: ACC/AHA guidelines for the management of patients with ST-elevation myocardial infarction (updating the 2004 guideline and 2007 focused update) and ACC/AHA/SCAI guidelines on percutaneous coronary intervention (updating the 2005 guideline and 2007 focused update) a report of the American College of Cardiology Foundation/American Heart Association Task Force on Practice Guidelines. J Am Coll Cardiol 2009;54:2205–41.

49. Stone GW, Ellis SG, O'Shaughnessy CD, et al. Paclitaxel-eluting stents vs vascular brachytherapy for in-stent restenosis within bare-metal stents: the TAXUS V ISR randomized trial. JAMA 2006;295:1253–63.

50. Holmes DR Jr, Teirstein P, Satler L, et al. Sirolimus-eluting stents vs vascular brachytherapy for in-stent restenosis within bare-metal stents: the SISR randomized trial. JAMA 2006;295:1264–73.

51. Unverdorben M, Vallbracht C, Cremers B, et al. Paclitaxel-coated balloon catheter versus paclitaxel-coated stent for the treatment of coronary in-stent restenosis: the three-year results of the PEPCAD II ISR study. EuroIntervention 2015;11:926–34.

52. Alfonso F, Perez-Vizcayno MJ, Cardenas A, et al. A randomized comparison of drug-eluting balloon versus everolimus-eluting stent in patients with bare-metal stent-in-stent restenosis: the RIBS V clinical trial (restenosis Intra-Stent of Bare Metal Stents: paclitaxel-eluting balloon vs. everolimus-eluting stent). J Am Coll Cardiol 2014;63:1378–86.

53. Byrne RA, Neumann FJ, Mehilli J, et al. Paclitaxel-eluting balloons, paclitaxel-eluting stents, and balloon angioplasty in patients with restenosis after implantation of a drug-eluting stent (ISAR-DESIRE 3): a randomised, open-label trial. Lancet 2013;381:461–7.

54. Kufner S, Cassese S, Valeskini M, et al. Long-term efficacy and safety of paclitaxel-eluting balloon for the treatment of drug-eluting stent restenosis: 3-year results of a randomized controlled trial. JACC Cardiovasc Interv 2015;8:877–84.

55. Lee JM, Park J, Kang J, et al. Comparison among drug-eluting balloon, drug-eluting stent, and plain balloon angioplasty for the treatment of in-stent restenosis: a network meta-analysis of 11 randomized, controlled trials. JACC Cardiovasc Interv 2015;8:382–94.

56. Mehran R, Dangas G, Mintz GS, et al. Treatment of in-stent restenosis with excimer laser coronary

angioplasty versus rotational atherectomy: comparative mechanisms and results. Circulation 2000;101: 2484–9.

57. Dahm JB, Kuon E. High-energy eccentric excimer laser angioplasty for debulking diffuse in-stent restenosis leads to better acute- and 6-month follow-up results. J Invasive Cardiol 2000;12: 335–42.

58. Litvack F, Eigler N, Margolis J, et al. Percutaneous excimer laser coronary angioplasty: results in the first consecutive 3,000 patients. the ELCA investigators. J Am Coll Cardiol 1994;23:323–9.

59. Stone GW, de Marchena E, Dageforde D, et al. Prospective, randomized, multicenter comparison of laser-facilitated balloon angioplasty versus stand-alone balloon angioplasty in patients with obstructive coronary artery disease. The Laser Angioplasty Versus Angioplasty (LAVA) Trial Investigators. J Am Coll Cardiol 1997;30:1714–21.

60. Reifart N, Vandormael M, Krajcar M, et al. Randomized comparison of angioplasty of complex coronary lesions at a single center. Excimer Laser, Rotational Atherectomy, and Balloon Angioplasty Comparison (ERBAC) study. Circulation 1997;96:91–8.

Antiplatelet Therapy in Percutaneous Coronary Intervention

Alexander C. Fanaroff, MD, Sunil V. Rao, MD*

KEYWORDS

- Antiplatelet agents • $P2Y12$ receptor antagonists • Glycoprotein IIb/IIIa inhibitors
- Percutaneous coronary intervention • Bleeding • Stent thrombosis

KEY POINTS

- Balancing the risks of stent thrombosis and major bleeding is key to the effective use of antiplatelet agents during and after percutaneous coronary intervention (PCI).
- The new oral $P2Y12$ inhibitors prasugrel and ticagrelor have onsets of action considerably faster than that of clopidogrel and reduce the incidence of recurrent ischemic events when administered to patients with acute coronary syndrome undergoing PCI.
- Despite the theoretic benefits of $P2Y12$ inhibitor preloading and platelet function testing–guided selection of antiplatelet agents, clinical trials have failed to show the benefit of these strategies.

INTRODUCTION

Dual antiplatelet therapy (DAPT) with aspirin and a $P2Y12$ inhibitor is the evidence-based, guideline-recommended cornerstone of antithrombotic therapy for patients undergoing percutaneous coronary intervention (PCI) across a spectrum of indications. Fundamental to DAPT use is the balance of bleeding with the risk of recurrent myocardial infarction (MI) and stent thrombosis.

Until recently, the only available $P2Y12$ inhibitors were clopidogrel and ticlopidine, both prodrugs metabolized into active metabolites that irreversibly bind the adenosine $P2Y12$ receptor on platelet surfaces, inhibiting platelet aggregation. Because of the requirement for first pass metabolism in the liver, neither drug achieves steady state levels of platelet inhibition for several hours following dosing, leaving a window of inadequate platelet inhibition during which post-PCI patients are theoretically vulnerable

to acute stent thrombosis if they are not loaded with a $P2Y12$ inhibitor before PCI.

Over the past 5 years, 3 highly potent, fast-acting $P2Y12$ inhibitors have been introduced to the market: prasugrel, ticagrelor, and cangrelor. Prasugrel and ticagrelor are oral agents, and cangrelor is an intravenous agent. These agents all achieve maximal platelet inhibition within 1 hour of loading dose in healthy volunteers. However, these drugs exhibit different pharmacokinetics in real-world patients undergoing PCI, especially patients with ST segment elevation MI (STEMI) and non–ST segment elevation acute coronary syndrome (NSTE-ACS), which may have important implications for their use as antiplatelet agents in urgent and primary PCI. These agents are additions to the antiplatelet armamentarium that also includes aspirin and glycoprotein IIb/IIIa inhibitors, creating an array of combinations available for use in patients undergoing PCI.

Funding sources: This article was prepared without external funding.
Disclosures: A.C. Fanaroff, none; S.V. Rao, consultant for Merck.
Duke Clinical Research Institute, 2400 Pratt Street, Durham, NC 27705, USA
* Corresponding author. 508 Fulton Street (111A), Durham, NC 27705.
E-mail address: sunil.rao@duke.edu

This article focuses on the pharmacokinetic and pharmacodynamics properties of the newer and older [P2Y]12 inhibitors as well as glycoprotein IIb/IIIa inhibitors, and the clinical trial evidence supporting the use of each of the available antiplatelet agents. Their effects on periprocedural major bleeding and early stent thrombosis are also discussed, as are the optimal combinations and usage to achieve the best clinical outcomes.

THE CENTRAL ROLE OF PLATELETS IN OUTCOMES AFTER PERCUTANEOUS CORONARY INTERVENTION: STENT THROMBOSIS AND BLEEDING

Platelets are integrally involved in the pathogenesis of adverse events after PCI. In particular, stent thrombosis is a platelet-mediated phenomenon, and the antithrombotic effect of antiplatelet therapy predisposes patients to bleeding complications. Inhibitors of platelet activation and aggregation are therapeutic options for patients undergoing PCI. **Fig. 1** shows potential receptor targets on the platelet surface, some of which are targets of available antiplatelet agents used for PCI.

In the immediate post-PCI period, acute stent thrombosis and periprocedural bleeding are events of concern. Both events are associated with increased mortality. Stent thrombosis can be grouped into acute (<24 hours after PCI), subacute (24 hours to 30 days), late (30 days to 1 year), and very late (>1 year). In an analysis of the Risk Model to Predict Adverse Outcomes after Primary PCI (RISK-PCI) clinical trial, the 30-day

risk-adjusted mortality was more than 5-fold higher in patients with early (acute or subacute) stent thrombosis than in those without, and 1-year risk-adjusted mortality was more than 4-fold higher.[1] In an analysis of the Drug Eluting Stent in Primary Angioplasty (DESERT) primary PCI registry, patients with stent thrombosis had a raw mortality of 23.6%, compared with 6% in those without stent thrombosis.[2] This increase in mortality with stent thrombosis persists in patients without STEMI: in an analysis of the Acute Catheterization and Urgent Intervention Triage Strategy (ACUITY) trial, which enrolled patients undergoing urgent PCI for NSTE-ACS, 30-day mortality was 24.7% in patients with stent thrombosis, compared with 0.5% in those without.[3]

Similarly, post-PCI bleeding has long been identified as an independent predictor of mortality in patients undergoing elective, urgent, and emergent PCI. In a pooled analysis of 3 clinical trials enrolling patients undergoing PCI for stable coronary artery disease (CAD), NSTE-ACS, and STEMI, post-PCI major bleeding increased risk-adjusted 1-year mortality 4.2-fold, an increase in mortality greater than that of recurrent MI within 30 days.[4] Analyses of the Global Registry of Acute Coronary Events (GRACE) and CathPCI registries found similar links between major bleeding and mortality,[5,6] with one CathPCI study showing an additional in-hospital death for every 29 patients with PCI-related major bleeding.[7]

Stent thrombosis carries a greater risk of death, but is rarer than bleeding, leading to differences in attributable deaths for the two

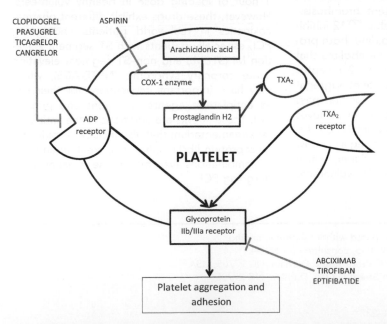

Fig. 1. Targets of antiplatelet agents used in patients undergoing PCI. Cyclooxygenase-1 (COX-1), the Adenosine diphosphate (ADP) receptor, and glycoprotein IIb/IIIa receptors are the targets of available antiplatelet agents. The ADP receptor and COX-1 mediate processes that activate the glycoprotein IIb/IIIa receptor, which is the major molecule mediating platelet aggregation and adhesion. TXA$_2$, thromboxane A$_2$.

events. Acute stent thrombosis occurs in about 0.4% of PCIs[8] and major bleeding occurs in about 1.7% to 2% in contemporary registries, depending on the definition.[7,9]

Importantly, both stent thrombosis and major bleeding are more common in patients with ACS than in those undergoing stenting for stable angina.[4] The rate of early stent thrombosis increases along the continuum from elective to primary PCI: 0.4% in elective PCI, 1.4% in urgent PCI for non–ST-elevation MI (NSTEMI), and 3.1% in primary PCI (Table 1).[10]

Beyond type of presentation, the strongest risk factors for PCI-related major bleeding include increasing age, female sex, preexisting anemia, and renal failure.[6,11] In clinical trials evaluating different antithrombotic strategies, like ACUITY, Harmonizing Outcomes with Revascularization and Stents in Acute Myocardial Infarction (HORIZONS-AMI), and Randomized Evaluation in PCI Linking Angiomax to Reduced Clinical Events (REPLACE-2), randomization to heparin plus routine glycoprotein IIb/IIIa inhibitors (compared with bivalirudin) was also a strong predictor of bleeding.[4]

The strongest predictor of stent thrombosis across multiple studies is premature cessation of DAPT. Other risk factors include presentation with STEMI, diabetes mellitus, complex CAD, and procedural factors like stent length, stent diameter, successful restoration of coronary artery flow, and lack of P2Y12 inhibitor treatment before stenting.[1-3,8,12,13] This fact highlights the central role of periprocedural antiplatelet therapy in both PCI-related major bleeding and early stent thrombosis.

ANTIPLATELET AGENTS
Ticlopidine
Ticlopidine is an oral thienopyridine molecule that requires metabolism in the liver into a biologically active form that irreversibly binds to, and inhibits, the P2Y12 subunit of the platelet adenosine diphosphate (ADP) receptor. Because

of this need for first pass metabolism, when given to healthy volunteers at a standard dose (250 mg twice daily), ticlopidine required 3 to 4 days to achieve maximal platelet inhibition.[14] However, despite favorable effects on platelets, ticlopidine's use is limited by its side effects, which include diarrhea, rash, and agranulocytosis.[15] Of these, the most serious is agranulocytosis, which develops in up to 2.4% of patients treated with ticlopidine, with the incidence increasing with longer duration of treatment.[15]

Clopidogrel
Clopidogrel is another oral thienopyridine that irreversibly inhibits the P2Y12 subunit of the ADP receptor on platelets. Clopidogrel is also a prodrug that is converted to its active form by the cytochrome 2C19 (CYP2C19) enzyme in the liver, with less than 15% of the prodrug being converted to active metabolite.[16] In healthy subjects treated with aspirin plus a loading dose of 300 mg of clopidogrel, inhibition of an ex vivo model of arterial thrombosis occurs within 1.5 hours, although the peak effect is delayed by 6 hours, consistent with clopidogrel's need to undergo first pass metabolism before taking effect.[17] Pharmacodynamic studies conducted in patients with stable CAD undergoing PCI similarly showed that platelet reactivity remained high 4 hours following a loading dose of 300 mg.[18]

Prasugrel
Prasugrel is another oral thienopyridine P2Y12 inhibitor that requires first pass metabolism into an active metabolite. However, unlike clopidogrel and ticlopidine, in which most of the absorbed drug is converted into molecules that have no effect on platelet aggregation, prasugrel is efficiently converted into its active metabolite, leading to a much higher likelihood of response and faster onset of action than clopidogrel.[19] In preclinical studies in healthy volunteers, prasugrel reaches peak platelet inhibition within 1 hour following administration, and reaches an

Table 1
Incidence of major bleeding and stent thrombosis by PCI indication

	Elective PCI (%)	Urgent PCI for NSTE-ACS (%)	Primary PCI for STEMI (%)
Major bleeding	0.7	1.8	2.6
Stent thrombosis	0.4	1.4	3.1

Adapted from Mehran R, Pocock S, Nikolsky E, et al. Impact of bleeding on mortality after percutaneous coronary intervention results from a patient-level pooled analysis of the REPLACE-2 (Randomized Evaluation of PCI Linking Angiomax to Reduced Clinical Events), ACUITY (Acute Catheterization and Urgent Intervention Triage Strategy), and HORIZONS-AMI (Harmonizing Outcomes with Revascularization and Stents in Acute Myocardial Infarction) trials. JACC Cardiovasc Interv 2011;4(6):657; and Cook S, Windecker S. Early stent thrombosis: past, present, and future. Circulation 2009;119(5):658.

equivalent level of platelet inhibition to clopidogrel's maximal platelet inhibition within 15 minutes.[20] These findings were similar in patients with stable CAD and those undergoing PCI, with maximal platelet inhibition reached within 2 hours after a loading dose of prasugrel 60 mg.[21,22]

Ticagrelor

Unlike prasugrel, clopidogrel, and ticlopidine, ticagrelor is an oral pentotriazolopyrimidine. Its development was precipitated by the discovery that adenosine triphosphate (ATP) reversibly inhibits the $P2Y12$ subunit of the ADP receptor at a site distinct from the thienopyridines.[19] Ticagrelor undergoes first pass metabolism in the liver, but both ticagrelor and its major metabolite inhibit platelet aggregation. Ticagrelor's rapidity of onset and potency were shown in the Randomized Double Blind Assessment of the ONSET and OFFSET of the Antiplatelet Effects of Ticagrelor Versus Clopidogrel in Patients with Stable Coronary Artery Disease (ONSET/OFFSET) trial, which randomized stable patients with CAD to a loading dose of ticagrelor or clopidogrel followed by maintenance dosing, and measured platelet function.[23] By 1 hour after loading, ticagrelor had already inhibited platelets more effectively than clopidogrel's peak effect, and 98% of patients had greater than 50% platelet inhibition after 2 hours. Other preclinical studies showed similar effects.[24]

Cangrelor

Like ticagrelor, cangrelor is an ATP analogue that is biologically active without any need for first pass metabolism and reversibly inhibits the $P2Y12$ subunit of the ADP receptor.[19] Unlike the previously discussed agents, cangrelor is administered intravenously. Because cangrelor does not require either gastrointestinal absorption or first pass metabolism, it inhibits platelets immediately at the start of its infusion. Unlike the oral $P2Y12$ inhibitors, which have plasma half-lives between 7 and 8.5 hours, cangrelor's plasma half-life is 3 minutes, and its antiplatelet effect lasts less than 30 minutes after the infusion is stopped.[19]

Glycoprotein IIb/IIIa Inhibitors: Tirofiban, Eptifibatide, and Abciximab

Unlike $P2Y12$ receptor antagonists, which inhibit platelet activation upstream of platelet aggregation, glycoprotein IIb/IIIa receptor antagonists exert their antiplatelet effect via blockade of the glycoprotein IIb/IIIa receptor, which is involved directly in binding fibrin and allows aggregation of adjacent platelets. First studied in the mid-1990s, these drugs, which include tirofiban, eptifibatide, and abciximab, inhibit platelet aggregation nearly completely within 15 minutes of intravenous bolus, theoretically making them ideal antiplatelet agents for use in PCI.[25] Abciximab, a fragment of a human-murine monoclonal antibody, irreversibly binds to and inactivates platelets; thus, even though abciximab has a short plasma half-life, it exerts its antiplatelet effect as long as abciximab-bound platelets remain in circulation. In contrast, tirofiban and eptifibatide are reversible inhibitors of the glycoprotein IIb/IIIa receptor with short plasma half-lives, with platelet aggregation returning to normal within 4 hours of cessation of an infusion.[26]

CLINICAL DATA

Ticlopidine

Pivotal randomized trials conclusively showed that coronary stents reduce the incidence of abrupt closure and restenosis compared with balloon angioplasty alone.[27–29] The disadvantages of stenting include neointimal hyperplasia (leading to in-stent restenosis) and stent thrombosis.[29] Subsequent clinical trials used aggressive antiplatelet treatment with aspirin and dipyridamole, and anticoagulation with heparin and warfarin. Despite these aggressive measures, stent thrombosis continued to complicate up to 3.5% of cases.[27,28]

The development of the potent antiplatelet agent ticlopidine and demonstration of its efficacy in registry studies and small clinical trials[30,31] led to the Stent Antithrombotic Regimen Study (STARS) trial, in which 1653 patients who underwent successful coronary stenting were randomized to aspirin alone, aspirin plus ticlopidine, or aspirin plus warfarin (Table 2).[32] Compared with aspirin alone, aspirin plus ticlopidine reduced the incidence of 30-day death, target vessel revascularization, angiographically evident stent thrombosis, or MI by 85% (0.5% vs 3.6%; relative risk [RR], 0.15; 95% confidence interval [CI], 0.05–0.43; $P<.001$). The rate of stent thrombosis was also reduced with ticlopidine (0.5% vs 2.9%; RR, 0.19; 95% CI, 0.06–0.57; $P = .005$). Compared with the combination of aspirin and warfarin, treatment with aspirin plus ticlopidine reduced the risk of the primary outcome to a slightly smaller degree (0.5% vs 2.7%; RR, 0.20; 95% CI, 0.07–0.61; $P = .01$); all clinical events in both groups were stent thromboses. The combination of aspirin and ticlopidine increased the rate of hemorrhagic complications 3-fold compared with aspirin alone (5.5% vs 1.8%; RR, 3.06; $P = .002$) but had a similar rate of hemorrhagic complications to the combination of aspirin plus warfarin. This trial established that stent thrombosis is a platelet-mediated phenomenon, and DAPT was essential to reduce adverse outcomes after PCI with stenting.

Clopidogrel

Despite ticlopidine's superior efficacy compared with aspirin alone, concerns persisted about its side effects, especially agranulocytosis, which was sometimes irreversible. Preclinical studies reported that clopidogrel was as efficacious as ticlopidine without similar safety concerns. The Clopidogrel Aspirin Stent International Cooperative Study (CLASSICS) trial was thus designed to compare the safety of several different regimens of aspirin plus clopidogrel with aspirin plus ticlopidine in a cohort of patients who had undergone successful stenting.[33] The primary end point of the study (major bleeding, neutropenia, thrombocytopenia, or treatment discontinuation caused by an adverse drug event at 28 days) occurred in 9.1% of the ticlopidine-treated cohort, compared with 4.6% of the clopidogrel cohort (RR, 0.50; 95% CI, 0.31–0.81; $P = .005$). This end point was driven almost entirely by discontinuation of ticlopidine for gastrointestinal reasons; only 1 of the 340 patients in the ticlopidine arm developed neutropenia, and bleeding risk was similar between the two groups. Although the study was not powered to detect a difference in cardiovascular events, patients treated with ticlopidine and clopidogrel had similar rates of major adverse cardiovascular events at 28 days.[33]

After other clinical trials showed comparable efficacy between clopidogrel and ticlopidine for the prevention of cardiovascular events,[15,34] and the long-term safety of clopidogrel was confirmed in the 19,000-patient Clopidogrel vs Aspirin in Patients at Risk of Ischemic Events (CAPRIE) study,[35] ticlopidine became less used because of its side effect profile.

Initially, trials of DAPT in patients undergoing stenting largely enrolled either populations with stable CAD or unselected populations. PCI-CURE was a substudy of patients undergoing PCI in the Clopidogrel in Unstable Angina to Prevent Recurrent Events (CURE) trial, which randomized patients with NSTE-ACS to clopidogrel or placebo, started immediately, and continued for 3 to 12 months.[36] Because the standard of care for patients undergoing stenting required DAPT for 4 weeks following stenting, all patients in PCI-CURE received clopidogrel following stenting; however, only the group randomized to clopidogrel received clopidogrel pretreatment before stenting.[37] Thus,

PCI-CURE's 30-day outcomes represent the findings of a clinical trial comparing clopidogrel pretreatment with no clopidogrel pretreatment. The clopidogrel group was loaded with 300 mg of clopidogrel and treated with 75 mg daily for a median of 6 days before PCI. Clopidogrel pretreatment reduced the rate of the primary end point of 30-day cardiovascular death, MI, or urgent target vessel revascularization by 30% (4.5% vs 6.4%; RR, 0.70; 95% CI, 0.50–0.97; $P = .03$); this reduction in the rate of the primary end point appeared as early as 2 days after PCI.[37] Major bleeding rates from the time of PCI to 30 days were comparable between the two groups (1.6% with clopidogrel vs 1.4% with placebo).

In the Clopidogrel as Adjunctive Reperfusion Therapy (CLARITY) trial, the benefit of clopidogrel plus aspirin for prevention of cardiovascular events after stenting was extended to patients with STEMI.[38,39] In CLARITY, patients with STEMI treated with fibrinolytics received clopidogrel (300-mg loading dose, followed by 75 mg daily) or placebo, before undergoing coronary angiography 2 to 8 days (median 3 days) after presentation.[38] PCI-CLARITY was a substudy enrolling patients undergoing PCI after coronary angiography. As in PCI-CURE, $P2Y12$ treatment as an adjunct to PCI had already been established as the standard of care, so 75% of patients in both the clopidogrel and placebo groups received a loading dose of clopidogrel or ticlopidine at the time of stenting, and 90% received maintenance $P2Y12$ inhibitor therapy.[39] Thus, PCI-CLARITY represents the results of a trial comparing clopidogrel pretreatment with no clopidogrel pretreatment in STEMI. Similar to PCI-CURE, pretreatment with clopidogrel reduced the risk of 30-day major adverse cardiovascular events (cardiovascular death, recurrent MI, or stroke) following PCI by 46% (3.6% vs 6.2%; odds ratio [OR] 0.54; 95% CI, 0.35–0.85; $P = .008$).[39] The rates of Thrombolysis in Myocardial Infarction (TIMI) major bleeding and overall bleeding were similar between the two groups (major bleeding, 0.5% with clopidogrel vs 1.1% with placebo; overall bleeding, 2% vs 1.9%).

After the Danish Trial In Acute Myocardial Infarction (DANAMI-2) and the Primary Angioplasty in Patients Transferred from General Community Hospitals to Specialized Percutaneous Transluminal Coronary Angioplasty Units With or Without Emergency Thrombolysis (PRAGUE-2) study (among other, smaller trials) showed the superiority of primary PCI to fibrinolytics in STEMI,[40,41] and multiple trials showed

Table 2
Major clinical trials evaluating antiplatelet agents in PCI

Trial		Number of Patients	Patient Population	IIb/IIIa Inhibitor (%)	P2Y12 Inhibitor	P2Y12 Inhibitor Treatment Before PCI	30-d Ischemic Events (%)	30-d Major Bleeding (%)
STARS[32]	Ticlopidine arm	546	Elective PCI	NA	Ticlopidine 250 mg BID	No	0.5	5.5
	Placebo arm	557		NA	None	NA	3.6	1.8
CLASSICS[33]	Clopidogrel 300/75 mg arm	345	Elective PCI	0	Clopidogrel 300 mg followed by 75 mg daily	No	1.2	1.5
	Clopidogrel 75 mg arm	335		0	Clopidogrel 75 mg daily	No	1.5	1.2
	Ticlopidine arm	340		0	Ticlopidine 250 mg BID	No	0.9	1.2
PCI-CURE[37]	Clopidogrel pretreatment arm	1313	NSTE-ACS	21	Clopidogrel 300 mg followed by 75 mg daily	Median 6 d before PCI	4.5	1.6
	Placebo arm	1345		27	None until after PCI	None	6.4	1.4
PCI-CLARITY[39]	Clopidogrel pretreatment arm	933	Fibrinolytic-treated STEMI	31	Clopidogrel 300 mg followed by 75 mg daily	Median 3 d before PCI	3.6	0.5
	Placebo arm	930		34	None until after PCI	None	6.2	1.1
CREDO[59]	Clopidogrel pretreatment arm	1053	Elective PCI	47	Clopidogrel 300 mg followed by 75 mg daily	3–24 h before PCI	6.8	4.8
	Placebo arm	1063		43	None until after PCI	None	8.3	3.8
CURRENT OASIS 7[44]	High-dose clopidogrel arm	8650	37% STEMI, 63% NSTE-ACS	41	600 mg clopidogrel	3.1 h in NSTE-ACS, 0.5 h in STEMI	3.9	1.6
	Low-dose clopidogrel arm	8703		40	300 mg clopidogrel	3.3 h in NSTE-ACS, 0.5 h in STEMI	4.5	1.1

Trial	Arm	N		Population	Regimen	Pretreatment		
ESPIRIT[72]	Eptifibatide arm	1040	100	50% elective, 50% NSTE-ACS within 180 d	Clopidogrel	NR	6.5	1.3
	Placebo arm	1024	0.04		Clopidogrel	NR	10.8	0.4
CHAMPION PHOENIX[54]	Clopidogrel arm	5470	3.5	11% STEMI, 25% NSTE-ACS, 57% elective	Clopidogrel 600 mg	63% before PCI	5.9	0.1
	Cangrelor arm	5472	2.3		Cangrelor, followed by clopidogrel 600 mg	63% before PCI	4.7	0.1
TRITON-TIMI 38[46]	Clopidogrel arm	—	55	26% STEMI, 74% NSTE-ACS	300 mg clopidogrel	No	7.2	1.8
	Prasugrel arm	—	54		60 mg prasugrel	No	5.6	2.4
PLATO[48]	Clopidogrel arm	9235	35	49% STEMI, 51% NSTE-ACS	300–600 mg clopidogrel	2.4 h in NSTE-ACS, 0.5 h in STEMI	5.4	5.8
	Ticagrelor arm	9186	35		180 mg ticagrelor	2.4 h in NSTE-ACS, 0.5 h in STEMI	4.8	5.8
ACCOAST[58]	Prasugrel pretreatment arm	1389	3.7	NSTE-ACS	30 mg prasugrel pretreatment, then 30 mg at the time of PCI	4.3 h before PCI	7.7	1.7
	No pretreatment arm	1372	3.9		60 mg prasugrel at the time of PCI	No	7.3	0.7
ATLANTIC[60]	Prehospital ticagrelor arm	908	30	STEMI	Prehospital ticagrelor 180 mg	63 min before PCI	4.5	1.3
	In-hospital ticagrelor arm	950	27		In-hospital ticagrelor, 180 mg	28 min before PCI	4.4	0.8

Abbreviations: ACCOAST, Comparison of Prasugrel at the Time of PCI or as Pre-Treatment at the Time of Diagnosis in Patients with NSTEMI; ATLANTIC, Administration of Ticagrelor in the Cath Lab or in the Ambulance for New STEMI to Open the Coronary Artery; BID, twice a day; CHAMPION PHOENIX, Clinical Trial Comparing Cangrelor to Clopidogrel Standard of Care Therapy in Patients Who Require PCI; CLASSICS, Clopidogrel Aspirin Stent International Cooperative Study; CREDO, Clopidogrel for the Reduction of Events During Observation; CURRENT OASIS-7, Clopidogrel and Aspirin Optimal Dose Usage to Reduce Recurrent Events; ESPRIT, Enhanced Suppression of the Platelet IIb/IIIa Receptor with Integrilin Therapy; NA, not available; NR, not reported; PCI-CLARITY, Clopidogrel as Adjunctive Reperfusion Therapy; PCI-CURE, Clopidogrel in Unstable Angina to Prevent Recurrent Events; PLATO, Platelet Inhibition and Patient Outcomes; TRITON-TIMI 38, Trial to Assess Improvement in Outcomes by Optimizing Platelet Inhibition with Prasugrel; STARS, Stent Antithrombotic Regimen Study.

Data from Refs. 32,33,37,39,44,46,48,54,58–60,72

the superiority of a routine invasive strategy in NSTE-ACS to a delayed, provisional strategy,[42] the practice of clopidogrel preloading followed by delayed PCI tested in PCI-CURE and PCI-CLARITY became inconsistent with contemporary clinical practice. Because treatment with P2Y12 inhibitors at the time of PCI was established as the standard of care, no trial has tested the efficacy of P2Y12 inhibitors versus placebo given immediately before PCI in patients with ACS. However, later trials of oral P2Y12 inhibitors in ACS compared either higher loading doses of clopidogrel with lower doses given within 8 hours of PCI or new P2Y12 inhibitors with clopidogrel.

In the Antiplatelet Therapy for Reduction of Myocardial Damage During Angioplasty (ARMYDA-2) trial, patients undergoing elective PCI who were randomized to a 600-mg loading dose of clopidogrel, given 4 to 8 hours before PCI, had a lower risk of death, periprocedural MI, or target vessel revascularization compared with the group randomized to the 300-mg loading dose (4% vs 12%; RR, 0.48).[43] Similarly, in Clopidogrel and Aspirin Optimal Dose Usage to Reduce Recurrent Events (CURRENT OASIS-7), patients with ACS (37% with STEMI) were randomized to a loading dose of 600 mg of clopidogrel followed by 150 mg daily or a loading dose of 300 mg followed by 75 mg daily. Among patients undergoing PCI, higher-dose clopidogrel reduced a primary end point of death, MI, or stroke by 14% (3.9% vs 4.5%; RR, 0.86; 95% CI, 0.76–0.99; $P = .039$), with most of that reduction driven by reduction in recurrent MI. Outcomes were consistent in the NSTE-ACS and STEMI subgroups, despite patients undergoing PCI for STEMI undergoing PCI at a median time of 0.5 hours following clopidogrel loading. Those patients treated with higher-dose clopidogrel also had a reduction in the rate of stent thrombosis occurring within 2 days of PCI, from 0.4% to 0.2%.[44] A subsequent meta-analysis of 7 studies investigating clinical outcomes in patients receiving 600-mg or 300-mg clopidogrel loading doses before PCI showed a 34% relative risk reduction in major adverse cardiac events in patients treated with a higher loading dose with no increase in major bleeding events.[45]

Prasugrel
In the Trial to Assess Improvement in Therapeutic Outcomes by Optimizing Platelet Inhibition with Prasugrel (TRITON-TIMI 38) trial, patients with moderate-risk to high-risk ACS (including both STEMI and NSTE-ACS) were randomized after diagnostic angiography to 300 mg of clopidogrel or 60 mg of prasugrel, with the loading dose

given any time between randomization and 1 hour after leaving the cardiac catheterization laboratory.[46] Because patients were not preloaded with a P2Y12 inhibitor, 55% received a glycoprotein IIb/IIIa inhibitor. Compared with clopidogrel, prasugrel reduced the incidence of death, nonfatal stroke, or nonfatal MI by 19% (9.9% vs 12.1%; Hazard Ratio (HR), 0.81; 95% CI, 0.73–0.90; $P<.001$) after 15 months. However, this reduction in ischemic events came at a cost of an increased risk of major bleeding, including fatal bleeding (2.4% vs 1.8%; HR, 1.32; 95% CI, 1.03–1.68; $P = .03$; with fatal bleeding 0.4% vs 0.1%; HR, 4.19; 95% CI, 1.58–11.11; $P = .002$). Prasugrel reduced the incidence of stent thrombosis by greater than 50% (1.1% vs 2.4%; RR, 0.48; 95% CI, 0.36–0.64; $P<.001$), with this reduction appearing as early as 3 days following stent implantation (0.33% vs 0.67%) and occurring regardless of stent type (drug-eluting or bare metal). The role of prasugrel in PCI for stable angina has not been studied.

Ticagrelor
In the Platelet Inhibition and Patient Outcomes (PLATO) trial, patients with ACS (STEMI and moderate-risk to high-risk NSTE-ACS) were randomized to either ticagrelor or clopidogrel. Patients were given a loading dose of either clopidogrel or ticagrelor; in patients who underwent PCI, the median time from loading dose to PCI was 15 minutes for STEMI and 4 hours for NSTE-ACS.[47] Roughly 35% of patients in both arms received glycoprotein IIb/IIIa inhibitors. Ticagrelor, compared with clopidogrel, reduced the rate of 12-month death, nonfatal MI, or stroke by 16% (9.0% vs 10.7%; RR, 0.84; 95% CI, 0.75–0.94; $P = .0025$) with no increase in major bleeding (7.9% in both arms). In addition, ticagrelor reduced cardiovascular and all-cause mortality (4.0% vs 5.1%; $P = .001$; 10.2% vs 12.3%; $P<.001$, respectively).[48] Definite stent thrombosis within 30 days was also reduced in the ticagrelor arm compared with the clopidogrel arm (1.3% vs 2.0%; RR, 0.64; 95% CI, 0.46–0.88; $P = .0054$).[48] However, there was no difference in the rate of definite or probable stent thrombosis seen in the first 24 hours after stent implantation (0.36% vs 0.37%).[49]

Glycoprotein IIb/IIIa Inhibitors
The efficacy of routine glycoprotein IIb/IIIa inhibitors for reducing early cardiovascular events following stent implantation was first conclusively established in the Evaluation of Platelet IIb/IIIa Inhibition in Stenting Trial (EPISTENT) trial, which randomized patients with stable

angina undergoing coronary stenting to abciximab or placebo, in addition to aspirin, ticlopidine, and heparin. The incidence of 30-day death, MI, or urgent target vessel revascularization was reduced by 52% with abciximab compared with placebo (5.3% vs 10.8%; HR, 0.48; 95% CI, 0.33–0.69; P<.001) without an increase in bleeding complications.[50] Although subsequent trials of glycoprotein IIb/IIIa inhibitors mostly showed similar reductions in ischemic complications, all have also shown an increase in bleeding events.

In a meta-analysis comparing glycoprotein IIb/IIIa inhibitors with placebo or usual care in patients undergoing PCI, use of glycoprotein IIb/IIIa inhibitors significantly reduced 30-day mortality by 21% (0.92% vs 1.33%; RR, 0.79; 95% CI, 0.64–0.97), and a combined end point of death or recurrent MI by 34% (5.05% vs 7.04%; RR, 0.66; 95% CI, 0.60–0.72).[51] The 30-day survival benefit was attenuated in patients with ACS (RR 0.71 in stable CAD, 0.79 in patients with NSTEMI, and 0.88 in patients with STEMI), and in those pretreated with clopidogrel (RR, 0.83). The reduction in ischemic events and mortality came at the cost of increased bleeding; glycoprotein IIb/IIIa inhibitor use increased the 30-day major bleeding rate by 39% (3.03% vs 2.23%; RR, 1.39; 95% CI, 1.21–1.61), an effect that persisted regardless of whether the patient had ACS or was pretreated with clopidogrel. Overall, treatment of 1000 patients with glycoprotein IIb/IIIa inhibitors would prevent 20 nonfatal MIs and 4 deaths at a cost of 8 excess bleeding events.[51] The availability of the newer, more potent oral antiplatelet agents and the trials showing better net clinical adverse outcomes with the direct thrombin inhibitor bivalirudin (and use of glycoprotein IIb/IIIa inhibitors for ischemic or angiographic bailout) has drastically diminished the role of glycoprotein IIb/IIIa inhibitors in clinical practice.

Cangrelor

The newest intravenous antiplatelet agent is the $^{P2Y}12$ inhibitor cangrelor. Its benefit in patients undergoing PCI was established by the Cangrelor Versus Standard Therapy to Achieve Optimal Management of Platelet Inhibition (CHAMPION) series of clinical trials. CHAMPION PLATFORM and CHAMPION PCI, the first two trials comparing cangrelor with clopidogrel and adequately powered to detect clinical outcomes, did not show a reduction in death, MI, or ischemia-driven revascularization (7.0% vs 8.7%; RR, 0.87; 95% CI, 0.71–1.07; P = .17 in CHAMPION PLATFORM; 7.5% vs 7.1%; RR,

1.05; 95% CI, 0.88–1.24; P = .67 in CHAMPION PCI).[52,53] However, cangrelor did reduce the incidence of acute stent thrombosis in both studies, and investigators hypothesized that cangrelor's failure to significantly reduce the primary end point in both studies could be explained by a definition of periprocedural MI that failed to distinguish true reinfarction in patients presenting with MI.

Subsequently, in the Clinical Trial Comparing Cangrelor to Clopidogrel Standard of Care Therapy in Patients Who Require PCI (CHAMPION PHOENIX) trial, investigators randomized patients undergoing PCI (57% elective, 25% urgent for NSTE-ACS, 18% primary PCI for STEMI) to cangrelor started before PCI, or clopidogrel given as a loading dose before PCI. Glycoprotein IIb/IIIa inhibitors were used infrequently. Patients in the cangrelor arm had a 22% lower rate of 48-hour death, MI, ischemia-driven revascularization, or stent thrombosis (4.7% vs 5.9%; OR, 0.78; 95% CI, 0.66–0.93; P = .005) with much of the difference accruing in the first 2 hours following PCI.[54] Similarly, cangrelor treatment reduced the rate of stent thrombosis (0.8% vs 1.4%; OR, 0.62; 95% CI, 0.43–0.90; P = .01), with much of the benefit in so-called intraprocedure stent thrombosis. The rate of 48-hour major bleeding was low, and similar in both groups (0.1%), and the benefits of cangrelor were similar in patients with and without STEMI.[54]

CONTROVERSIES: PRELOADING AND PLATELET FUNCTION TESTING

Preloading with $^{P2Y}12$ Inhibitors Before Percutaneous Coronary Intervention

Given the rapid onset of action of prasugrel and ticagrelor in healthy volunteers, both drugs should have shown early benefit in the prevention of acute stent thrombosis. However, neither prasugrel nor ticagrelor work as rapidly in patients with ACS as they do in healthy volunteers.[55] In the Rapid Activity of Platelet Inhibitor Drugs (RAPID) trial, investigators randomized 50 patients with STEMI, all treated with bivalirudin monotherapy, to prasugrel or ticagrelor and measured platelet activity at 2, 4, 8, and 12 hours.[56] After 2 hours, high residual platelet activity was found in 44% of prasugrel-treated patients and 60% of ticagrelor-treated patients; 35% of ticagrelor-treated patients still had high residual platelet activity 4 hours after the loading dose. This delayed onset of action in patients with ACS may be partially explained by the frequent use of morphine sulfate to treat angina pain because the absorption of both ticagrelor and prasugrel is delayed when morphine is administered.[57]

Given the delayed onset of antiplatelet effect with oral [P2Y]12 inhibitors, especially in patients with ACS, and the high risk of bleeding with glycoprotein IIb/IIIa inhibitors, early administration of oral [P2Y]12 inhibitors may theoretically provide a benefit. Earlier administration of clopidogrel, prasugrel, or ticagrelor would allow their antiplatelet activity to take effect before stent deployment, limiting the need for the adjunctive antiplatelet activity of glycoprotein IIb/IIIa inhibitors. Moreover, in patients with STEMI, early, potent platelet inhibition could limit continued intracoronary thrombosis, potentially restoring patency to the infarct-related artery and limiting total ischemic time. These hypotheses were tested in a series of clinical trials examining the effect of early [P2Y]12 inhibitor administration.[37,58–60] However, despite the theoretic benefits of [P2Y]12 inhibitor preloading, none of these trials has shown a conclusive benefit to this strategy.

Although PCI-CURE and PCI-CLARITY showed that clopidogrel preloading reduced 30-day ischemic events in patients with ACS, patients enrolled in PCI-CURE and PCI-CLARITY underwent PCI at a median of 6 and 3 days following the start of clopidogrel loading, respectively; a time course that is inconsistent with modern clinical practice, but better aligned with clopidogrel's pharmacokinetics.[37,39] the Clopidogrel for the Reduction of Events During Observation (CREDO) trial, which randomized patients with stable CAD undergoing elective PCI in the next 3 to 24 hours to clopidogrel or placebo pretreatment, may be a better approximation of modern clinical practice.[59] In CREDO, clopidogrel pretreatment had no significant effect on the 28-day rate of cardiovascular death, MI, or urgent target vessel revascularization (6.8% with pretreatment vs 8.3% without pretreatment, RR, 0.81; 95% CI, 0.58–1.14; $P = .23$). However, consistent with clopidogrel pharmacokinetics, a prespecified subset analysis in patients pretreated with clopidogrel at least 6 hours before stent implantation showed a marginally significant 39% reduction in the primary end point (RR, 0.61; 95% CI, 0.37–1.02; $P = .051$).[59]

A meta-analysis of 9 trials comparing clopidogrel pretreatment with no clopidogrel pretreatment (including CREDO, PCI-CURE, and PCI-CLARITY) reported that pretreatment reduced the incidence of major cardiovascular events by 23% (9.8% vs 12.4%; OR, 0.77%; 95% CI, 0.66–0.89; $P<.001$).[61] In subset analyses, pretreatment reduced cardiovascular events in patients with ACS, but not in those with stable angina. Importantly, most of the trials included evaluated a preloading strategy with a delay of 4 to 6 hours or more from loading to PCI.

Despite the fact that the theoretic advantages of [P2Y]12 pretreatment should be accentuated with the new oral [P2Y]12 inhibitors prasugrel and ticagrelor because of their favorable pharmacokinetics compared with clopidogrel, trials examining preloading with these agents have also failed to show a clear clinical benefit.

In the Comparison of Prasugrel at the Time of PCI or as Pre-Treatment at the Time of Diagnosis in Patients with NSTEMI (ACCOAST) trial, investigators examined the potential benefits and harms of pretreatment with prasugrel in patients with NSTE-ACS. Patients were randomized to receive either 30 mg of prasugrel at the time of diagnosis followed by another 30 mg after angiography but before PCI, or to receive 60 mg of prasugrel after angiography but before PCI (the strategy used in TRITON-TIMI 38).[58] Pretreatment with prasugrel did not significantly reduce the incidence of the primary end point, 7-day cardiovascular death, MI, stroke, urgent revascularization, or glycoprotein IIb/IIIa inhibitor bail-out (10% vs 9.8%; HR, 1.02; 95% CI, 0.84–1.25; $P = .81$), but did increase the incidence of 7-day non–CABG-related TIMI major bleeding by 3-fold (1.3% vs 0.5%; HR, 2.95; 95% CI, 1.39–6.28; $P = .003$).

In the Administration of Ticagrelor in the Cath Lab or in the Ambulance for New STEMI to Open the Coronary Artery (ATLANTIC) trial, investigators attempted an alternative strategy to achieve earlier platelet inhibition with [P2Y]12 inhibitors, randomizing patients with STEMI to ticagrelor loading in the ambulance en route to the hospital or on hospital arrival.[60] The group receiving ticagrelor in the ambulance received it 31 minutes earlier than the group receiving it at the hospital and 63 minutes before PCI. Although the primary end point of infarct artery patency on arrival at the catheter laboratory did not differ between the two arms, the rate of acute stent thrombosis was lower in the prehospital ticagrelor arm compared with the in-hospital ticagrelor arm (0% vs 0.8%; $P = .008$). TIMI major bleeding at 30 days was 1.3% in both groups. In a pharmacodynamic substudy involving 37 patients, there were no significant differences between the 2 groups in mean platelet inhibition at any time. However, platelet inhibition was numerically greater in the prehospital group than the in-hospital group at the end of PCI and at 1 hour after PCI.[60] These data suggest that preloading with ticagrelor may reduce stent thrombosis. Confirmatory studies are needed, especially because the pre-hospital group had higher mortality than the in-hospital group (3.3% vs 2.0%; OR, 1.68; 95% CI, 0.94–3.01).

Another strategy used by investigators to quickly reduce platelet activity in patients with STEMI was used in the Mashed or Just Integral Tablets of Ticagrelor (MOJITO) trial, in which 82 patients undergoing primary PCI for STEMI were randomized to a loading dose of crushed or whole ticagrelor tablets.[62] Although the study was not powered to detect clinical end points, this strategy led to reduced platelet activity in the group receiving crushed ticagrelor at 1 hour after PCI (35% vs 63%). Ticagrelor's package insert notes that tablets may be crushed, mixed with water, and drunk.

Platelet Function Testing

When given a loading dose of clopidogrel, healthy individuals with polymorphisms of the gene encoding a CYP2C19 enzyme with reduced function have 34% less exposure to clopidogrel's active metabolite and 9% less of a reduction in platelet activity than individuals without CYP2C19 polymorphisms.[63] In patients with ACS (STEMI and NSTE-ACS) randomized to clopidogrel in TRITON-TIMI 38, a reduced-function CYP2C19 allele was associated with an increased risk of cardiovascular death (2% vs 0.4%; OR, 4.79) and stent thrombosis (2.7% vs 0.8%; OR, 3.33).[63] Nearly all of the increased risk of stent thrombosis was concentrated in the first few days following PCI. This finding has also been shown in multiple registry studies,[64] including the Platelet Reactivity and Clinical Outcomes of Coronary Artery Implantation of Drug-Eluting Stents (ADAPT-DES) registry, in which patients with high on-clopidogrel platelet reactivity had a 3-fold increased risk of early stent thrombosis, and high on-treatment platelet reactivity explained 60% of early stent thrombosis events.[65]

Recognizing this heterogeneity in clopidogrel responsiveness among different patients and the higher incidence of stent thrombosis and adverse cardiovascular events among clopidogrel nonresponders,[64] there has been a series of clinical investigations exploring a strategy involving platelet function testing and escalation of antiplatelet therapy based on the results. This strategy theoretically ensures that clopidogrel nonresponders receive an effective dose of antiplatelet therapy, while avoiding the use of more potent antiplatelet regimens and their attendant higher bleeding risk in patients whose platelet function is effectively inhibited by standard dosing of clopidogrel.

The Assessment with a Double Randomization of a Fixed Dose Versus a Monitoring-Guided Dose of Aspirin and Clopidogrel After DES Implantation and Treatment Interruption Versus Continuation (ARCTIC) trial randomized patients undergoing PCI for stable angina to standard therapy or to platelet reactivity testing after diagnostic angiography; all patients were supposed to receive a loading dose of clopidogrel at least 6 hours before angiography.[66] If platelet reactivity was high despite the loading dose of clopidogrel, then these patients received glycoprotein IIb/IIIa inhibitors at the time of PCI, and either a larger loading dose of clopidogrel (≥600 mg) or a loading dose of 60 mg of prasugrel. High platelet reactivity was identified in 34.5% of patients in the platelet function testing arm; 80.2% of these patients received another loading dose of clopidogrel, 3.3% received a loading dose of prasugrel, and 87.1% received glycoprotein IIb/IIIa inhibitors.[66] Patients with high platelet reactivity, either at the time of stenting or 2 to 4 weeks later, also received higher maintenance doses of clopidogrel. Despite more aggressive antiplatelet therapy in the platelet function testing–guided arm, this group had a numerically higher incidence of the primary efficacy end point of 1-year death, MI, stent thrombosis, stroke, or urgent revascularization (34.6% vs 31.1%; HR, 1.13; 95% CI, 0.98–1.29; $P = .10$).

Other trials have approached the question of adjusting antiplatelet therapy based on platelet function testing through different means, but have nevertheless failed to show any benefit with this strategy. The Testing Platelet Reactivity in Patients Undergoing Elective Stent Placement on Clopidogrel to Guide Alternative Therapy with Prasugrel (TRIGGER-PCI) trial, which randomized patients who had undergone successful drug-eluting stent implantation for stable angina and had high platelet reactivity to either continued clopidogrel or more aggressive antiplatelet therapy with prasugrel, was stopped early because of a low rate of outcome events.[67] The Gauging Responsiveness with a VerifyNow Assay – Impact on Thrombosis and Safety (GRAVITAS) trial, which had a similar design but randomized patients with high on-clopidogrel platelet reactivity to higher-dose clopidogrel, also failed to show that more aggressive antiplatelet therapy reduced cardiovascular events in clopidogrel nonresponders.[68] In the Treatment with ADP Receptor Inhibitors: Longitudinal Treatment Patterns and Events after ACS – Prospective, Open Label

Table 3 Guideline recommendations		
Recommendation	**ACC/AHA/SCAI**	**ESC/EACTS**
Stable Angina		
A loading dose of clopidogrel (600 mg) should be given to patients undergoing PCI with stenting	Class I, LOE B	Class I, LOE A
Clopidogrel should be loaded once anatomy is known and decision is made to proceed with PCI, preferably 2 hours or more before the procedure	—	Class I, LOE A
It is reasonable to administer a glycoprotein IIb/IIIa inhibitor in patients undergoing elective PCI treated with UFH and not adequately pretreated with clopidogrel	Class IIa, LOE B	—
It may be reasonable to administer a glycoprotein IIb/IIIa inhibitor to patients undergoing elective PCI treated with UFH and adequately pretreated with clopidogrel	Class IIb, LOE B	—
Glycoprotein IIb/IIIa inhibitors should be considered only for bail-out	—	Class IIa, LOE C
NSTE-ACS		
A loading dose of clopidogrel (600 mg), prasugrel (60 mg), or ticagrelor (60 mg) should be given to patients undergoing PCI with stenting	Class I, LOE B	—
A loading dose of prasugrel (60 mg) should be given to patients in whom coronary anatomy is known and who are proceeding to PCI if no contraindications	—	Class I, LOE B
A loading dose of ticagrelor (180 mg) should be given to patients at moderate to high risk of ischemic events if no contraindications	—	Class I, LOE B
Clopidogrel should be used only when prasugrel and ticagrelor are unavailable or contraindicated	—	Class I, LOE B
Prasugrel should not be used in patients in whom coronary anatomy is not known	Class III, LOE B	Class III, LOE B
It is useful to administer a glycoprotein IIb/IIIa bolus at the time of PCI to patients with high-risk features treated with UFH and not adequately pretreated with clopidogrel	Class I, LOE A	—
It is reasonable to administer a glycoprotein IIb/IIIa inhibitor at the time of PCI to patients with high-risk features treated with UFH	Class IIa, LOE B	—
Glycoprotein IIb/IIIa inhibitors should be considered for bail-out situation or thrombotic complications	—	Class IIa, LOE C
Pretreatment with glycoprotein IIb/IIIa inhibitors is not recommended	—	Class III, LOE A
STEMI		
A loading dose of clopidogrel (600 mg), prasugrel (60 mg), or ticagrelor (60 mg) should be given to patients undergoing PCI with stenting	Class I, LOE B	—
A loading dose of prasugrel (60 mg) should be given to patients in whom coronary anatomy is known and who are proceeding to PCI if no contraindications	—	Class I, LOE B
A loading dose of ticagrelor (180 mg) should be given to patients at moderate-to-high risk of ischemic events if no contraindications	—	Class I, LOE B

(continued on next page)

Table 3
(continued)

Recommendation	ACC/AHA/SCAI	ESC/EACTS
Clopidogrel should be used only when prasugrel and ticagrelor are unavailable or contraindicated	—	Class I, LOE B
It is reasonable to administer a glycoprotein IIb/IIIa inhibitor in patients treated with UFH not pretreated with clopidogrel	Class IIa, LOE A	—
It is reasonable to administer a glycoprotein IIb/IIIa inhibitor in patients treated with UFH pretreated with clopidogrel	Class IIa, LOE C	—
Glycoprotein IIb/IIIa inhibitors should be considered for bail-out or evidence of no-reflow, or evidence of a thrombotic complication	—	Class IIa, LOE C

Abbreviations: EACTS, European Association for Cardiothoracic Surgery; UFH, unfractionated heparin.
Adapted from Levine GN, Bates ER, Blankenship JC, et al. 2011 ACCF/AHA/SCAI guideline for percutaneous coronary intervention: a report of the American College of Cardiology Foundation/American Heart Association Task Force on Practice Guidelines and the Society for Cardiovascular Angiography and Interventions. Catheter Cardiovasc Interv 2013;82(4):E266–355; and Windecker S, Kolh P, Alfonso F, et al. 2014 ESC/EACTS guidelines on myocardial revascularization. Eur Heart J 2014;35(37):2541–619.

Antiplatlet Therapy Study (TRANSLATE-POPS), hospitals were randomized to either no-cost platelet function testing or standard care.[69] In hospitals randomized to receive no-cost platelet function testing, 66.9% of patients underwent platelet function testing before discharge compared with 1.4% at control hospitals, and patients undergoing coronary stenting more frequently had their antiplatelet agent adjusted before discharge (14.8% vs 10.5%; OR, 1.68; 95% CI, 1.18–2.64; P = .004). However, cardiovascular events and major bleeding at 30-day follow-up were similar in both groups (OR, 0.94; 95% CI, 0.66–1.34 for cardiovascular events; and OR, 0.86; 95% CI, 0.55–1.34 for major bleeding).

Based on these trials, the use of routine genotype or platelet function testing to guide antiplatelet therapy cannot be recommended.

GUIDELINES RECOMMENDATIONS

In patients undergoing PCI for stable angina, the American College of Cardiology Foundation (ACCF)/American Heart Association (AHA)/Society for Cardiovascular Angiography and Interventions (SCAI) and European Society of Cardiology (ESC) guidelines recommend clopidogrel 600 mg (class I, level of evidence [LOE] B in the ACC/AHA guidelines, LOE A in the ESC guidelines) (Table 3).[70,71] The ESC guidelines add that clopidogrel loading should preferably occur at least 2 hours before the procedure (class I, LOE A).[71] The ACCF/AHA/SCAI guidelines note that it is reasonable to use glycoprotein IIb/IIIa inhibitors in patients undergoing PCI for stable angina who have

not been preloaded with clopidogrel (class IIa, LOE B) or in patients who have been preloaded with clopidogrel (class IIb, LOE B).[70] The ESC guidelines recommend reserving glycoprotein IIb/IIIa inhibitors only for bail-out (class IIa, LOE C).[71]

In patients undergoing PCI for an ACS indication, the ACCF/AHA/SCAI guidelines recommend a loading dose of either 600 mg of clopidogrel, 60 mg of prasugrel, or 180 mg of ticagrelor (class I, LOE B).[70] The ESC guidelines recommend either prasugrel or ticagrelor, with clopidogrel reserved for situations in which the newer $P2Y12$ agents are not available or contraindicated (class I, LOE A for NSTE-ACS, LOE B for STEMI).[71] The ACCF/AHA/SCAI guidelines recommend the use of glycoprotein IIb/IIIa inhibitors in patients with high-risk NSTE-ACS treated with heparin and not adequately pretreated with clopidogrel (class I, LOE A), and note that glycoprotein IIb/IIIa inhibitors are reasonable in these patients even if they are adequately pretreated with clopidogrel (class IIa, LOE B).[70] In contrast, the ESC guidelines recommend considering glycoprotein IIb/IIIa inhibitors during PCI for NSTE-ACS only for bail-out, or with thrombotic complications (class IIa, LOE C).[71] In all patients undergoing primary PCI for STEMI, the ACCF/AHA/SCAI guidelines allow for the consideration of glycoprotein IIb/IIIa inhibitors (class IIa, LOE A in patients not pretreated with clopidogrel, LOE C in patients pretreated with clopidogrel).[70] The ESC guidelines recommend reserving glycoprotein IIb/IIIa inhibitors for bail-out, thrombotic complications, or no-reflow (class IIa, LOE C).[71]

Neither set of guidelines issues formal recommendations with regard to platelet function testing, and, as of this writing, a set of recommendations regarding cangrelor has not been developed.

SUMMARY

The introduction in the past 5 years of the potent and fast-acting $P2Y12$ inhibitors prasugrel, ticagrelor, and cangrelor has provided interventional cardiologists with new agents for inhibiting platelet activity and preventing thrombotic events following stent implantation. However, significant questions still exist regarding the optimal antiplatelet strategy. Increased potency of antiplatelet effect is associated with an increased bleeding risk, particularly in vulnerable populations like the elderly and those with prior stroke or transient ischemic attack. It remains unclear whether pretreatment is beneficial in patients undergoing PCI. Genotype or platelet reactivity testing has not been proved to be beneficial. As PCI continues to evolve, these issues will be important to resolve in order to improve outcomes.

REFERENCES

1. Mrdovic I, Savic L, Lasica R, et al. Usefulness of the RISK-PCI score to predict stent thrombosis in patients treated with primary percutaneous coronary intervention for ST-segment elevation myocardial infarction: a substudy of the RISK-PCI trial. Heart Vessels 2013;28(4):424–33.
2. De Luca G, Dirksen MT, Spaulding C, et al. Time course, predictors and clinical implications of stent thrombosis following primary angioplasty. Insights from the DESERT cooperation. Thromb Haemost 2013;110(4):826–33.
3. Palmerini T, Dangas G, Mehran R, et al. Predictors and implications of stent thrombosis in non-ST-segment elevation acute coronary syndromes: the ACUITY Trial. Circ Cardiovasc Interv 2011;4(6):577–84.
4. Mehran R, Pocock S, Nikolsky E, et al. Impact of bleeding on mortality after percutaneous coronary intervention results from a patient-level pooled analysis of the REPLACE-2 (Randomized Evaluation of PCI Linking Angiomax to Reduced Clinical Events), ACUITY (Acute Catheterization and Urgent Intervention Triage Strategy), and HORIZONS-AMI (Harmonizing Outcomes with Revascularization and Stents in Acute Myocardial Infarction) trials. JACC Cardiovasc Interv 2011;4(6):654–64.
5. Moscucci M, Fox KA, Cannon CP, et al. Predictors of major bleeding in acute coronary syndromes: the Global Registry of Acute Coronary Events (GRACE). Eur Heart J 2003;24(20):1815–23.
6. Rao SV, Dai D, Subherwal S, et al. Association between periprocedural bleeding and long-term outcomes following percutaneous coronary intervention in older patients. JACC Cardiovasc Interv 2012;5(9):958–65.
7. Chhatriwalla AK, Amin AP, Kennedy KF, et al. Association between bleeding events and in-hospital mortality after percutaneous coronary intervention. JAMA 2013;309(10):1022–9.
8. D'Ascenzo F, Bollati M, Clementi F, et al. Incidence and predictors of coronary stent thrombosis: evidence from an international collaborative meta-analysis including 30 studies, 221,066 patients, and 4276 thromboses. Int J Cardiol 2013;167(2):575–84.
9. Marso SP, Amin AP, House JA, et al. Association between use of bleeding avoidance strategies and risk of periprocedural bleeding among patients undergoing percutaneous coronary intervention. JAMA 2010;303(21):2156–64.
10. Cook S, Windecker S. Early stent thrombosis: past, present, and future. Circulation 2009;119(5):657–9.
11. Mehran R, Pocock SJ, Nikolsky E, et al. A risk score to predict bleeding in patients with acute coronary syndromes. J Am Coll Cardiol 2010;55(23):2556–66.
12. Iqbal J, Sumaya W, Tatman V, et al. Incidence and predictors of stent thrombosis: a single-centre study of 5,833 consecutive patients undergoing coronary artery stenting. EuroIntervention 2013;9(1):62–9.
13. Aoki J, Lansky AJ, Mehran R, et al. Early stent thrombosis in patients with acute coronary syndromes treated with drug-eluting and bare metal stents: the Acute Catheterization and Urgent Intervention Triage Strategy trial. Circulation 2009;119(5):687–98.
14. Di Perri T, Pasini F, Frigerio C, et al. Pharmacodynamics of ticlopidine in man in relation to plasma and blood cell concentration. Eur J Clin Pharmacol 1991;41(5):429–34.
15. Moussa I, Oetgen M, Roubin G, et al. Effectiveness of clopidogrel and aspirin versus ticlopidine and aspirin in preventing stent thrombosis after coronary stent implantation. Circulation 1999;99(18):2364–6.
16. Yousuf O, Bhatt DL. The evolution of antiplatelet therapy in cardiovascular disease. Nature reviews. Cardiology 2011;8(10):547–59.
17. Cadroy Y, Bossavy J-P, Thalamas C, et al. Early potent antithrombotic effect with combined aspirin and a loading dose of clopidogrel on experimental arterial thrombogenesis in humans. Circulation 2000;101(24):2823–8.
18. Angiolillo DJ, Fernandez-Ortiz A, Bernardo E, et al. Is a 300 mg clopidogrel loading dose sufficient to inhibit platelet function early after coronary stenting? A platelet function profile study. J Invasive Cardiol 2004;16(6):325–9.

19. Ferri N, Corsini A, Bellosta S. Pharmacology of the new P2Y12 receptor inhibitors: insights on pharmacokinetic and pharmacodynamic properties. Drugs 2013;73(15):1681–709.

20. Brandt JT, Payne CD, Wiviott SD, et al. A comparison of prasugrel and clopidogrel loading doses on platelet function: magnitude of platelet inhibition is related to active metabolite formation. Am Heart J 2007;153(1):66.e9–16.

21. Braun O, Johnell M, Varenhorst C, et al. Greater reduction of platelet activation markers and platelet-monocyte aggregates by prasugrel compared to clopidogrel in stable coronary artery disease. Thromb Haemost 2008;100(4):626–33.

22. Wiviott SD, Trenk D, Frelinger AL, et al. Prasugrel compared with high loading-and maintenance-dose clopidogrel in patients with planned percutaneous coronary intervention: the Prasugrel in Comparison to Clopidogrel for Inhibition of Platelet Activation and Aggregation–Thrombolysis in Myocardial Infarction 44 trial. Circulation 2007;116(25):2923–32.

23. Gurbel PA, Bliden KP, Butler K, et al. Randomized double-blind assessment of the ONSET and OFFSET of the antiplatelet effects of ticagrelor versus clopidogrel in patients with stable coronary artery disease: the ONSET/OFFSET study. Circulation 2009;120(25):2577–85.

24. Husted S, Emanuelsson H, Heptinstall S, et al. Pharmacodynamics, pharmacokinetics, and safety of the oral reversible P2Y12 antagonist AZD6140 with aspirin in patients with atherosclerosis: a double-blind comparison to clopidogrel with aspirin. Eur Heart J 2006;27(9):1038–47.

25. Harrington RA, Kleiman NS, Kottke-Marchant K, et al. Immediate and reversible platelet inhibition after intravenous administration of a peptide glycoprotein IIb/IIIa inhibitor during percutaneous coronary intervention. Am J Cardiol 1995;76(17):1222–7.

26. Tcheng JE. Clinical challenges of platelet glycoprotein IIb/IIIa receptor inhibitor therapy: bleeding, reversal, thrombocytopenia, and retreatment. Am Heart J 2000;139(2):s38–45.

27. Serruys PW, de Jaegere P, Kiemeneij F, et al. A comparison of balloon-expandable-stent implantation with balloon angioplasty in patients with coronary artery disease. N Engl J Med 1994;331(8):489–95.

28. Fischman DL, Leon MB, Baim DS, et al. A randomized comparison of coronary-stent placement and balloon angioplasty in the treatment of coronary artery disease. N Engl J Med 1994;331(8):496–501.

29. Serruys PW, Strauss BH, Beatt KJ, et al. Angiographic follow-up after placement of a self-expanding coronary-artery stent. N Engl J Med 1991;324(1):13–7.

30. Serruys PW, Emanuelsson H, Van Der Giessen W, et al. Heparin-coated Palmaz-Schatz stents in human coronary arteries early outcome of the Benestent-II pilot study. Circulation 1996;93(3):412–22.

31. Schömig A, Neumann F-J, Kastrati A, et al. A randomized comparison of antiplatelet and anticoagulant therapy after the placement of coronary-artery stents. N Engl J Med 1996;334(17):1084–9.

32. Leon MB, Baim DS, Popma JJ, et al. A clinical trial comparing three antithrombotic-drug regimens after coronary-artery stenting. N Engl J Med 1998;339(23):1665–71.

33. Bertrand ME, Rupprecht H-J, Urban P, et al. Double-blind study of the safety of clopidogrel with and without a loading dose in combination with aspirin compared with ticlopidine in combination with aspirin after coronary stenting: the Clopidogrel Aspirin Stent International Cooperative Study (CLASSICS). Circulation 2000;102(6):624–9.

34. Taniuchi M, Kurz HI, Lasala JM. Randomized comparison of ticlopidine and clopidogrel after intracoronary stent implantation in a broad patient population. Circulation 2001;104(5):539–43.

35. CAPRIE Steering Committee. A randomised, blinded, trial of clopidogrel versus aspirin in patients at risk of ischaemic events (CAPRIE). Lancet 1996;348(9038):1329–39.

36. Yusuf S, Fox K, Tognoni G, et al. Effects of clopidogrel in addition to aspirin in patients with acute coronary syndromes without ST-segment elevation. N Engl J Med 2001;345(7):494–502.

37. Mehta SR, Yusuf S, Peters RJ, et al. Effects of pretreatment with clopidogrel and aspirin followed by long-term therapy in patients undergoing percutaneous coronary intervention: the PCI-CURE study. Lancet 2001;358(9281):527–33.

38. Sabatine MS, Cannon CP, Gibson CM, et al. Addition of clopidogrel to aspirin and fibrinolytic therapy for myocardial infarction with ST-segment elevation. N Engl J Med 2005;352(12):1179–89.

39. Sabatine MS, Cannon CP, Gibson CM, et al. Effect of clopidogrel pretreatment before percutaneous coronary intervention in patients with ST-elevation myocardial infarction treated with fibrinolytics: the PCI-CLARITY study. JAMA 2005;294(10):1224–32.

40. Andersen HR, Nielsen TT, Rasmussen K, et al. A comparison of coronary angioplasty with fibrinolytic therapy in acute myocardial infarction. N Engl J Med 2003;349(8):733–42.

41. Widimsky P, Budesinsky T, Vorac D, et al, PRAGUE Study Group Investigators. Long distance transport for primary angioplasty vs immediate thrombolysis in acute myocardial infarction: final results of the randomised national multicentre trial–PRAGUE-2. Eur Heart J 2003;24(1):94–104.

42. Mehta SR, Cannon CP, Fox KA, et al. Routine vs selective invasive strategies in patients with acute coronary syndromes: a collaborative meta-analysis of randomized trials. JAMA 2005;293(23):2908–17.

43. Patti G, Colonna G, Pasceri V, et al. Randomized trial of high loading dose of clopidogrel for reduction of periprocedural myocardial infarction in patients undergoing coronary intervention: results from the ARMYDA-2 (Antiplatelet therapy for Reduction of MYocardial Damage during Angioplasty) study. Circulation 2005;111(16):2099–106.

44. Mehta SR, Tanguay JF, Eikelboom JW, et al. Double-dose versus standard-dose clopidogrel and high-dose versus low-dose aspirin in individuals undergoing percutaneous coronary intervention for acute coronary syndromes (CURRENT-OASIS 7): a randomised factorial trial. Lancet 2010;376(9748): 1233–43.

45. Siller-Matula JM, Huber K, Christ G, et al. Impact of clopidogrel loading dose on clinical outcome in patients undergoing percutaneous coronary intervention: a systematic review and meta-analysis. Heart 2011;97(2):98–105.

46. Wiviott SD, Braunwald E, McCabe CH, et al. Prasugrel versus clopidogrel in patients with acute coronary syndromes. N Engl J Med 2007;357(20):2001–15.

47. Wallentin L, Becker RC, Budaj A, et al. Ticagrelor versus clopidogrel in patients with acute coronary syndromes. N Engl J Med 2009;361(11):1045–57.

48. Cannon CP, Harrington RA, James S, et al. Comparison of ticagrelor with clopidogrel in patients with a planned invasive strategy for acute coronary syndromes (PLATO): a randomised double-blind study. Lancet 2010;375(9711):283–93.

49. Steg PG, Harrington RA, Emanuelsson H, et al. Stent thrombosis with ticagrelor versus clopidogrel in patients with acute coronary syndromes: an analysis from the prospective randomized PLATO trial. Circulation 2013;128(10):1055–65.

50. Topol EJ, EPISTENT Investigators. Randomised placebo-controlled and balloon-angioplasty-controlled trial to assess safety of coronary stenting with use of platelet glycoprotein-IIb/IIIa blockade. Lancet 1998;352(9122):87–92.

51. Bosch X, Marrugat J, Sanchis J. Platelet glycoprotein IIb/IIIa blockers during percutaneous coronary intervention and as the initial medical treatment of non-ST segment elevation acute coronary syndromes. Cochrane Database Syst Rev 2010;(9):CD002130.

52. Bhatt DL, Lincoff AM, Gibson CM, et al. Intravenous platelet blockade with cangrelor during PCI. N Engl J Med 2009;361(24):2330–41.

53. Harrington RA, Stone GW, McNulty S, et al. Platelet inhibition with cangrelor in patients undergoing PCI. N Engl J Med 2009;361(24):2318–29.

54. Bhatt DL, Stone GW, Mahaffey KW, et al. Effect of platelet inhibition with cangrelor during PCI on ischemic events. N Engl J Med 2013;368(14):1303–13.

55. Michelson AD, Frelinger AL, Braunwald E, et al. Pharmacodynamic assessment of platelet inhibition by prasugrel vs. clopidogrel in the TRITON-TIMI 38 trial. Eur Heart J 2009;30(14):1753–63.

56. Parodi G, Valenti R, Bellandi B, et al. Comparison of prasugrel and ticagrelor loading doses in ST-segment elevation myocardial infarction patients: RAPID (Rapid Activity of Platelet Inhibitor Drugs) primary PCI study. J Am Coll Cardiol 2013;61(15):1601–6.

57. Parodi G, Bellandi B, Xanthopoulou I, et al. Morphine is associated with a delayed activity of oral antiplatelet agents in patients with ST-elevation acute myocardial infarction undergoing primary percutaneous coronary intervention. Circulation 2015;8(1):e001593.

58. Montalescot G, Bolognese L, Dudek D, et al. Pretreatment with prasugrel in non–ST-segment elevation acute coronary syndromes. N Engl J Med 2013; 369(11):999–1010.

59. Steinhubl SR, Berger PB, Mann JT III, et al. Early and sustained dual oral antiplatelet therapy following percutaneous coronary intervention: a randomized controlled trial. JAMA 2002;288(19): 2411–20.

60. Montalescot G, van't Hof AW, Lapostolle F, et al. Prehospital ticagrelor in ST-segment elevation myocardial infarction. N Engl J Med 2014;371(11): 1016–27.

61. Bellemain-Appaix A, O'Connor SA, Silvain J, et al. Association of clopidogrel pretreatment with mortality, cardiovascular events, and major bleeding among patients undergoing percutaneous coronary intervention: a systematic review and meta-analysis. JAMA 2012;308(23):2507–16.

62. Parodi G, Xanthopoulou I, Bellandi B, et al. Ticagrelor crushed tablets administration in STEMI patients: The MOJITO study. J Am Coll Cardiol 2015;65(5):511–2.

63. Mega JL, Close SL, Wiviott SD, et al. Cytochrome p-450 polymorphisms and response to clopidogrel. N Engl J Med 2009;360(4):354–62.

64. Aradi D, Storey RF, Komócsi A, et al. Expert position paper on the role of platelet function testing in patients undergoing percutaneous coronary intervention. Eur Heart J 2014;35(4):209–15.

65. Stone GW, Witzenbichler B, Weisz G, et al. Platelet reactivity and clinical outcomes after coronary artery implantation of drug-eluting stents (ADAPT-DES): a prospective multicentre registry study. Lancet 2013;382(9892):614–23.

66. Collet J-P, Cuisset T, Rangé G, et al. Bedside monitoring to adjust antiplatelet therapy for coronary stenting. N Engl J Med 2012;367(22):2100–9.

67. Trenk D, Stone GW, Gawaz M, et al. A randomized trial of prasugrel versus clopidogrel in patients with high platelet reactivity on clopidogrel after elective percutaneous coronary intervention with implantation of drug-eluting stents: results of the TRIGGER-PCI (Testing Platelet Reactivity In

Patients Undergoing Elective Stent Placement on Clopidogrel to Guide Alternative Therapy With Prasugrel) study. J Am Coll Cardiol 2012;59(24): 2159–64.

68. Price MJ, Berger PB, Teirstein PS, et al. Standard-vs high-dose clopidogrel based on platelet function testing after percutaneous coronary intervention: the GRAVITAS randomized trial. JAMA 2011; 305(11):1097–105.

69. Wang TY, Henry TD, Effron MB, et al. Cluster-randomized clinical trial examining the impact of platelet function testing on practice the treatment with adenosine diphosphate receptor inhibitors: longitudinal assessment of treatment patterns and events after acute coronary syndrome prospective open label antiplatelet therapy study. Circulation 2015;8(6):e001712.

70. Levine GN, Bates ER, Blankenship JC, et al. 2011 ACCF/AHA/SCAI guideline for percutaneous coronary intervention: a report of the American College of Cardiology Foundation/American Heart Association Task Force on Practice Guidelines and the Society for Cardiovascular Angiography and Interventions. Catheter Cardiovasc Interv 2013;82(4): E266–355.

71. Windecker S, Kolh P, Alfonso F, et al. 2014 ESC/EACTS guidelines on myocardial revascularization. Eur Heart J 2014;35(37):2541–619.

72. ESPRIT Investigators, Enhanced Suppression of the Platelet IIb/IIIa Receptor with Integrilin Therapy. Novel dosing regimen of eptifibatide in planned coronary stent implantation (ESPRIT): a randomised, placebo-controlled trial. Lancet 2000; 356(9247):2037.

Antithrombotic Therapy in Percutaneous Coronary Intervention

Xiaoyu Yang, MD, Joanna Ghobrial, MD,
Duane S. Pinto, MD, MPH*

KEYWORDS

- Antithrombotics • Anticoagulation • Percutaneous coronary intervention • Acute coronary syndrome • Stable coronary artery disease

KEY POINTS

- Despite lack of randomized data compared with placebo, unfractionated heparin is the most commonly used antithrombotic agent in percutaneous coronary intervention. Dose adjustment based on activated clotting time and use of antiplatelet therapy are crucial when using unfractionated heparin.
- Low-molecular-weight heparin is more difficult to monitor than unfractionated heparin in percutaneous coronary intervention. Bleeding rates are higher when switching between low-molecular-weight heparin and unfractionated heparin.
- Fondaparinux is useful among patients being medically managed for acute coronary syndromes. Use of fondaparinux during percutaneous coronary intervention is limited by the occurrence of catheter-related thrombosis.
- Bivalirudin is associated with similar ischemic outcomes compared with heparin and glycoprotein IIb/IIIa receptor inhibitors as well as fewer bleeding complications. It is likely associated with higher rates of acute stent thrombosis.

INTRODUCTION

Antithrombotic therapy is a crucial component in the management of patients undergoing percutaneous coronary intervention (PCI). These drugs target various points in the coagulation cascade to ultimately prevent thrombin activation, which converts fibrinogen to fibrin, activates platelets, stimulates platelet aggregation, and may lead to catastrophic clot formation. Antithrombotic and antiplatelet therapies for PCI have undergone considerable evolution since the early days of balloon angioplasty. The ideal combination of agents minimizes ischemic complications while limiting bleeding risk.

The main goal of antithrombotic therapy during PCI is to avoid the adverse consequences related to thrombus formation from vascular injury and intravascular foreign bodies, including catheters, wires, and stents. Vascular injury exposes tissue factor, which activates the coagulation cascade. In addition, plaque rupture from balloon inflation or stent deployment exposes the thrombogenic lipid core, inciting an influx of coagulation factors causing thrombosis.

A large body of evidence supports the use of a variety of agents in the setting of stable

Disclosures: Drs X. Yang and J. Ghobrial have no disclosures. Dr D.S. Pinto is a consultant for the Medicines Company.
Division of Cardiovascular Medicine, Department of Medicine, Beth Israel Deaconess Medical Center, Harvard Medical School, Boston, MA, USA
* Corresponding author. Division of Cardiology, Beth Israel Deaconess Medical Center, 1 Deaconess Road, Boston, MA 02115.
E-mail address: dpinto@bidmc.harvard.edu

Intervent Cardiol Clin 5 (2016) 239–247
http://dx.doi.org/10.1016/j.iccl.2015.12.008

coronary artery disease (CAD), non-ST elevation acute coronary syndrome (NSTE-ACS), and ST-elevation myocardial infarction (STEMI). This review describes antithrombotic therapies used in PCI, including unfractionated heparin (UFH), low-molecular-weight heparin (LMWH), factor Xa inhibitors, and direct thrombin inhibitors, and summarizes their pharmacokinetics and evidence supporting their clinical use.

ANTITHROMBOTIC AGENTS

Unfractionated Heparin

UFH is the most commonly used antithrombotic agent for PCI. UFH is easy to administer and has a rapid onset when used with initial bolus, and the degree of anticoagulation is easily monitored with activated partial thromboplastin time or activated clotting time (ACT). In the absence of randomized data compared with placebo, the first antithrombotic agent used for PCI, UFH, became the standard of care. Therefore, current dosing regimens are empiric and based on clinical experience. In a pooled analysis of data from the UFH control arms of 6 randomized clinical trials, ischemic events with relationship to ACT followed a U-shaped curve. An ACT of 350 to 375 seconds yielded the lowest 7-day composite ischemic event rate, although bleeding rates were the lowest with ACT of 300 to 325 seconds.[1] A substudy of the STEEPLE trial[2] noted the ACT range with the lowest ischemic outcome, and major bleeding was 300 to 350 seconds, with bleeding increasing significantly with ACT greater than 325 seconds, but ischemic events increasing with ACT less than 325 seconds. Available data do not support the use of prolonged heparin infusions after PCI whereby excess bleeding events and length of stay are not offset by a reduction in ischemic events.[3]

Anticoagulation using UFH alone appears insufficient to optimally protect against ischemic events in patients undergoing PCI. Aggressive antiplatelet therapy is necessary to further prevent platelet activation and/or aggregation. The use of P2Y12 platelet inhibitors and/or glycoprotein IIb/IIIa receptor inhibitors (GPI) along with UFH reduces periprocedural ischemic complications.[4-6] The high ACTs used in early studies are no longer necessary when UFH is given with antiplatelet agents. A meta-analysis of 4 large clinical trials with high use of clopidrogrel or GPI showed that ACT in the lowest quartile (<256 seconds) group was associated with the lowest bleeding rates without an increased ischemic rate.[7] Current guidelines recommend using a 50 to 70 U/kg bolus for goal ACT of

200 to 250 seconds when GPI is used and a bolus of 70 to 100 U/kg for goal ACT of 250 to 300 seconds when UFH is used alone[8] (Table 1).

During PCI, major limitations of UFH include its narrow therapeutic window, unpredictable individual response, and a risk for heparin-induced thrombocytopenia (HIT).[9] In addition, clot-bound thrombin is resistant to inhibition by the heparin-antithrombin complex and can continue to serve as a nidus to propagate thrombus upon discontinuation of heparin. To address these limitations, other agents have been developed.

Low-Molecular-Weight Heparin

Low-molecular-weight heparin (LMWH) is produced by depolymerization of UFH, resulting in fragments with a low mean molecular weight. These agents have a greater activity against factor Xa than against thrombin and a lower incidence of HIT. They have more predictable and consistent anticoagulation because there is less plasma protein binding. LMWHs are cleared renally and have a longer half-life than UFH. LMWH dosing cannot be reliably adjusted using the ACT (see Table 1).

Enoxaparin is the most studied LMWH. An observational study of 803 patients with ACS treated with 1 mg/kg twice daily enoxaparin subcutaneously showed that 30-day mortality was closely linked with anti-Xa levels,[10] and anti-Xa levels greater than 0.5 U/mL are considered therapeutic for enoxaparin.[11] However, because of logistical challenges, anti-Xa levels are not commonly measured during PCI, although they are occasionally measured in medically treated patients.

The CRUISE[12] trial randomized 261 patients undergoing elective or urgent PCI to intravenous (IV) enoxaparin 1 mg/kg or UFH, with all patients also receiving eptifibatide. There was no difference in the primary endpoint of bleeding as well as vascular access site complications, angiographic complications, or ischemic endpoints, although the study was underpowered to detect these differences. The STEEPLE[11] trial evaluated 3528 elective PCI patients who were randomized to IV enoxaparin (0.5 or 0.75 mg/kg) or UFH and stratified according to the use of GPI. GPI and P2Y12 inhibitors were used in 40% and 95% of patients, respectively. Compared with UFH, the 0.5 mg/kg enoxaparin arm had a lower bleeding rate at 48 hours (5.9% vs 8.5%; P = .01), and the 0.75 mg/kg enoxaparin arm had a nonsignificantly lower bleeding rate (6.5% vs 8.5%, P = .051). The trial was not

Table 1
Overview and dosing for antithrombin agents

	Dose in PCI[34]	Half-Life	Note	Trials
Heparins				
UFH	Without IV GPI: 70–100 U/kg bolus to maintain ACT 250–300 s for HemoTec or 300–350 s for Hemochron With GPI: 50–70 U/kg IV bolus to maintain ACT 200–250	1 h	Contraindicated with HIT Avoid switching to LMWH Continue if planned CABG May use with fibrinolytic therapy, although enoxaparin and fondaparinux superior	—
Enoxaparin	0.5–0.75 mg/kg IV bolus 0.3 mg/kg IV bolus if last SQ dose >8 h or <2 doses administered	4.5 h	Reduce dose (1 mg per kg every 24 h) with renal failure (CrCl <30 mL/min) Avoid switch to UFH Avoid if CABG <24 h; discontinue 12–24 h before CABG and dose with UFH	ESSENCE/TIMI-11B SYNERGY ACUTE-II INTERACT A to Z ExTRACT-TIMI 25 CRUISE STEEPLE
Factor Xa inhibitor				
Fondaparinux	2.5 mg IV Additional anticoagulant with anti-IIa activity should be administered due to risk of catheter thrombosis when used as single agent	17–21 h	Contraindicated with renal failure (CrCl <30 mL/min) Significantly lower incidence of HITS compared with heparins. Discontinue enoxaparin 12–24 h before CABG and dose with UFH	ASPIRE OASIS-5 OASIS-6
Direct thrombin inhibitors				
Bivalirudin	0.75 mg/kg IV bolus, then 1.75 mg/kg/h With prior UFH, wait 30 min, then give 0.75 mg/kg IV bolus and 1.75 mg/kg/h	25 min	Reduced with renal failure (0.25 mg/kg/h IV for hemodialysis) Caution with GFR <30 mL/h Discontinue bivalirudin 3 h before CABG and dose with UFH	ACUITY REPLACE-2 ISAR-REACT-3 ISAR-REACT-4 HORIZONS-AMI EUROMAX NAPLES-III BRIGHT HEAT-PPCI MATRIX
Argatroban	350 µg/kg IV bolus, then 15 µg/kg/min With prior anticoagulation, 200 µg/kg IV bolus then 15 µg/kg/min	50 min	Caution with hepatic impairment	—

Abbreviations: GFR, glomerular filtration rate; SQ, subcutaneous.

large enough to provide a definitive comparison of efficacy in prevention of ischemic events.

The ESSENCE[13] and TIMI 11-B[14] studies examined the potential advantages of enoxaparin in the setting of high-risk NSTE-ACS. In a post-hoc analysis of these 2 trials,[15] in medically managed patients who did not undergo PCI, enoxaparin was superior to UFH. This finding is likely due to the more consistent anticoagulation achieved by enoxaparin as compared with UFH, which resulted in lower death and myocardial infarction (MI). In contrast, treatment with enoxaparin was not superior to heparin in the short term in patients who underwent PCI.

The SYNERGY[16] trial compared subcutaneous enoxaparin and UFH in 9987 high-risk NSTE-ACS patients undergoing early PCI. There were no differences in rates of death and MI, unsuccessful PCI, abrupt closure, or emergency coronary artery bypass grafting between the 2 groups. There was a significantly higher rate of TIMI major bleeding in patients receiving enoxaparin, but no significant difference in the rate of GUSTO severe bleeding or blood transfusions. Additional analysis showed that excessive bleeding was particularly high in patients who switched from UFH to LMWH or vice versa.[17]

The ATOLL[18] trial enrolled 910 STEMI patients who were anticoagulant naïve and randomized to UFH or IV enoxaparin. The IV enoxaparin group received 0.5 mg/kg infusion without monitoring. Most of the patients were loaded with clopidogrel; 80% received GPIs, and 66% of the cases were performed via radial access. The primary composite endpoint of 30-day death, complications of MI, procedural failure, or bleeding was nonsignificantly lower in the enoxaparin group (28% vs 34%, $P = .06$). However, enoxaparin reduced the secondary composite ischemic endpoint of 30-day death, recurrent ACS, or urgent revascularization (7% vs 11%, $P = .015$).

A meta-analysis of 13 trials comparing LMWH with UFH showed that an LMWH was associated with significant reduction in major bleeding (odds ratio 0.57; 95% confidence interval [CI] 0.40–0.82), with no difference in death, MI, or target vessel revascularization (TVR).[19] Overall, the use of IV enoxaparin during PCI is associated with a better safety profile than weight-adjusted UFH with no additional risk of ischemic events. However, given the inability to easily monitor therapeutic levels during PCI and the need for dose adjustment among patients with renal dysfunction, enoxaparin is infrequently used during PCI. Enoxaparin should be used with caution and the dose should be adjusted for patients with severe renal impairment. A creatinine clearance (CrCl) less than 30 mL/min is often used, but the degree of renal impairment required before LMWH will bioaccumulate is unknown.[20]

Factor Xa Inhibitor/Fondaparinux

Newer agents have been developed to specifically inhibit factor Xa, as an alternative to UFH. Fondaparinux, a pentasaccharide, is a synthetic indirect inhibitor of factor Xa that mimics the action of heparin through its interaction with antithrombin. The half-life is approximately 20 hours, allowing daily dosing.[21] It is primarily renally cleared and is contraindicated in patients with renal insufficiency (see Table 1).

The OASIS-5[22] trial compared fondaparinux and enoxaparin in 20,078 patients with ACS. Sixty percent of patients underwent coronary angiography, and the use of UFH during PCI was left at the discretion of the operator. The primary ischemic composite endpoint of death, MI, or refractory ischemia at 9 days was similar (5.8% vs 5.7%; $P = .007$ for noninferiority). The rate of major bleeding was lower with fondaparinux (2.2% vs 4.1%; $P<.001$), particularly with patients undergoing PCI (2.3% vs 5.1%). The overall 30-day mortality was significantly reduced with fondaparinux (2.9% vs 3.5%; $P = .02$), and 61 of the 64 excess deaths in the enoxaparin group were attributed to bleeding complications. However, 30-day mortality was not different in the 34.3% of patients who underwent PCI (2.0% vs 2.1%; $P = $ NS). Fondaparinux was associated with a small but significant increase in catheter-related thrombus in patients undergoing PCI (0.9% vs 0.4%; $P = .001$). The protocol was modified during the course of the study to ensure use of UFH with fondaparinux, which mitigated the catheter-related thrombotic events but also reduced the advantage for fondaparinux in avoiding bleeding events.

The subsequent OASIS-6[23] trial evaluated fondaparinux versus UFH in 12,092 STEMI patients, with 3789 patients undergoing primary PCI. The rate of the primary end point of death or reinfarction (9.7% vs 11.2%; $P = .008$) and rate of death (7.8% vs 8.9%; $P = .03$) both favored fondaparinux. However, there was no benefit with fondaparinux among the 3789 patients who underwent primary PCI. Again, in the fondaparinux group, there was a higher rate of catheter thrombosis (0 vs 22; $P<.001$) and coronary complications (225 vs 270; $P = .04$). As a result, fondaparinux is suggested for use among patients being treated medically for ACS and has a limited role in PCI (Table 2).

Table 2
Recommendations for antithrombin use

	Recommendation	Class of Recommendation	Level of Evidence	Guideline
UFH	IV UFH is an useful agent and dosing should be based on whether GPI is coadministered	I	C	PCI
	UFH should not be given to patients who received SC enoxaparin <12 h	III	B	PCI
Enoxaparin	Additional 0.3 mg/mg IV dose if last SQ dose >8–12 h or <2 doses administered	I	B	PCI
	Enoxaparin may be reasonable in patients either treated with "upstream" subcutaneous enoxaparin for UA/NSTEMI or who have not received prior antithrombin therapy and are administered IV enoxaparin at the time of PCI	IIa	B	PCI
Fondaparinux	Fondaparinux should not be used as the sole anticoagulant to support PCI. An additional anticoagulant with anti-IIa activity should be used because of catheter thrombosis risk	III	C	PCI
Bivalirudin	Bivalirudin is useful as an anticoagulant with or without prior treatment with UFH	I	B	PCI
	With HIT, bivalirudin or argatroban should be used instead of UFH	I	B	PCI
Argatroban	With HIT, bivalirudin or argatroban should be used instead of UFH	I	B	PCI

Abbreviations: SQ, subcutaneous; UA/NSTEMI, unstable angina/non-ST segment myocardial infarction.

Director Thrombin Inhibition/Bivalirudin

The most studied direct thrombin inhibitor in PCI is bivalirudin. Bivalirudin is a synthetic small molecule consisting of 20 amino acids. It binds directly to thrombin in both its free and its clot-bound forms, unlike the heparin drug class, which only binds to free thrombin. Thrombin-induced platelet aggregation is essentially obliterated by bivalirudin. The half-life is approximately 25 minutes; no laboratory monitoring is required, and there is no risk of HIT.

A large body of evidence supports the use of bivalirudin in ACS patients. In the ACUITY[24] trial, 13,819 patients with NSTE-ACS undergoing early invasive PCI strategy were randomized to bivalirudin monotherapy versus bivalirudin and GPI versus heparin or enoxaparin and GPI, although 64% received heparin or enoxaparin before randomization. Overall, bivalirudin alone

was noninferior to heparin plus GPI for ischemic endpoints of death, MI, or urgent revascularization at 30 days. Bivalirudin reduced major bleeding at 30 days by 47% (3.0% vs 5.7%; P<.001).

The HORIZONS-AMI[25] trial assessed 3602 STEMI patients and reported a mortality benefit at 30 days in the bivalirudin monotherapy group as compared with a heparin plus GPI group (cardiac death 1.8% vs 2.9%; P = .03; all-cause mortality 2.1% vs 3.1%; P = .047). In the trial, 71% of patients received UFH before randomization. The 30-day rate of net adverse clinical events was lower in the bivalirudin group due to a lower rate of major bleeding (4.9% vs 8.3%; P<.001). Acute stent thrombosis rate was higher in the bivalirudin alone group (1.3% vs 0.3%; P<.001) but was not significantly different at 30 days (2.5% vs 1.9%; P = .30).

To evaluate the use of upstream bivalirudin in STEMI, the EUROMAX[26] trial randomized 2218 STEMI patients who were being transported for primary PCI to bivalirudin (0.75 mg/kg bolus followed by 1.75 mg/kg/h infusion) or UFH or enoxaparin with optional GPI. At 30 days, bivalirudin reduced the rate of the primary endpoint of death or non-coronary artery bypass graft surgery (CABG)-related major bleeding by 40% as well as the principal secondary endpoint of death, reinfarction, and major bleeding by approximately 25%. Major bleeding was decreased by approximately 60%. This benefit was present regardless of whether radial or femoral access was used and regardless of which P2Y12 inhibitor was used. The risk of definite stent thrombosis was higher with bivalirudin compared with heparin (1.6% vs 0.5%; $P = .02$).

In the BRIGHT[27] trial, 2194 STEMI patients were randomized to bivalirudin with a post-PCI infusion for a median of 3 hours, heparin alone, or heparin plus tirofiban with a post-PCI infusion. With the primary endpoint of death, MI, TVR, or stroke, any bleeding at 30 days occurred in 8.8% of the bivalirudin group, 13.2% of the heparin-only group, and 17% of the heparin plus tirofiban group ($P<.001$). This difference was driven entirely by reduction in bleeding complications (4.1% vs 7.5% vs 12.3%; $P<.001$), with no difference in death or ischemic events.

The HEAT-PPCI[28] trial, a single-center UK trial of 1812 patients undergoing primary PCI randomized to bivalirudin or UFH, demonstrated outcomes that differed from previous studies. The primary efficacy endpoint of all-cause mortality, cerebrovascular accident, reinfarction, and TVR occurred in 8.7% of the bivalirudin group and 5.7% of the heparin group ($P = .01$). The difference was driven by a higher rate of definite stent thrombosis in the bivalirudin group (3.3% vs 0.7%; $P = .001$). The primary safety outcome of major bleeding occurred in 3.5% of the bivalirudin group and 3.1% in the heparin group ($P = .59$). Approximately 90% of patients were loaded with prasugrel or ticagrelor, and 80% of patients had radial access. The use of GPI was similar in each arm (13% and 15%). These factors likely explain the lesser bleeding advantage observed for bivalirudin compared with other trials. Furthermore, the median door to balloon time was only 29 minutes, and bivalirudin infusion was stopped at the end of the case. As such, higher rates of stent thrombosis may be explained by the short duration exposure to the antithrombin and withdrawal before antiplatelet medication had achieved therapeutic levels.

The MATRIX[29] trial compared bivalirudin to UFH in 7213 patients with ACS. UFH dose was 70 to 100 U/kg or 50 to 70 U/kg if used with concurrent GPI (25.9% in UFH group, 4.6% in bivalirudin group). Major adverse cardiovascular events were not significantly lower with bivalirudin compared with UFH nor was the rate of net adverse clinical events (11.2% and 12.4%, respectively; relative risk, 0.89; 95% CI, 0.78–1.03; $P = .12$). The rate of definite stent thrombosis was higher with bivalirudin (1.0% vs 0.6%; rate ratio, 1.71; 95% CI, 1.00–2.93; $P = .048$). Bivalirudin was associated with a lower all-cause mortality rate (1.7% vs 2.3%; rate ratio, 0.71; 95% CI, 0.51–0.99; $P = .04$).

The bivalirudin group was further randomized to immediate discontinuation of bivalirudin at the end of the procedure or extended post-PCI bivalirudin infusion at full dose (1.75 mg/kg/h) or at a reduced dose of 0.25 mg/kg/h. The coprimary endpoint of death, MI, or stroke was similar in the post-PCI infusion group and no infusion group (10.2% vs 10.5%; rate ratio 0.96; 95% CI 0.77–1.18; $P = .67$). The coprimary endpoint of death, MI, or stroke plus major bleeding was also similar in the 2 groups (10.7% vs 11.7%, rate ratio 0.90; 95% CI 0.73–1.10; $P = .31$). Although extended bivalirudin infusion post-PCI did not decrease definite stent thrombosis, subanalysis showed that high-dose extended infusion resulted in no stent thrombosis.[29]

In patients with stable CAD undergoing elective PCI, the REPLACE-2[30] and the ISAR-REACT-3[31,32] trials reported that bivalirudin was associated with lower bleeding events. In the REPLACE-2 trial,[30] 6010 low- to moderate-risk patients undergoing urgent (44%) or elective PCI (56%) were randomized to heparin with planned GPI or bivalirudin with provisional GPI. At 30 days, there was no significant difference in composite endpoint of death, MI, urgent revascularization, or major bleeding between the groups (9.2% in bivalirudin group vs 10.0% in heparin plus GPI group). In-hospital major bleeding rates were significantly reduced by bivalirudin (2.4% vs 4.1%; $P<.001$). However, the higher major bleeding rates in the heparin group may be explained by planned use of GPI, which is infrequently used in elective PCI. In the ISAR-REACT-3 trial,[31,32] 4570 troponin-negative patients treated with aspirin and clopidogrel at least 2 hours before planned PCI were randomized to 140 U/kg UFH or bivalirudin. Although the primary endpoint of death, MI, urgent TVR, or major bleeding at 30 days was similar with UFH and bivalirudin (8.7% vs 8.3%; $P = .57$), UFH was associated with a significantly higher risk of major (4.6% vs

3.1%; $P = .008$) and minor bleeding (9.9% vs 6.8%; $P = .001$). A major criticism is that UFH dosing was higher than used in contemporary practice and the currently recommended dose of 70 to 100 U/kg when GPI are not used.[8]

The NAPLES-III[33] trial, which randomized 837 biomarker-negative patients with increased bleeding risk undergoing elective transfemoral PCI, reported that the primary endpoint of in-hospital bleeding was similar between the bivalirudin and heparin arms (3.3% vs 2.6%; $P = .54$). Clinical endpoints at 30 days were also similar with regard to major adverse cardiovascular events (6.5% vs 4.3%; $P = .17$), death (2.4% vs 1.4%), MI (0.2% vs 0%), stent thrombosis (0.5% vs 0.5%), and 1-year outcomes. Notably, the lack of difference in bleeding events likely stems from the fact that the patient population was at low risk for bleeding, and UFH dosing was at 70 U/kg with GPI use reserved for only bailout indications.

Overall, there is considerable heterogeneity in the many trials comparing bivalirudin to heparin with respect to upstream heparin exposure, heparin dosing, P2Y12 inhibitor use, and concurrent GPI use. Taken together, these trials suggest that bivalirudin is a reasonable alternative to UFH alone or in combination with GPI in patients undergoing PCI, especially in patients with high bleeding risk or when using femoral artery access. However, several of the ACS trials showed a higher rate of acute stent thrombosis associated with bivalirudin use, which may be alleviated using a variety of strategies. For elective PCI patients, bivalirudin has no bleeding advantage over standard dose heparin alone, but can lower bleeding when compared with high-dose heparin, or heparin with GPI.

OTHER AGENTS

Argatroban is a direct thrombin inhibitor used for prophylaxis and treatment of thrombosis associated with HIT, including during PCI and cardiopulmonary bypass. The half-life is approximately 50 minutes and is metabolized in the liver. It can be used in the setting of renal failure, but not in those with significant hepatic dysfunction. Novel oral anticoagulants such as rivaroxaban and apixaban have been studied for extended anticoagulation after recent ACS. Their role in PCI remains uncertain and will require more evidence.

SUMMARY

Antithrombotic strategies during PCI have evolved over recent decades, and numerous agents are now available to target key components of the coagulation cascade. Along with improvements in PCI technique and antiplatelet agents, refinements in antithrombotic agents have led to reductions in both ischemic and bleeding events. In PCI for ACS, bleeding reduction with bivalirudin over UFH with or without GPI must be weighed against the increased risk of stent thrombosis. The bleeding risk with UFH may be reduced with dosing in accordance with the current PCI guidelines, more judicious use of concurrent GPI, and radial artery access. The mainstay for anticoagulation in PCI for patients with stable CAD remains UFH, with selective use of additional IV antiplatelet agents, but LMWH and direct thrombin inhibitors, either alone or in combination with heparins, have a variety of benefits, particularly in patients with a high risk of bleeding. In the era of new antithrombotic and antiplatelet agents, finding the appropriate combination of these medications has the potential to dramatically improve outcomes but remains an enormously challenging task for future investigations.

REFERENCES

1. Chew DP, Bhatt DL, Lincoff AM, et al. Defining the optimal activated clotting time during percutaneous coronary intervention: aggregate results from 6 randomized, controlled trials. Circulation 2001;103:961–6.
2. Montalescot G, Cohen M, Salette G, et al, STEEPLE Investigators. Impact of anticoagulation levels on outcomes in patients undergoing elective percutaneous coronary intervention: insights from the STEEPLE trial. Eur Heart J 2008;29:462–71.
3. Rabah M, Mason D, Muller DW, et al. Heparin after percutaneous intervention (HAPI): a prospective multicenter randomized trial of three heparin regimens after successful coronary intervention. J Am Coll Cardiol 1999;34:461–7.
4. Valgimigli M, Percoco G, Barbieri D, et al. The additive value of tirofiban administered with the high-dose bolus in the prevention of ischemic complications during high-risk coronary angioplasty: the ADVANCE trial. J Am Coll Cardiol 2004;44:14–9.
5. Randomised placebo-controlled and balloon-angioplasty-controlled trial to assess safety of coronary stenting with use of platelet glycoprotein-IIb/IIIa blockade. Lancet 1998;352:87–92.
6. ESPRIT Investigators. Enhanced Suppression of the Platelet IIb/IIIa Receptor with Integrilin Therapy. Novel dosing regimen of Eptifibatide in Planned Coronary Stent Implantation (ESPRIT): a randomised, placebo-controlled trial. Lancet 2000;356: 2037–44.

7. Brener SJ, Moliterno DJ, Lincoff AM, et al. Relationship between activated clotting time and ischemic or hemorrhagic complications: analysis of 4 recent randomized clinical trials of percutaneous coronary intervention. Circulation 2004; 110:994–8.

8. Levine GN, Bates ER, Blankenship JC, et al. 2011 ACCF/AHA/SCAI guideline for percutaneous coronary intervention: a report of the American college of cardiology foundation/American heart association task force on practice guidelines and the society for cardiovascular angiography and interventions. Circulation 2011;124:e574–651.

9. Hirsh J, Fuster V. Guide to anticoagulant therapy. Part 1: heparin. American Heart Association. Circulation 1994;89:1449–68.

10. Montalescot G, Collet JP, Tanguy ML, et al. Anti-Xa activity relates to survival and efficacy in unselected acute coronary syndrome patients treated with enoxaparin. Circulation 2004;110:392–8.

11. Montalescot G, White HD, Gallo R, et al. Enoxaparin versus unfractionated heparin in elective percutaneous coronary intervention. N Engl J Med 2006;355:1006–17.

12. Bhatt DL, Lee BI, Casterella PJ, et al, CRUISE Study Investigators. Safety of concomitant therapy with eptifibatide and enoxaparin in patients undergoing percutaneous coronary intervention: results of the Coronary Revascularization Using Integrilin and Single Bolus Enoxaparin Study. J Am Coll Cardiol 2003;41:20–5.

13. Goodman SG, Cohen M, Bigonzi F, et al. Randomized trial of low molecular weight heparin (enoxaparin) versus unfractionated heparin for unstable coronary artery disease: one-year results of the ESSENCE study. Efficacy and Safety of Subcutaneous Enoxaparin in Non-Q wave Coronary Events. J Am Coll Cardiol 2000;36:693–8.

14. Antman EM, McCabe CH, Gurfinkel EP, et al. Enoxaparin prevents death and cardiac ischemic events in unstable angina/non-Q-wave myocardial infarction. Results of the Thrombolysis In Myocardial Infarction (TIMI) 11B trial. Circulation 1999;100: 1593–601.

15. Fox KA, Antman EM, Cohen M, et al, ESSENCE Investigators. Comparison of enoxaparin versus unfractionated heparin in patients with unstable angina pectoris/non-ST-segment elevation acute myocardial infarction having subsequent percutaneous coronary intervention. Am J Cardiol 2002; 90:477–82.

16. SYNERGY Trial Investigators. Enoxaparin vs unfractionated heparin in high-risk patients with non-ST-segment elevation acute coronary syndromes managed with an intended early invasive strategy: primary results of the SYNERGY randomized trial. JAMA 2004;292:45–54.

17. Cohen M, Mahaffey KW, Pieper K, et al, SYNERGY Trial Investigators. A subgroup analysis of the impact of prerandomization antithrombin therapy on outcomes in the SYNERGY trial: enoxaparin versus unfractionated heparin in non-ST-segment elevation acute coronary syndromes. J Am Coll Cardiol 2006;48:1346–54.

18. Montalescot G, Zeymer U, Silvain J, et al, ATOLL Investigators. Intravenous enoxaparin or unfractionated heparin in primary percutaneous coronary intervention for ST-elevation myocardial infarction: the International Randomised Open-label ATOLL Trial. Lancet 2011;378:693–703.

19. Dumaine R, Borentain M, Bertel O, et al. Intravenous low-molecular-weight heparins compared with unfractionated heparin in percutaneous coronary intervention: quantitative review of randomized trials. Arch Intern Med 2007;167:2423–30.

20. Farooq V, Hegarty J, Chandrasekar T, et al. Serious adverse incidents with the usage of low molecular weight heparins in patients with chronic kidney disease. Am J Kidney Dis 2004;43:531–7.

21. Mehta SR, Steg PG, Granger CB, et al. Randomized, blinded trial comparing fondaparinux with unfractionated heparin in patients undergoing contemporary percutaneous coronary intervention: Arixtra Study in Percutaneous Coronary Intervention: a Randomized Evaluation (ASPIRE) Pilot Trial. Circulation 2005;111:1390–7.

22. Fifth Organization to Assess Strategies in Acute Ischemic Syndromes Investigators, Yusuf S, Mehta SR, et al. Comparison of fondaparinux and enoxaparin in acute coronary syndromes. N Engl J Med 2006;354:1464–76.

23. Yusuf S, Mehta SR, Chrolavicius S, et al. Effects of fondaparinux on mortality and reinfarction in patients with acute ST-segment elevation myocardial infarction: the OASIS-6 randomized trial. JAMA 2006;295:1519–30.

24. Stone GW, McLaurin BT, Cox DA, et al, Acuity Investigators. Bivalirudin for patients with acute coronary syndromes. N Engl J Med 2006;355:2203–16.

25. Stone GW, Witzenbichler B, Guagliumi G, et al, HORIZONS-AMI Trial Investigators. Bivalirudin during primary PCI in acute myocardial infarction. N Engl J Med 2008;358:2218–30.

26. Steg PG, van 't Hof A, Hamm CW, et al, EUROMAX Investigators. Bivalirudin started during emergency transport for primary PCI. N Engl J Med 2013;369: 2207–17.

27. Han Y, Guo J, Zheng Y, et al, BRIGHT Investigators. Bivalirudin vs heparin with or without tirofiban during primary percutaneous coronary intervention in acute myocardial infarction: the BRIGHT randomized clinical trial. JAMA 2015;313:1336–46.

28. Shahzad A, Kemp I, Mars C, et al, HEAT-PPCI Trial Investigators. Unfractionated heparin versus

bivalirudin in primary percutaneous coronary intervention (HEAT-PPCI): an open-label, single centre, randomised controlled trial. Lancet 2014;384: 1849–58.

29. Valgimigli M, Frigoli E, Leonardi S, et al, MATRIX Investigators. Bivalirudin or unfractionated heparin in acute coronary syndromes. N Engl J Med 2015; 373:997–1009.

30. Lincoff AM, Bittl JA, Harrington RA, et al, REPLACE-2 Investigators. Bivalirudin and provisional glycoprotein IIb/IIIa blockade compared with heparin and planned glycoprotein IIb/IIIa blockade during percutaneous coronary intervention: REPLACE-2 randomized trial. JAMA 2003; 289:853–63.

31. Schulz S, Mehilli J, Ndrepepa G, et al, ISAR-REACT 3 Trial Investigators. Bivalirudin vs. unfractionated heparin during percutaneous coronary interventions in patients with stable and unstable angina pectoris: 1-year results of the ISAR-REACT 3 trial. Eur Heart J 2010;31:582–7.

32. Kastrati A, Neumann FJ, Mehilli J, et al, ISAR-REACT Trial Investigators. Bivalirudin versus unfractionated heparin during percutaneous coronary intervention. N Engl J Med 2008;359:688–96.

33. Briguori C, Visconti G, Focaccio A, et al. Novel approaches for preventing or limiting events (Naples) III trial: randomized comparison of bivalirudin versus unfractionated heparin in patients at increased risk of bleeding undergoing transfemoral elective coronary stenting. JACC Cardiovasc Interv 2015;8:414–23.

34. Levine GN, Bates ER, Blankenship JC, et al, American College of Cardiology Foundation, American Heart Association Task Force on Practice Guidelines, Society for Cardiovascular Angiography and Interventions. 2011 ACCF/AHA/SCAI guideline for percutaneous coronary intervention. A report of the American College of Cardiology Foundation/American Heart Association Task Force on practice guidelines and the Society for Cardiovascular Angiography and Interventions. J Am Coll Cardiol 2011;58:e44–122.

Risk Stratification for Percutaneous Coronary Intervention

Davide Capodanno, MD, PhD*

KEYWORDS

• SYNTAX score • Risk stratification • Percutaneous coronary intervention • Risk scores

---

KEY POINTS

- The Synergy Between Percutaneous Coronary Intervention with Taxus and Cardiac Surgery (SYNTAX) score is the most-studied risk model in the setting of percutaneous coronary intervention (PCI).
- Several validation studies have proved the SYNTAX score to be an effective prognostic tool in multiple clinical scenarios.
- Proofs-of-concept studies have shown the predictive ability of the SYNTAX score to be significantly improved by the addition of clinical variables or functional information into the original angiographic model.
- The SYNTAX score II incorporates clinical and angiographic variables into logistic formulas for 4-year mortality estimation after PCI and coronary artery bypass grafting.

INTRODUCTION

In patients with coronary artery disease referred for percutaneous coronary intervention (PCI), anticipating the risk of the procedure to fail at long-term follow-up is important for several reasons. First, patients at high risk of recurrent events after PCI may be considered for alternative treatments (ie, coronary artery bypass grafting [CABG]). Second, patients and their families get a better understanding of the prognostic implications of PCI and provide their consent on a more objective basis. Third, forecasting the risk of PCI assists quality-of-care monitoring and facilitates comparing the outcomes of procedures performed in different hospitals or settings.

Risk stratification for PCI is a relatively young field of interest, fueled in recent years by the introduction of several specific risk models and scores. The 2014 guidelines for myocardial revascularization issued by the European Society of Cardiology recommend 3 clinical scores (European System for Cardiac Operative Risk Evaluation [EuroSCORE] II, Age, Creatinine, Ejection Fraction [ACEF], and National Cardiovascular data Registry [NCDR] PCI) for risk stratification of in-hospital or 30-day mortality.[1] However, the grade of recommendation for these 3 scores is only IIb, reflecting the scarcity of validation studies and the weaker implication of anticipating periprocedural mortality in the PCI setting. In contrast, one score (Synergy Between Percutaneous Coronary Intervention with Taxus and Cardiac Surgery [SYNTAX] score) has been given a class I, and 3 scores (Logistic Clinical SYNTAX score, SYNTAX score II, and ACCF and STS Database Collaboration on the Comparative Effectiveness of Revascularization Strategies [ASCERT] PCI) have been given a class IIa degree of recommendation for assessing the risk of medium- to long-term (≥1 year) outcomes. Indeed, anticipating medium-to long-term outcomes is more reasonable for a procedure like PCI, which is not burdened by excessive perioperative

---

Disclosures: none.
Dipartimento Cardio-Toraco-Vasculare, Ferrarotto Hospital, University of Catania, Via Citelli, 6, Catania 95124, Italy
* Corresponding author. Cardiology Department, Ferrarotto Hospital, University of Catania, Via Citelli 6, Catania 95124, Italy.
E-mail address: dcapodanno@gmail.com

Intervent Cardiol Clin 5 (2016) 249–257
http://dx.doi.org/10.1016/j.iccl.2015.12.009
2211-7458/16/$ – see front matter © 2016 Elsevier Inc. All rights reserved.

mortality. Notably, this is quite different from other settings like CABG, whereby the individual early risk of the intervention must be weighted against the benefits expected in the longer term.

With more than 50 validation studies, the SYNTAX score is the most-studied risk model in the setting of PCI. In this article, the evolutionary journey of the SYNTAX score is reviewed, with emphasis on its sequential modifications and adaptations, now culminated in the development and validation of the SYNTAX score II.

THE SYNERGY BETWEEN PERCUTANEOUS CORONARY INTERVENTION WITH TAXUS AND CARDIAC SURGERY SCORE
Calculation and Variability
The SYNTAX score can be calculated online at www.syntaxscore.com. The calculation begins by defining the coronary dominance. Second, a single lesion is characterized with regard to the number and location of the branches involved. The third step requires a detailed description of the angiographic features of the lesion (ie, chronic total occlusion, trifurcation, bifurcation, vessel tortuosity, lesion length, heavy calcification, and thrombus). This process is reiterated for each lesion with a visual stenosis more than 50% in vessels of at least 2 mm in diameter. Finally, once all lesions have been scored, the calculator requires indicating whether there are segments that fulfill the criteria for small vessel disease (Fig. 1). A significant issue that comes from this quite cumbersome process[2] is the moderate interobserver variability of the SYNTAX score, with the scoring of bifurcations lesions representing the

Left Main
• Segment 5	10 points
• Segment 6	7 points
• Segment 11	3 points
• Medina 1,1,1	2 points
• Heavy Calcification	1 point

Obtuse Marginal
• Segment 12a	2 points
• Severe Tortuosity	2 points

Right Coronary Artery
• Segment 2	2 points
• Length >20 mm	1 points

SYNTAX score	**31 points**

Fig. 1. Case example of SYNTAX score calculation. The grading process to obtain the SYNTAX score is illustrated for a patient with atherosclerotic disease of the left main, the obtuse marginal, and the right coronary artery.

main source of inconsistency.[3–9] The level of agreement improves after adequate training but remains generally more satisfactory in a core-laboratory setting than in daily routine.[7,8,10]

Derivation and Validation
The SYNTAX score was not developed from a PCI dataset, but rather built based on expert consensus by merging several preexisting angiographic schemes.[11,12] At that time, the idea behind the creation of a new and more comprehensive angiographic scoring system was not to apply it for risk stratification but to use it merely as a catheterization laboratory tool to assess the equipoise of PCI and CABG as a prerequisite for randomization in the SYNTAX trial.[13,14] The score sought to surpass the old concept of 3-vessel disease as representing ipso facto the worst degree of coronary burden, introducing a pragmatic instrument to appreciate the substantial differences in lesion complexity that exist even in patients with 3 coronary vessels involved. Subsequently and post hoc, the score proved to work properly as a risk stratification tool either in the SYNTAX trial itself or in early external validation studies conducted in patients with 3-vessel[15] or left main disease.[16]

Over time, the SYNTAX score has proved to be highly transportable to other clinical scenarios, including all-comers PCI,[17–19] PCI with newer-generation drug-eluting stents,[18,20] acute coronary syndromes with[21–30] and without[31–34] ST-segment elevation, and even transcatheter aortic valve implantation.[35,36]

In parallel, studies have demonstrated the ability of the score to assess the risk of other end points softer than mortality or major adverse cardiac events, such as

- No reflow[37,38]
- Distal embolization[39]
- Left ventricle thrombus development[40]
- Culprit vessel vulnerability[41]
- Periprocedural myocardial infarction[42]
- Contrast-induced nephropathy[43,44]

Multiple studies have also proved the (mostly nonindependent) association of the SYNTAX score with blood markers and components, which include

- Fasting glucose[45]
- Hemoglobin A_{1c}[46]
- Creatinine[47,48]
- Albumin[49]
- Lipoprotein (a)[50]
- N-terminal pro-brain natriuretic peptide[51]
- High-sensitivity troponin T[52]

- High-sensitivity C-reactive protein[53]
- Endothelial progenitor cells[54]
- CD4 T cells[55]
- Neutrophil to lymphocyte ratio[56]

Finally, the SYNTAX score has been correlated with multiple imaging metrics:

- Myocardial performance index and other systolic/diastolic echocardiographic parameters[57,58]
- Myocardial defect scores at single-photon emission computed tomography[59]
- Delayed enhancement at cardiac magnetic resonance[60]
- Carotid artery intima-media thickness[61–63]
- Arterial stiffness[64]

The Synergy Between Percutaneous Coronary Intervention with Taxus and Cardiac Surgery Score as a Tool for Decision Making

An intrinsic characteristic of the SYNTAX score is its inability to prognostically stratify patients who ultimately undergo CABG.[65–67] One potential explanation for this finding is that the issue of coronary complexity becomes less problematic and prognostically important at long-term follow-up if a graft is placed to protect an entire vessel.[68] Indeed, when a comparison is undertaken between PCI and CABG across SYNTAX score tertiles, the score stratifies the risk of PCI but does not do the same for CABG, which typically generates a progressive separation of the estimated outcomes of the two procedures as far as the coronary complexity increases.[13,14] Therefore, the SYNTAX score can also be used as a meaningful tool for decision making between PCI and CABG, particularly in that it represents a plausible indirect indicator of the ability of each procedure to achieve the goal of complete anatomic revascularization.[69]

Adaptations of the Synergy Between Percutaneous Coronary Intervention with Taxus and Cardiac Surgery Score and Proofs of Concept

Defining the coronary anatomy with regard to lesion and technical complexity has an established prognostic significance. However, there are many potential clinical variables that also jeopardize the prognosis of a patient undergoing PCI. For this reason, it was originally postulated that adding clinical variables to the SYNTAX boosts significantly its accuracy.[70] This line of research, now culminated into the development of the SYNTAX score II, has had many intermediate steps[71–76] (Fig. 2). The Global Risk classification subdivided patients into combinations of SYNTAX score and EuroSCORE categories, a strategy that proved to improve the discrimination of the SYNTAX score taken alone.[70,77–79] Subsequently, the Clinical SYNTAX score achieved the same goal by combining the SYNTAX score with only 3 clinical variables (age, creatinine, and ejection fraction).[19,80–82] The Clinical SYNTAX score has currently been adapted into a logistic form for prediction of 1-year[83,84] and 3-year[85] mortality, at the price of a slightly more complex calculation also involving the use of a nomogram.[84,86,87]

Interestingly, the SYNTAX score has also been modified over time in proof-of-concept studies by incorporating information coming from fractional flow reserve[88–90] and computed tomography.[91–96] Finally, the score has been adapted to the post-PCI (Residual SYNTAX score[97–102]) and CABG (CABG-SYNTAX score[103,104]) setting, proving the common perception that residual coronary artery disease

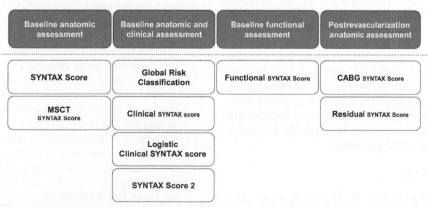

Fig. 2. SYNTAX score and SYNTAX score–based models for prognostic stratification and decision making. MSCT, multi-slice computed tomography.

(ie, incomplete revascularization) keeps prognostic significance even after revascularization has been partially already achieved.

The Synergy Between Percutaneous Coronary Intervention with Taxus and Cardiac Surgery Score II

The SYNTAX score II has been derived by using data from the SYNTAX trial.[105] In contrast to the classic SYNTAX score, the new model incorporates clinical variables into 2 logistic formulas for estimating 4-year mortality after PCI and CABG, respectively. As such, the score serves as a tool for selecting the appropriate revascularization strategy based on individual clinical and angiographic risk. At the time of writing this article, an online calculator is not available, which makes the workability of the SYNTAX score II suboptimal in daily practice. The score has been validated retrospectively in patients with left main disease[105,106] and those undergoing all-comers PCI.[107] However, one may advocate that for a score that acts as a decision-making tool, retrospective validation is insufficient (ie, a decision for a procedure over another has already been taken) and prospective validation is necessary (ie, the score should demonstrate the ability to assist in taking appropriate decisions that positively impact on the outcomes of patients selected for PCI or CABG).[108] Validation of the SYNTAX score II is prespecified as an end point in the ongoing randomized Evaluation of the Xience Everolimus-Eluting Stent Versus Coronary Artery Bypass Surgery for Effectiveness of Left Main Revascularization [EXCEL] trial and the planned SYNTAX trial II, which will use the SYNTAX score II to recruit patients on the grounds of patient safety.[109,110]

SUMMARY

Risk stratification is key in predicting the medium- to long-term success of PCI. The SYNTAX score is currently endorsed by clinical practice guidelines as the most meaningful tool for selecting left main or 3-vessel disease candidates to PCI. The SYNTAX score II is just the most recent (but not the only and possibly not the final) attempt in the process of refining the predictive ability of the SYNTAX score to forecast later events and select the most appropriate revascularization strategy for patients with complex coronary artery disease.

REFERENCES

1. Windecker S, Kolh P, Alfonso F, et al. 2014 ESC/EACTS guidelines on myocardial revascularization: the task force on myocardial revascularization of the European Society of Cardiology (ESC) and the European Association for Cardio-thoracic Surgery (EACTS) developed with the special contribution of the European Association of Percutaneous Cardiovascular Interventions (EAPCI). Eur Heart J 2014;35:2541–619.

2. Capodanno D, Tamburino C. Does the SYNTAX score get on your nerves? Practical considerations on how and when avoiding it to maximize its usefulness with no waste of time. Int J Cardiol 2012; 159:165–8.

3. Serruys PW, Onuma Y, Garg S, et al. Assessment of the SYNTAX score in the Syntax study. EuroIntervention 2009;5:50–6.

4. Garg S, Girasis C, Sarno G, et al. The SYNTAX score revisited: a reassessment of the SYNTAX score reproducibility. Catheter Cardiovasc Interv 2010;75:946–52.

5. Morrison DA. How much delta does your kappa make to my patients? Putting the SYNTAX score into clinical context. Catheter Cardiovasc Interv 2010;75:953–6.

6. Tanboga IH, Ekinci M, Isik T, et al. Reproducibility of syntax score: from core lab to real world. J Interv Cardiol 2011;24:302–6.

7. Genereux P, Palmerini T, Caixeta A, et al. SYNTAX score reproducibility and variability between interventional cardiologists, core laboratory technicians, and quantitative coronary measurements. Circ Cardiovasc Interv 2011;4:553–61.

8. Zhang YJ, Iqbal J, Campos CM, et al. Prognostic value of site SYNTAX score and rationale for combining anatomic and clinical factors in decision making: insights from the SYNTAX trial. J Am Coll Cardiol 2014;64:423–32.

9. Shiomi H, Tamura T, Niki S, et al. Inter- and intra-observer variability for assessment of the synergy between percutaneous coronary intervention with TAXUS and cardiac surgery (SYNTAX) score and association of the SYNTAX score with clinical outcome in patients undergoing unprotected left main stenting in the real world. Circ J 2011;75:1130–7.

10. Garot P, Tafflet M, Kumar S, et al. Reproducibility and factors influencing the assessment of the SYNTAX score in the left main Xience study. Catheter Cardiovasc Interv 2012;80:231–7.

11. Sianos G, Morel MA, Kappetein AP, et al. The SYNTAX score: an angiographic tool grading the complexity of coronary artery disease. EuroIntervention 2005;1:219–27.

12. Capodanno D, Tamburino C. Integrating the synergy between percutaneous coronary intervention with Taxus and cardiac surgery (SYNTAX) score into practice: use, pitfalls, and new directions. Am Heart J 2011;161:462–70.

13. Serruys PW, Morice MC, Kappetein AP, et al. Percutaneous coronary intervention versus coronary-

artery bypass grafting for severe coronary artery disease. N Engl J Med 2009;360:961–72.

14. Mohr FW, Morice MC, Kappetein AP, et al. Coronary artery bypass graft surgery versus percutaneous coronary intervention in patients with three-vessel disease and left main coronary disease: 5-year follow-up of the randomised, clinical SYNTAX trial. Lancet 2013;381:629–38.

15. Valgimigli M, Serruys PW, Tsuchida K, et al. Cyphering the complexity of coronary artery disease using the syntax score to predict clinical outcome in patients with three-vessel lumen obstruction undergoing percutaneous coronary intervention. Am J Cardiol 2007;99:1072–81.

16. Capodanno D, Di Salvo ME, Cincotta G, et al. Usefulness of the SYNTAX score for predicting clinical outcome after percutaneous coronary intervention of unprotected left main coronary artery disease. Circ Cardiovasc Interv 2009;2:302–8.

17. Wykrzykowska JJ, Garg S, Girasis C, et al. Value of the SYNTAX score for risk assessment in the all-comers population of the randomized multicenter LEADERS (Limus Eluted from A Durable versus Erodable Stent coating) trial. J Am Coll Cardiol 2010;56:272–7.

18. Wykrzykowska JJ, Garg S, Onuma Y, et al. Implantation of the biodegradable polymer biolimus-eluting stent in patients with high SYNTAX score is associated with decreased cardiac mortality compared to a permanent polymer sirolimus-eluting stent: two year follow-up results from the "all-comers" LEADERS trial. EuroIntervention 2011;7:605–13.

19. Girasis C, Garg S, Raber L, et al. SYNTAX score and clinical SYNTAX score as predictors of very long-term clinical outcomes in patients undergoing percutaneous coronary interventions: a substudy of SIRolimus-eluting stent compared with pacliTAXel-eluting stent for coronary revascularization (SIRTAX) trial. Eur Heart J 2011;32:3115–27.

20. Garg S, Serruys PW, Silber S, et al. The prognostic utility of the SYNTAX score on 1-year outcomes after revascularization with zotarolimus- and everolimus-eluting stents: a substudy of the RESOLUTE all comers trial. JACC Cardiovasc Interv 2011;4:432–41.

21. Garg S, Sarno G, Serruys PW, et al. Prediction of 1-year clinical outcomes using the SYNTAX score in patients with acute ST-segment elevation myocardial infarction undergoing primary percutaneous coronary intervention: a substudy of the STRATEGY (single high-dose bolus tirofiban and sirolimus-eluting stent versus abciximab and bare-metal stent in acute myocardial infarction) and MULTISTRATEGY (multicenter evaluation of single high-dose bolus tirofiban versus abciximab with sirolimus-eluting stent or bare-metal stent in acute myocardial infarction study) trials. JACC Cardiovasc Interv 2011;4:66–75.

22. Magro M, Nauta S, Simsek C, et al. Value of the SYNTAX score in patients treated by primary percutaneous coronary intervention for acute ST-elevation myocardial infarction: the MI SYNTAX score study. Am Heart J 2011;161:771–81.

23. Scherff F, Vassalli G, Surder D, et al. The SYNTAX score predicts early mortality risk in the elderly with acute coronary syndrome having primary PCI. J Invasive Cardiol 2011;23:505–10.

24. Yang CH, Hsieh MJ, Chen CC, et al. SYNTAX score: an independent predictor of long-term cardiac mortality in patients with acute ST-elevation myocardial infarction. Coron Artery Dis 2012;23:445–9.

25. Kul S, Akgul O, Uyarel H, et al. High SYNTAX score predicts worse in-hospital clinical outcomes in patients undergoing primary angioplasty for acute myocardial infarction. Coron Artery Dis 2012;23:542–8.

26. Yang CH, Hsieh MJ, Chen CC, et al. The prognostic significance of SYNTAX score after early percutaneous transluminal coronary angioplasty for acute ST elevation myocardial infarction. Heart Lung Circ 2013;22:341–5.

27. Brown AJ, McCormick LM, Gajendragadkar PR, et al. Initial SYNTAX score predicts major adverse cardiac events after primary percutaneous coronary intervention. Angiology 2014;65:408–12.

28. Akgun T, Oduncu V, Bitigen A, et al. Baseline SYNTAX Score and long-term outcome in patients with ST-segment elevation myocardial infarction undergoing primary percutaneous coronary intervention. Clin Appl Thromb Hemost 2014;21(8):712–9.

29. Ayca B, Akin F, Celik O, et al. Does SYNTAX score predict in-hospital outcomes in patients with ST elevation myocardial infarction undergoing primary percutaneous coronary intervention? Kardiol Pol 2014;72:806–13.

30. Su MI, Tsai CT, Yeh HI, et al. The impact of SYNTAX score of non-infarct-related artery on long-term outcome among patients with acute ST segment elevation myocardial infarction undergoing primary percutaneous coronary intervention. PLoS One 2014;9:e109828.

31. Palmerini T, Genereux P, Caixeta A, et al. Prognostic value of the SYNTAX score in patients with acute coronary syndromes undergoing percutaneous coronary intervention: analysis from the ACUITY (acute catheterization and urgent intervention triage strategy) trial. J Am Coll Cardiol 2011;57:2389–97.

32. Caixeta A, Genereux P, Palmerini T, et al. Prognostic utility of the SYNTAX score in patients with single versus multivessel disease undergoing percutaneous coronary intervention (from the acute catheterization and urgent intervention triage strategy [ACUITY] trial). Am J Cardiol 2014;113:203–10.

33. Yadav M, Genereux P, Palmerini T, et al. SYNTAX score and the risk of stent thrombosis after percutaneous coronary intervention in patients with non-ST-segment elevation acute coronary syndromes: an ACUITY trial substudy. Catheter Cardiovasc Interv 2015;85:1–10.

34. Palmerini T, Calabro P, Piscione F, et al. Impact of gene polymorphisms, platelet reactivity, and the SYNTAX score on 1-year clinical outcomes in patients with non-ST-segment elevation acute coronary syndrome undergoing percutaneous coronary intervention: the GEPRESS study. JACC Cardiovasc Interv 2014;7:1117–27.

35. Stefanini GG, Stortecky S, Cao D, et al. Coronary artery disease severity and aortic stenosis: clinical outcomes according to SYNTAX score in patients undergoing transcatheter aortic valve implantation. Eur Heart J 2014;35:2530–40.

36. Khawaja MZ, Asrress KN, Haran H, et al. The effect of coronary artery disease defined by quantitative coronary angiography and SYNTAX score upon outcome after transcatheter aortic valve implantation (TAVI) using the Edwards bioprosthesis. EuroIntervention 2015;11:450–5.

37. Magro M, Nauta ST, Simsek C, et al. Usefulness of the SYNTAX score to predict "no reflow" in patients treated with primary percutaneous coronary intervention for ST-segment elevation myocardial infarction. Am J Cardiol 2012;109:601–6.

38. Sahin DY, Gur M, Elbasan Z, et al. SYNTAX score is a predictor of angiographic no-reflow in patients with ST-elevation myocardial infarction treated with a primary percutaneous coronary intervention. Coron Artery Dis 2013;24:148–53.

39. Biyik I, Akturk IF, Ozturk D, et al. Can syntax score predict angiographically visible distal embolization during primary percutaneous coronary intervention? Minerva Cardioangiol 2015. [Epub ahead of print].

40. Gokdeniz T, Boyaci F, Hatem E, et al. SYNTAX score predicts the left ventricle thrombus development in patients undergoing primary percutaneous coronary intervention for first anterior myocardial infarction. Clin Appl Thromb Hemost 2014;20:698–705.

41. Saka K, Hibi K, Kozuma K, et al. Relation between the SYNTAX score and culprit vessel vulnerability in non-ST-segment elevation acute coronary syndrome. JACC Cardiovasc Imaging 2015;8:496–8.

42. Tandjung K, Lam MK, Sen H, et al. Value of the SYNTAX score for periprocedural myocardial infarction according to WHO and the third universal definition of myocardial infarction: insights from the TWENTE trial. EuroIntervention 2015;11. [Epub ahead of print].

43. Oduncu V, Erkol A, Karabay CY, et al. Relation of the severity of contrast induced nephropathy to SYNTAX score and long term prognosis in patients treated with primary percutaneous coronary intervention. Int J Cardiol 2013;168:3480–5.

44. Madhavan MV, Genereux P, Rubin J, et al. Usefulness of the SYNTAX score to predict acute kidney injury after percutaneous coronary intervention (from the acute catheterization and urgent intervention triage strategy trial). Am J Cardiol 2014;113:1331–7.

45. Yang X, Liu H, Yang F, et al. Elevated risk of an intermediate or high SYNTAX score in subjects with impaired fasting glucose. Intern Med 2015;54:439–44.

46. Arbel Y, Zlotnik M, Halkin A, et al. Admission glucose, fasting glucose, HbA1c levels and the SYNTAX score in non-diabetic patients undergoing coronary angiography. Clin Res Cardiol 2014;103:223–7.

47. Yan LQ, Cao XF, Zheng Y, et al. Association of cystatin C-based glomerular filtration rate with SYNTAX score in patients with diabetes. Exp Clin Endocrinol Diabetes 2013;121:455–60.

48. Ucar H, Gur M, Seker T, et al. Impaired kidney function is associated with SYNTAX score in patients with stable coronary artery disease. Turk Kardiyol Dern Ars 2014;42:621–8.

49. Kurtul A, Murat SN, Yarlioglues M, et al. Usefulness of serum albumin concentration to predict high coronary SYNTAX score and in-hospital mortality in patients with acute coronary syndrome. Angiology 2016;67:34–40.

50. Ashfaq F, Goel PK, Moorthy N, et al. Lipoprotein(a) and SYNTAX score association with severity of coronary artery atherosclerosis in north India. Sultan Qaboos Univ Med J 2012;12:465–72.

51. Sahin DY, Gur M, Elbasan Z, et al. NT-proBNP is associated with SYNTAX score and aortic distensibility in patients with stable CAD. Herz 2013;38:922–7.

52. Altun B, Turkon H, Tasolar H, et al. The relationship between high-sensitive troponin T, neutrophil lymphocyte ratio and SYNTAX score. Scand J Clin Lab Invest 2014;74:108–15.

53. Karadeniz M, Duran M, Akyel A, et al. High sensitive CRP level is associated with intermediate and high syntax score in patients with acute coronary syndrome. Int Heart J 2015;56:377–80.

54. Chi J, Hong X, Wang Y, et al. Inverse correlation between circulating endothelial progenitor cells with CD34+CD133+ and the severity of coronary atherosclerosis assessed by Syntax score. Am J Med Sci 2014;347:457–62.

55. Kim JD, Lee SH, Seo EH, et al. Role of Th1 and Th17 cells in the development and complexity of coronary artery disease: comparison analysis by

the methods of flow cytometry and SYNTAX score. Coron Artery Dis 2015;26(7):604–11.

56. Kurtul S, Sarli B, Baktir AO, et al. Neutrophil to lymphocyte ratio predicts SYNTAX score in patients with non-ST segment elevation myocardial infarction. Int Heart J 2015;56:18–21.

57. Sahin DY, Gur M, Elbasan Z, et al. Relationship between myocardial performance index and severity of coronary artery disease assessed with SYNTAX score in stable coronary artery disease. Echocardiography 2013;30:385–91.

58. Liu S, Moussa M, Wassef AW, et al. The utility of systolic and diastolic echocardiographic parameters for predicting coronary artery disease burden as defined by the SYNTAX score. Echocardiography 2015. [Epub ahead of print].

59. Tanaka H, Chikamori T, Hida S, et al. Relationship of SYNTAX score to myocardial ischemia as assessed on myocardial perfusion imaging. Circ J 2013;77:2772–7.

60. van Gaal WJ, Ponnuthurai FA, Selvanayagam J, et al. The Syntax score predicts peri-procedural myocardial necrosis during percutaneous coronary intervention. Int J Cardiol 2009;135:60–5.

61. Ikeda N, Kogame N, Iijima R, et al. Impact of carotid artery ultrasound and ankle-brachial index on prediction of severity of SYNTAX score. Circ J 2013;77:712–6.

62. Ikeda N, Saba L, Molinari F, et al. Automated carotid intima-media thickness and its link for prediction of SYNTAX score in Japanese coronary artery disease patients. Int Angiol 2013;32:339–48.

63. Ikeda N, Kogame N, Iijima R, et al. Carotid artery intima-media thickness and plaque score can predict the SYNTAX score. Eur Heart J 2012;33:113–9.

64. Xiong Z, Zhu C, Zheng Z, et al. Relationship between arterial stiffness assessed by brachial-ankle pulse wave velocity and coronary artery disease severity assessed by the SYNTAX score. J Atheroscler Thromb 2012;19:970–6.

65. Lemesle G, Bonello L, de Labriolle A, et al. Prognostic value of the Syntax score in patients undergoing coronary artery bypass grafting for three-vessel coronary artery disease. Catheter Cardiovasc Interv 2009;73:612–7.

66. Holzhey DM, Luduena MM, Rastan A, et al. Is the SYNTAX score a predictor of long-term outcome after coronary artery bypass surgery? Heart Surg Forum 2010;13:E143–8.

67. Gannot S, Fefer P, Kopel E, et al. Higher syntax score is not predictive of late mortality in "real-world" patients with multivessel coronary artery disease undergoing coronary artery bypass grafting. Isr Med Assoc J 2014;16:764–7.

68. Feldman T. The SYNTAX score in practice: an aid for patient selection for complex PCI. Catheter Cardiovasc Interv 2009;73:618–9.

69. Capodanno D, Capranzano P, Di Salvo ME, et al. Usefulness of SYNTAX score to select patients with left main coronary artery disease to be treated with coronary artery bypass graft. JACC Cardiovasc Interv 2009;2:731–8.

70. Capodanno D, Miano M, Cincotta G, et al. Euro-SCORE refines the predictive ability of SYNTAX score in patients undergoing left main percutaneous coronary intervention. Am Heart J 2010; 159:103–9.

71. Farooq V, Brugaletta S, Serruys PW. The SYNTAX score and SYNTAX-based clinical risk scores. Semin Thorac Cardiovasc Surg 2011;23:99–105.

72. Capodanno D. Beyond the SYNTAX score–advantages and limitations of other risk assessment systems in left main percutaneous coronary intervention. Circ J 2013;77:1131–8.

73. Farooq V, Head SJ, Kappetein AP, et al. Widening clinical applications of the SYNTAX score. Heart 2014;100:276–87.

74. Yadav M, Palmerini T, Caixeta A, et al. Prediction of coronary risk by SYNTAX and derived scores: synergy between percutaneous coronary intervention with taxus and cardiac surgery. J Am Coll Cardiol 2013;62:1219–30.

75. Chen SL, Chen JP, Mintz G, et al. Comparison between the NERS (new risk stratification) score and the SYNTAX (synergy between percutaneous coronary intervention with taxus and cardiac surgery) score in outcome prediction for unprotected left main stenting. JACC Cardiovasc Interv 2010;3: 632–41.

76. Chen SL, Han YL, Zhang YJ, et al. The anatomic- and clinical-based NERS (new risk stratification) score II to predict clinical outcomes after stenting unprotected left main coronary artery disease: results from a multicenter, prospective, registry study. JACC Cardiovasc Interv 2013;6: 1233–41.

77. Capodanno D, Caggegi A, Miano M, et al. Global risk classification and clinical SYNTAX (synergy between percutaneous coronary intervention with TAXUS and cardiac surgery) score in patients undergoing percutaneous or surgical left main revascularization. JACC Cardiovasc Interv 2011;4: 287–97.

78. Capodanno D, Capranzano P, Tamburino C. A post-hoc analysis of the CUSTOMIZE Registry on the differential impact of EuroSCORE and SYNTAX score in left main patients with intermediate global risk. Int J Cardiol 2011;150:116–7.

79. Serruys PW, Farooq V, Vranckx P, et al. A global risk approach to identify patients with left main or 3-vessel disease who could safely and efficaciously be treated with percutaneous coronary intervention: the SYNTAX trial at 3 years. JACC Cardiovasc Interv 2012;5:606–17.

80. Garg S, Sarno G, Garcia-Garcia HM, et al. A new tool for the risk stratification of patients with complex coronary artery disease: the clinical SYNTAX score. Circ Cardiovasc Interv 2010;3:317–26.

81. Jou YL, Lu TM, Chen YH, et al. Comparison of the predictive value of EuroSCORE, SYNTAX score, and clinical SYNTAX score for outcomes of patients undergoing percutaneous coronary intervention for unprotected left main coronary artery disease. Catheter Cardiovasc Interv 2012; 80:222–30.

82. Hara H, Aoki J, Tanabe K, et al. Impact of the clinical syntax score on 5-year clinical outcomes after sirolimus-eluting stents implantation. Cardiovasc Interv Ther 2013;28:258–66.

83. Farooq V, Vergouwe Y, Raber L, et al. Combined anatomical and clinical factors for the long-term risk stratification of patients undergoing percutaneous coronary intervention: the Logistic Clinical SYNTAX score. Eur Heart J 2012;33:3098–104.

84. Farooq V, Vergouwe Y, Genereux P, et al. Prediction of 1-year mortality in patients with acute coronary syndromes undergoing percutaneous coronary intervention: validation of the logistic clinical SYNTAX (synergy between percutaneous coronary interventions with taxus and cardiac surgery) score. JACC Cardiovasc Interv 2013;6:737–45.

85. Iqbal J, Vergouwe Y, Bourantas CV, et al. Predicting 3-year mortality after percutaneous coronary intervention: updated logistic clinical SYNTAX score based on patient-level data from 7 contemporary stent trials. JACC Cardiovasc Interv 2014;7: 464–70.

86. Capodanno D. Lost in calculation: the clinical SYNTAX score goes logistic. Eur Heart J 2012; 33:3008–10.

87. Capodanno D, Giacoppo D, Dipasqua F, et al. Usefulness of the logistic clinical SYNTAX score for predicting 1-year mortality in patients undergoing percutaneous coronary intervention of the left main coronary artery. Catheter Cardiovasc Interv 2013;82:E446–52.

88. Nam CW, Mangiacapra F, Entjes R, et al. Functional SYNTAX score for risk assessment in multivessel coronary artery disease. J Am Coll Cardiol 2011;58:1211–8.

89. Novara M, D'Ascenzo F, Gonella A, et al. Changing of SYNTAX score performing fractional flow reserve in multivessel coronary artery disease. J Cardiovasc Med (Hagerstown) 2012;13:368–75.

90. Dehnee A, Gerula C, Mazza V, et al. The functional SYNTAX score - a huge step forward or research in motion? J Invasive Cardiol 2012;24:304–5.

91. Tanboga IH, Aksakal E, Kurt M, et al. Computed tomography-based SYNTAX score: a case report. Eurasian J Med 2013;45:65–7.

92. Papadopoulou SL, Girasis C, Dharampal A, et al. CT-SYNTAX score: a feasibility and reproducibility study. JACC Cardiovasc Imaging 2013;6:413–5.

93. Kerner A, Abadi S, Abergel E, et al. Direct comparison between coronary computed tomography and invasive angiography for calculation of SYNTAX score. EuroIntervention 2013;8:1428–34.

94. Ugur M, Uluganyan M, Cicek G, et al. The reliability of computed tomography-derived SYNTAX score measurement. Angiology 2015;66:150–4.

95. Suh YJ, Hong YJ, Lee HJ, et al. Prognostic value of SYNTAX score based on coronary computed tomography angiography. Int J Cardiol 2015;199:460–6.

96. Wolny R, Jastrzebski J, Szubielski M, et al. Coronary computed tomography angiography for the assessment of the SYNTAX score. Kardiol Pol 2015. [Epub ahead of print].

97. Genereux P, Palmerini T, Caixeta A, et al. Quantification and impact of untreated coronary artery disease after percutaneous coronary intervention: the residual SYNTAX (Synergy Between PCI with Taxus and Cardiac Surgery) score. J Am Coll Cardiol 2012;59:2165–74.

98. Capodanno D, Chisari A, Giacoppo D, et al. Objectifying the impact of incomplete revascularization by repeat angiographic risk assessment with the residual SYNTAX score after left main coronary artery percutaneous coronary intervention. Catheter Cardiovasc Interv 2013;82:333–40.

99. Schwietz T, Spyridopoulos I, Pfeiffer S, et al. Risk stratification following complex PCI: clinical versus anatomical risk stratification including "post PCI residual SYNTAX-score" as quantification of incomplete revascularization. J Interv Cardiol 2013;26:29–37.

100. Malkin CJ, George V, Ghobrial MS, et al. Residual SYNTAX score after PCI for triple vessel coronary artery disease: quantifying the adverse effect of incomplete revascularisation. EuroIntervention 2013;8:1286–95.

101. Farooq V, Serruys PW, Bourantas CV, et al. Quantification of incomplete revascularization and its association with five-year mortality in the synergy between percutaneous coronary intervention with taxus and cardiac surgery (SYNTAX) trial validation of the residual SYNTAX score. Circulation 2013;128:141–51.

102. Witberg G, Lavi I, Assali A, et al. The incremental impact of residual SYNTAX score on long-term clinical outcomes in patients with multivessel coronary artery disease treated by percutaneous coronary interventions. Catheter Cardiovasc Interv 2015;86:3–10.

103. Farooq V, Girasis C, Magro M, et al. The CABG SYNTAX Score - an angiographic tool to grade the complexity of coronary disease following coronary artery bypass graft surgery: from the SYNTAX left

main angiographic (SYNTAX-LE MANS) substudy. EuroIntervention 2013;8:1277–85.

104. Farooq V, Girasis C, Magro M, et al. The coronary artery bypass graft SYNTAX score: final five-year outcomes from the SYNTAX-LE MANS left main angiographic substudy. EuroIntervention 2013;9: 1009–10.

105. Farooq V, van Klaveren D, Steyerberg EW, et al. Anatomical and clinical characteristics to guide decision making between coronary artery bypass surgery and percutaneous coronary intervention for individual patients: development and validation of SYNTAX score II. Lancet 2013;381:639–50.

106. Xu B, Genereux P, Yang Y, et al. Validation and comparison of the long-term prognostic capability of the SYNTAX score-II among 1,528 consecutive patients who underwent left main percutaneous coronary intervention. JACC Cardiovasc Interv 2014;7:1128–37.

107. Campos CM, Garcia-Garcia HM, van Klaveren D, et al. Validity of SYNTAX score II for risk stratification of percutaneous coronary interventions: a patient-level pooled analysis of 5,433 patients enrolled in contemporary coronary stent trials. Int J Cardiol 2015;187:111–5.

108. Tajik P, Oude Rengerink K, Mol BW, et al. SYNTAX score II. Lancet 2013;381:1899.

109. Campos CM, Stanetic BM, Farooq V, et al. Risk stratification in 3-vessel coronary artery disease: applying the SYNTAX score II in the heart team discussion of the SYNTAX II trial. Catheter Cardiovasc Interv 2015;86(6):E229–38.

110. Campos CM, van Klaveren D, Farooq V, et al. Long-term forecasting and comparison of mortality in the evaluation of the Xience everolimus eluting stent vs. coronary artery bypass surgery for effectiveness of left main revascularization (EXCEL) trial: prospective validation of the SYNTAX score II. Eur Heart J 2015;36:1231–41.

Acute Myocardial Infarction/Thrombectomy

Jonathan Soverow, MD, MPH*, Manish A. Parikh, MD

KEYWORDS

- Thrombectomy • Cardiogenic shock • Acute myocardial infarction • Culprit lesion

---

KEY POINTS

- Although the benefits of routine upfront thrombectomy are uncertain, aspiration may be necessary in bailout situations.
- Recent randomized trials suggest complete revascularization should be considered during the index hospitalization for ST-segment myocardial infarction.
- Few data support the use of intra-aortic balloon pump in acute myocardial infarction complicated by shock; newer devices may offer essential hemodynamic support in select cases.

THROMBECTOMY

The histopathologic hallmark of acute myocardial infarction (AMI) is plaque rupture and attendant thrombus formation, which can either be occlusive (leading to ST-elevation MI [STEMI]) or partially occlusive (unstable angina or non-STEMI). The goal of thrombectomy during AMI is to debulk intraluminal thrombus to prevent its downstream embolization and to improve flow and visualization (Fig. 1). Theoretically, this should enhance myocardial perfusion and facilitate procedural success. In fact, observational studies associate high thrombus burden with worse outcomes and higher stent thrombosis rates.[1]

Early trials supported this concept and even demonstrated a mortality advantage to upfront routine thrombectomy in STEMI. However, later evidence and a large randomized controlled trial published in 2015 have dimmed enthusiasm. Despite these recent data, a full discussion of thrombectomy and available devices is warranted, because interventionalists need familiarity with them for use, at minimum, as a bailout adjunct to AMI cases where heavy thrombus burden forestalls successful achievement of thrombolysis in MI (TIMI) grade 3 flow.

Mechanical Thrombectomy

Mechanical thrombectomy devices use moving, machine-driven parts to macerate and aspirate clot. Although they succeed at debulking large-volume thrombus, the evidence supporting their routine use is lacking. Previous devices included the Transluminal Extraction Catheter (InterVentional Technologies, Inc., San Diego, CA) and X-Sizer (eV3, White Bear Lake, MN). Currently, the only Food and Drug Administration (FDA)-approved mechanical thrombectomy device for AMI, Angiojet (Boston Scientific, Marlborough, MA), uses rheolytic thrombectomy (RT) to break up and remove thrombus. The 6F catheter–compatible system is intended for use in vessels larger than 2 mm in diameter with angiographic evidence of thrombus. High-velocity saline jets in the device's nose-cone fire into the diseased region, physically tearing the thrombus apart and creating a low-pressure vacuum via the Venturi-Bernoulli effect to aspirate debris (Fig. 2).

Angiojet was approved in 1999 based on a saphenous vein graft study (VEGAS-2) that demonstrated superiority to intragraft urokinase infusion.[2] It was later studied in two larger randomized trials (AiMI [AngioJet Rheolytic Thrombectomy in Patients Undergoing Primary

Disclosure Statement: The authors have nothing to disclose.
Center for Interventional Vascular Therapy, Columbia-Presbyterian Hospital, 161 Fort Washington Avenue, Herbert Irving Pavilion, 6th Floor, New York, NY 10032, USA
* Corresponding author.
E-mail address: jonathan.soverow@gmail.com

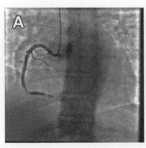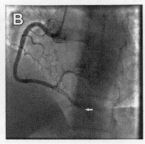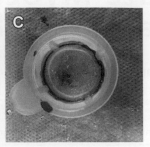

Fig. 1. Acute thrombotic occlusion of right coronary artery before (A) and after thrombectomy (B). Residual, distal thrombus (*arrow*) could not be recovered. (C) Thrombus retrieved using manual aspiration thrombectomy. (*Courtesy of* Jonathan Soverow, MD, MPH, Columbia-Presbyterian Hospital, New York, NY.)

Angioplasty for Acute Myocardial Infarction] and JETSTENT [AngioJet Rheolytic Thrombectomy Before Direct Infarct Artery Stenting in Patients Undergoing Primary PCI for Acute Myocardial Infarction]), which raised concerns about the device's safe use in the setting of AMI.

The AiMI trial randomized 480 patients presenting within 12 hours with STEMI by electrocardiogram (EKG) criteria to RT versus percutaneous coronary intervention (PCI) alone.[3] Of note, visible thrombus was not required for enrollment. Patients with high-risk features, such as cardiogenic shock, ejection fraction less than 35%, and recent stroke, were excluded. The primary end point, infarct size as measured by sestamibi imaging at 14 to 28 days, was higher in the RT group. There were no differences in tissue myocardial perfusion blush or ST-segment resolution. In addition, 30-day major adverse cardiac event (MACE) was higher in the RT group (6.7% vs 1.7%; $P = .01$), driven primarily by higher mortality rates (4.6% vs 0.8%; $P = .02$). Only around 20% of patients had moderate-high thrombus burden at baseline, but use of RT in this subset did not reduce infarct size compared with PCI alone. Nearly 60% of patients in the RT group had upfront temporary pacing wires placed. In their discussion, the

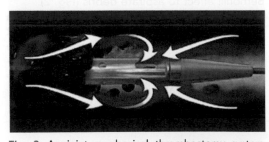

Fig. 2. Angiojet mechanical thrombectomy system. High-pressure saline jets create a vacuum effect that allows maceration and aspiration of large-volume thrombus. (Image provided *courtesy of* Boston Scientific. © 2016 Boston Scientific Corporation or its affiliates. All rights reserved.)

study investigators highlighted that introduction of the device into the artery takes longer and may embolize debris. In addition, the study itself was not powered to detect differences in mortality, which had an extremely low rate in the PCI-alone group (0.8%) at 1 month and became nonsignificant at 6 months (5.8% vs 2.1%; $P = .06$).

The JETSTENT trial attempted to redress these outcomes by refocusing the target population.[4] The JETSTENT trial randomized 501 patients with STEMI in a greater than 2.5-mm vessel and with visible thrombus to RT versus direct stenting. Moreover, in contrast to AiMI, the JETSTENT protocol required the device be activated before crossing the lesion. Although ST-segment resolution, 6-month MACE (11.2% vs 19.4%; $P = .011$), and 12-month event-free survival rates (85.2% vs 75.0%; $P = .009$) were improved with Angiojet, there was no difference again in infarct size. These results may emphasize the need for stricter patient selection, suggesting that those most likely to benefit have significant thrombus burden in larger diameter vessels, and the need to turn on the device before advancing through the lesion. Of note, temporary pacemaker was rarely needed (0.7%) despite prior experience suggesting high rates of bradycardia with the use of AngioJet.

Another mechanical thrombectomy device, the X-Sizer, received FDA approval for PCI and was evaluated in AMI, but is not currently available in most markets. The X-Sizer was a dual-lumen over-the-wire device that used a motorized, helical cutter to dislodge thrombus paired with an aspiration port attached to a vacuum. The X AMINE ST trial (X-Sizer in AMI for Negligible Embolization and Optimal ST Resolution) randomized 201 patients with STEMI and TIMI 0 to 1 grade flow to X-Sizer thrombectomy versus PCI alone.[5] Use of the device was associated with improved ST-segment resolution and a reduction in the occurrence of distal embolization, but without significant differences in TIMI flow grade, myocardial blush, and 6-month major adverse cardiac and cerebrovascular events. The device was compared with manual aspiration in a small trial randomizing 201 patients with AMI; overall outcomes were similar, but the X-Sizer proved difficult to deploy and traverse lesions.[6]

Manual Thrombectomy

Manual aspiration thrombectomy uses a dual-lumen catheter in either rapid exchange or over-the-wire format with a second port attached to a vacuum syringe that is activated by the operator on reaching the target lesion. The catheters are available in a variety of sizes, shapes, and crossing profiles, each with specific characteristics designed to address a diverse set of lesions. Beyond thrombectomy, these catheters may be used off-label to deliver medications (eg, vasodilators, such as nitroprusside, nicardipine, and adenosine) to a distal coronary target, particularly in the case of distal embolization with no reflow.

The foundational evidence informing use of manual aspiration rests on three large randomized trials: TAPAS (Thrombus Aspiration during Percutaneous Coronary Intervention in Acute Myocardial Infarction Study; 2008), TASTE (Thrombus Aspiration in ST-Elevation Myocardial Infarction in Scandinavia; 2013), and TOTAL (Trial of Routine Aspiration Thrombectomy with PCI versus PCI Alone in Patients with EKG-defined STEMI; 2015) (Table 1).

TAPAS was a single-center, prospective randomized trial conducted at the University Medical Center Groningen, the Netherlands.[7] The study randomized 1071 patients with EKG criteria for STEMI to manual aspiration with the 6F catheter Export catheter (Medtronic, Minneapolis, MN) versus PCI alone. Thrombus burden and vessel size were not part of enrollment criteria. The primary end point was the frequency of myocardial blush grade 0 to 1, with secondary end points including TIMI flow grade, target vessel revascularization, and MACE at 30 days. Manual aspiration improved ST-segment resolution (56.6% vs 44.2%; $P < .001$) and myocardial blush grade (17.1% vs 26.3%; $P < .001$). There was no statistical difference in MACE at 30 days (6.8% vs 9.4%; $P = .12$), but in those patients who achieved myocardial blush grade 0 to 1, which was more common in the aspiration group, MACE and overall mortality were significantly reduced, a finding that persisted out to 1-year follow-up.[8] Limitations of this trial include its single-center enrollment and fact that it was powered to detect differences in a surrogate end point, not major clinical events. A meta-analysis of nine randomized trials including a total of 2417 patients (with TAPAS contributing 1071 of those) reported improved TIMI 3 flow, myocardial blush grade, and a reduction in 30-day mortality (1.7% vs 3.1%; $P = .04$) with use of manual aspiration thrombectomy.[9]

However, a large randomized trial conducted within a prospective registry did not corroborate these findings. The TASTE trial was a multicenter, prospective, open-label, randomized trial conducted within the Swedish Coronary Angiography and Angioplasty Registry.[10] A total of 7244 patients with EKG-validated STEMI were randomized to manual thrombus aspiration versus PCI alone; the trial was powered to detect a mortality difference. At 30 days, there was no significant difference in the rate of MACE or its composite end points, including mortality and stroke, or stent thrombosis. These trends persisted to 1 year of follow-up, including null findings in overall MACE, death, stent thrombosis, and rehospitalization for MI.[11] Limitations of TASTE include its nested study design, lack of blinding, and of centralized event adjudication.

To clarify these mixed data, a dedicated, large, multicenter, randomized controlled trial was designed and powered to address a primary

Table 1 Manual aspiration thrombectomy: major RCTs					
Trial	Publication Date	Size	Device	30-d MACE Thrombectomy Arm	30-d MACE Control Arm
TAPAS	2008	1071	Export	6.8%	9.4%
TASTE	2013	7244	Multiple	3.3%[a]	3.9%[a]
TOTAL	2015	10,732	Export	6.9%	7.0%

Abbreviations: RCT, randomized controlled trial; TAPAS, Thrombus Aspiration During Percutaneous Coronary Intervention in Acute Myocardial Infarction study; TASTE, Thrombus Aspiration in ST-Elevation Myocardial Infarction in Scandinavia trial; TOTAL, Trial of Routine Aspiration Thrombectomy with PCI versus PCI Alone in Patients with EKG-defined STEMI.
[a] Mortality or myocardial infarction.

composite outcome of cardiovascular death, shock, or heart failure with a primary safety outcome of stroke within 30 days. The TOTAL randomized 10,732 patients with STEMI to upfront aspiration using the Export catheter versus PCI alone.[12] There were no significant differences in the rates of the primary outcome (6.9% vs 7.0%; P = .86) or of cardiovascular death (3.1% vs 3.5%; P = .34), stent thrombosis, or target vessel revascularization at 180 days. However, there was a suggestion of possible harm, because 30-day stroke rates were higher in the thrombectomy group (0.7% vs 0.3%; P = .02).

This increased stroke risk had been observed in prior meta-analyses of thrombectomy.[13] This has led to concern that the device may be a source of embolus (either thrombus or air). However, studies have shown an increase in acute and subacute (30–180 days) stroke rates, although there were immediate differences within the immediate 48-hour window.[14] In any case, these findings emphasize the need to fully aspirate the guide catheter after the thrombectomy device is removed. Of note, a follow-up substudy of 214 patients in TOTAL showed no reduction in culprit thrombus volume as assessed by optical coherence tomography.[15]

The 2013 American College of Cardiology Foundation/American Heart Association (ACCF/AHA) STEMI guidelines had already downgraded the use of aspiration thrombectomy to IIa and a 2015 update further downgraded it to class III (no benefit or harm).[16] Based on available data, aspiration thrombectomy has thus been relegated to bailout in cases of heavy thrombus burden and poor flow, which occurred in 7.1% of cases in the PCI-only arm of TOTAL. Given that frequency, familiarity with thrombectomy devices is important. However, attention to proper technique and meticulous guide aspiration to prevent device-related embolism are warranted.

MULTIVESSEL CORONARY DISEASE

Approximately 40% to 65% patients presenting with AMI have significant nonculprit coronary artery disease.[17,18] The 2013 ACCF/AHA STEMI guidelines rate PCI of nonculprit lesions in a hemodynamically stable patient class III.[19] These prior guidelines draw on case-control studies that suggest complete revascularization increases mortality during the index procedure.[20–22] However, because these studies are largely observational, they are subject to significant residual confounding. A series of new, prospective randomized trials challenge these data

and have led to a revision in the 2015 guidelines, upgrading noninfarct intervention to a class IIb recommendation.[16]

The PRAMI (Prevention Angioplasty in Acute Myocardial Infarction) trial randomized 465 patients with STEMI to culprit-only versus complete revascularization during the index procedure of all lesions with greater than 50% stenosis.[23] After a mean follow-up of 23 months, a significant mortality benefit in the complete revascularization arm (hazard ratio, 0.34; P < .001) resulted in early study termination. Rates of nonfatal MI and refractory angina were also significantly improved by upfront nonculprit intervention.

Although early termination threatens the precision of clinical trials, two additional randomized trials support the concept of early complete revascularization following STEMI. The CvLPRIT (Complete versus Lesion-only Primary PCI Trial) randomized 296 patients with STEMI to culprit-only or complete revascularization.[24] Nonculprit PCI was performed either during the index procedure or later during the same hospitalization. The composite of death, MI, heart failure, and ischemia-driven revascularization at 12 months favored early complete revascularization (10.0% vs 21.2%; P = .009), although the individual end points were nonsignificant. Similarly, the DANAMI-3-PRIMULTI (Third Danish Study of Optimal Acute Treatment of Patients with ST-segment Elevation Myocardial Infarction Primary PCI in Multivessel Disease) trial randomized 627 patients with STEMI to culprit-alone or fractional flow reserve–guided complete revascularization and demonstrated a 44% reduction in the composite end point of death, MI, or revascularization at 12 months.[25]

A meta-analysis including these trials and just over 1000 patients found a summary relative risk ratio of 0.57 (P = .02) for all-cause mortality favoring multivessel PCI during the index hospitalization.[26] Although an individualized approach should be undertaken to any patient presenting with AMI and multivessel disease, these data suggest nonculprit PCI should be considered in the appropriately selected patient. Based on current data, it is unclear if it should be performed at the index procedure or staged later in the initial hospitalization and whether to use a fractional flow reserve–guided strategy. Further direction should come from a large multicenter randomized trial, the COMPLETE (Culprit-only Revascularization to Treat Multivessel Disease After Primary PCI for STEMI) trial (NCT01740479), which intends to randomize 4000 patients with STEMI to culprit-only versus complete revascularization.

CARDIOGENIC SHOCK

In most trials, cardiogenic shock requires a systolic blood pressure less than 90 mm Hg with evidence of end-organ damage, a cardiac index less than 2.2 L/min/m^2, and a pulmonary capillary wedge pressure greater than 15.[27,28] Cardiogenic shock complicates 5% to 8% of AMI and is associated with a 59% to 66% mortality rate at 3 to 6 years.[29] Prompt revascularization, as demonstrated by the SHOCK trial, improves mortality with a 13% absolute risk reduction at 6 months that extends out to 1 year of follow-up.[30]

There is a paucity of data to guide treatment decisions otherwise. Minimal evidence supports one pressor or inotropic medication over others, although the SOAP II (Sepsis Occurrence in Acutely Ill Patients) trial in patients with septic shock suggests that dopamine may be more arrhythmogenic compared with norepinephrine.[31,32] Although clinical trials advocating the use of percutaneous ventricular support devices provide mixed results, these devices can provide essential backup cardiac output in cardiogenic shock.

The most widely available options include intra-aortic balloon pump (IABP), Impella (Abiomed, Inc, Danvers, MA), TandemHeart (CardiacAssist, Inc, Pittsburgh, PA), and extracorporeal membrane oxygenation (ECMO). Precise indications for hemodynamic support do not exist, but each device offers a variety of strengths and weaknesses (Table 2).

Intra-aortic Balloon Pump

The fastest to place of the devices listed, IABP augments diastolic coronary blood flow and reduces afterload, leading to a compensatory reduction in left ventricular end-diastolic pressure, wall tension, cardiac work, and heart rate. At best, physiologic studies demonstrate modest unloading of the left ventricle with a rise in mean arterial blood pressure, but the exact impact on coronary flow past a physiologically significant lesion is controversial.[33]

An IABP may be inserted via femoral or axillary approaches with 7.5F to 8.0F catheter sheath and is contraindicated in cases of severe peripheral arterial disease, aortic dissection, or aortic insufficiency. Major complications encompass vascular access, limb ischemia, infection, stroke, and renal failure; daily rounds on a patient with IABP should include assessment of ongoing need for the device, location, anticoagulation, and the pressure waveform to ensure appropriate timing, diastolic augmentation, and systolic unloading.

These untoward risks may counterbalance the benefits of IABP. The device was used in greater than 80% of patients in both arms of the SHOCK trial, and retrospective analysis suggested that it conferred a reduction in mortality.[34] However, little overall benefit was found in AMI in the two randomized trials of IABP: CRISP-AMI (Counter-pulsation to Reduce Infarct Size Pre-PCI Acute Myocardial Infarction) and IABP-SHOCK II (Intraaortic Balloon Pump Shock II).

The CRISP-AMI trial randomized 337 patients with anterior MI without cardiogenic shock to IABP within 6 hours versus standard care.[35] Although it was powered to assess a primary end point of mean infarct size using cardiac MRI 3 to 5 days postintervention, there was no differences in this or other major clinical end points, including ejection fraction, vascular complications, bleeding, or 6-month MACE. The crossover rate was 8.5% from PCI-only to IABP-assisted arm. Critics argue that randomized patients were less sick and with little to gain from IABP.

Table 2
Percutaneous ventricular support devices

Device	Cardiac Support (L/min)	Arterial Sheath/ Cannula Size	Advantages	Disadvantages
IABP	0.5–1.0	7–8F catheter	Rapid placement	Minimal support Negative outcomes data
Impella	2.5–5.0	12F (2.5) catheter 14F (4.0) catheter 21F (5.0) catheter	Rapid placement Low profile	Multiple contraindications Expense
TandemHeart	2.0–5.0	15F–19F catheter	VSD Aortic insufficiency	Laborious placement Expense
ECMO	>3.0	15F–17F catheter	Rapid placement	Requires perfusion team Does not unload LV

Abbreviations: LV, left ventricle; VSD, ventricular septal defect.

The IABP-SHOCK II trial randomized 598 patients with AMI and cardiogenic shock to IABP versus primary PCI alone.[36] Inclusion criteria included systolic blood pressure less than 90 mm Hg for 30 minutes or requiring infusion of catecholamines, pulmonary edema, and presence of end-organ damage as evidenced by altered mental status, cool extremities, oliguria, or elevated lactate. Patients were excluded if they had a mechanical cause of cardiogenic shock (acute mitral regurgitation or ventricular septal defect), moderate aortic regurgitation, or severe peripheral vascular disease (in addition to usual exclusion criteria of age and overall health status). Crossover from control group was permitted only if mechanical complications developed following enrollment. At 30 days, there was no difference in mortality (39.7% vs 41.3%; $P = .69$) in the IABP and primary PCI groups, respectively. Furthermore, length of stay, dose and duration of pressors, kidney function, or serum lactate levels were not significantly different. However, there were no differences with regard to harm; rates of major bleeding (3.3% vs 4.4%; $P = .51$), peripheral ischemic complications (4.3% vs 3.4%; $P = .53$), sepsis, and stroke were similar. Unfortunately, the crossover rate was 10%, most of which constituted protocol violations. That said, the findings persisted to 6 and 12 months followup, and a per-protocol analysis of IABP use revealed no advantage to the device.[37] Although the study was powered to detect an absolute difference of 12% in the primary outcome between groups, and the event rate was lower than expected (calling into question the inclusion criteria), the nearly identical number of deaths in both groups suggest that a larger study would be unlikely to reveal a significant benefit. Results of the primary end points revealed no benefit in all prespecified and post hoc subgroups.

These data mirror the BCIS-1 (Balloon Pump-Assisted Coronary Intervention Study-1), which reported no benefit to prophylactic IABP use for high-risk elective PCI in the initial 30 days.[38] Of note, subsequent long-term analysis did find a mortality benefit. However, these results are difficult to interpret given the study's initial primary outcome.[39]

Overall, interest in IABP use has waned, with use in AMI complicated by cardiogenic shock in only 24.8% of cases and an even lower rate in high-risk PCI (10.5%).[40,41] The 2013 ACCF/AHA STEMI and 2014 ACCF/AHA non-STEMI guidelines provide IABP a class IIa recommendation, with the suggestion it be limited to those who "do not quickly stabilize with pharmacologic therapy."[19,42] In each of the trials discussed previously, the crossover rate from the control group was approximately 10%. However, given the lack of clinical benefit seen with IABP, including in meta-analyses, it may be advisable to use higher levels of support in patients with refractory shock.[43]

Impella

Impella is a nonpulsatile axial flow device inserted retrograde across the aortic valve into the left ventricle (Figs. 3 and 4). It is FDA-approved in multiple flavors, the most common being Impella 2.5 and Impella CP. The 2.5 variety offers 2.5 L/min output (12F catheter sheath), whereas CP offers up to 4.0 L/min (14F catheter sheath). Absolute contraindications include presence of an aortic mechanical valve, left ventricular thrombus, and severe peripheral artery disease (PAD); aortic stenosis, ventricular septal defect, and mitral regurgitation represent relative contraindications.

Major complications include vascular, limb ischemia, stroke, and hemolysis. Some clinicians prefer to advance the device across the aortic valve without a wire, as with standard pigtail

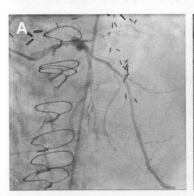 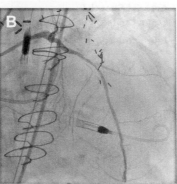

Fig. 3. (*A, B*) Percutaneous intervention of severe left main coronary artery disease in a patient with cardiogenic shock and occlusion of a left internal mammary to mid-left anterior descending artery. Placement of Impella CP device led to immediate improvement in blood pressure and symptoms. The device was removed at the end of the case and the arteriotomy closed with double Perclose sutures.

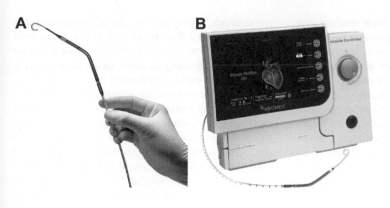

Fig. 4. Impella CP device (A) with controller (B). (*Courtesy of* Abiomed, Inc, Danvers, MA; with permission.)

catheter. Although this approach may avoid entrapment within the mitral apparatus and ensuing mitral regurgitation, the FDA Maude database has reported catheter kinking, requiring surgical removal.[44]

Most trials pitting IABP against Impella suggest greater cardiac output with the latter, without any difference in hard clinical end points. The ISAR-SHOCK study was a small, pilot study randomizing 25 patients to IABP versus Impella 2.5 and demonstrated a significant increase in cardiac index (0.49 L/min/m^2 vs 0.11 L/min/m^2; P = .02) in patients with cardiogenic shock, but with a higher incidence of hemolysis.[45]

The PROTECT II (Prospective Randomized Clinical Trial of Hemodynamic Support with Impella 2.5) trial randomized 452 patients with three-vessel disease or unprotected left main and reduced ejection fraction (<35%) to IABP versus Impella 2.5.[46] The trial intended to enroll greater than 600 patients, but was terminated early because of slow enrollment and futility at an interim data assessment. The primary composite end point of death, MI, stroke, repeat revascularization, renal insufficiency, intraprocedural hypotension, cardiac arrest, and procedure failure was similar between Impella and IABP at 30 and 90 days, respectively (35.1% vs 40.1%, P = .23; 40.6% vs 49.3%, P = .07) in the intention-to-treat analysis. However, the per-protocol analysis suggested benefit at the 90-day mark (40.0% vs 51.0%; P = .02).

An ongoing trial randomizing patients with AMI and CS to Impella versus IABP (IMPella vs IABP Reduces mortality in STEMI patients [IMPRESS; NTR3450]) will report results on a small number of participants (N = 48) once enrollment has finished.

Compared with IABP, Impella seems to offer more support at the expense of larger sheath size, increased complexity in terms of insertion and monitoring, and higher cost of the catheter. However, PROTECT II did not find a risk of increased adverse events compared with IABP. Although further data are pending, it is a reasonable alternative for cardiogenic shock and AMI. If possible, the access site should be "pre-closed" with two crisscrossed Perclose sutures so the device may be taken out in the laboratory and the arteriotomy closed.

In addition to stand-alone use in AMI and high-risk PCI, Impella may be used to "vent" or off load the left ventricle during ECMO. For patients with right ventricular failure or unstable arrhythmias, a new version of the device, Impella RP, has received limited approval from the FDA under humanitarian exemption; it was studied in a single arm trial, RECOVER-RIGHT, which demonstrated safety in 30 patients with acute right ventricular failure.[47]

TandemHeart

TandemHeart is an external centrifugal pump with intake cannula resting in the left atrium and output in the iliac artery. It can provide 3.5-5 L/min output depending on which arterial cannula is selected, 15F or 19F catheter. These larger sheath sizes in addition to a 21F catheter venous sheath, needed for transseptal access, and complex postprocedure maintenance with an experienced perfusion team make insertion of the TandemHeart more laborious than Impella for little additional support. Both devices have been used for extensive periods (up to 30 days or more), but have similar FDA approval for only up to 6 days. One advantage of Tandem-Heart is its use in decompensated aortic regurgitation or ventricular septal defect because it can circumvent flow across the ventricular septum, whereas the Impella cannula may theoretically worsen right-to-left shunting. The device requires right ventricular function or ventricular assist device support to ensure left atrium filling.

TandemHeart has not been well-studied in a prospective fashion. A single-center open-label study randomized 33 patients with cardiogenic shock to IABP or TandemHeart and found improvements in hemodynamic parameters with TandemHeart (decreased pulmonary capillary wedge pressure, increased cardiac index) but no difference in mortality.[48] Another randomized trial of IABP versus TandemHeart in 41 patients AMI with cardiogenic shock also demonstrated no benefit, but high rates of vascular complications with TandemHeart (7 of 20 patients had limb ischemia).[49]

Extracorporeal Membrane Oxygenation

Similar to bypass, ECMO can provide full cardiopulmonary support via shunting venous blood through an oxygenator and pump, but with the advantage of percutaneous access. Permutations include venovenous for pure oxygenation, venoarterial for hemodynamic support, and venoarterial-venous for hemodynamic and added oxygenation support. Typically used to bridge patients off cardiopulmonary bypass, ECMO is used in AMI complicated by cardiogenic shock or recurrent cardiac arrest with an otherwise viable health status and expected long-term need for support. ECMO requires large-bore arterial access (15F–17F catheter), an experienced perfusion team, and availability of the device, which now has smaller formats that enable interhospital transfer. In addition, therapeutic hypothermia/tight temperature control may be instituted through the circuit.

Registry and case series data reveal overall expected mortality of 51% to 73% for patients with cardiogenic shock treated with ECMO.[50–52] Compared with historical control subjects, early institution of ECMO in AMI with cardiogenic shock seems to improve 30-day mortality. However, prospective randomized trials evaluating its effectiveness have not been conducted.[53]

SUMMARY

Therapy for AMI continues to emerge. It has become clear that efficient and timely reperfusion of the culprit vessel is paramount. Primary PCI performed in a timely manner with experienced operators has yielded the best results for patients. The emphasis on door-to-balloon times is reasonable, and the method of reperfusion has many variables. The goal is restoration of flow and minimizing injury to the distal vascular bed. Guideline-based use of current anticoagulants and antiplatelet agents is paramount. Although the use of thrombectomy during primary PCI does not seem to benefit across large randomized trials the use must be tailored individually to each case. When flow is not restored with a guidewire or simple balloon inflation it is critical to assess the vessel and determine the reason for flow disruption. Simple aspiration thrombectomy in some cases facilitates restoration of flow and allows adequate decision-making regarding size and length of stents required to complete the case. Although primary PCI is not available in all geographies globally the authors do believe that certain key procedural elements should be maintained. Adequate assessment of left ventricular function and mechanical complications should be assessed as part of the STEMI index procedure and must not be overlooked during the race against the door-to-balloon time. The need for mechanical circulatory support devices has a growing body of literature and experience and should be considered in cases of cardiogenic shock or failed PCI in the AMI setting.

REFERENCES

1. Sianos G, Papafaklis MI, Daemen J, et al. Angiographic stent thrombosis after routine use of drug-eluting stents in ST-segment elevation myocardial infarction: the importance of thrombus burden. J Am Coll Cardiol 2007;50(7):573–83.
2. Kuntz RE, Baim DS, Cohen DJ, et al. A trial comparing rheolytic thrombectomy with intracoronary urokinase for coronary and vein graft thrombus (the Vein Graft AngioJet Study [VeGAS 2]). Am J Cardiol 2002;89(3):326–30.
3. Ali A, Cox D, Dib N, et al. Rheolytic thrombectomy with percutaneous coronary intervention for infarct size reduction in acute myocardial infarction: 30-day results from a multicenter randomized study. J Am Coll Cardiol 2006;48(2):244–52.
4. Migliorini A, Stabile A, Rodriguez AE, et al. Comparison of AngioJet rheolytic thrombectomy before direct infarct artery stenting with direct stenting alone in patients with acute myocardial infarction. The JETSTENT trial. J Am Coll Cardiol 2010;56(16):1298–306.
5. Lefevre T, Garcia E, Reimers B, et al. X-sizer for thrombectomy in acute myocardial infarction improves ST-segment resolution: results of the X-sizer in AMI for negligible embolization and optimal ST resolution (X AMINE ST) trial. J Am Coll Cardiol 2005;46(2):246–52.
6. Vink MA, Patterson MS, van Etten J, et al. A randomized comparison of manual versus mechanical thrombus removal in primary percutaneous coronary intervention in the treatment of

ST-segment elevation myocardial infarction (TREAT-MI). Catheter Cardiovasc Interv 2011;78(1):14–9.

7. Svilaas T, Vlaar PJ, van der Horst IC, et al. Thrombus aspiration during primary percutaneous coronary intervention. N Engl J Med 2008;358(6):557–67.

8. Vlaar PJ, Svilaas T, van der Horst IC, et al. Cardiac death and reinfarction after 1 year in the Thrombus Aspiration during Percutaneous coronary intervention in Acute myocardial infarction Study (TAPAS): a 1-year follow-up study. Lancet 2008;371(9628): 1915–20.

9. De Luca G, Dudek D, Sardella G, et al. Adjunctive manual thrombectomy improves myocardial perfusion and mortality in patients undergoing primary percutaneous coronary intervention for ST-elevation myocardial infarction: a meta-analysis of randomized trials. Eur Heart J 2008;29(24): 3002–10.

10. Frobert O, Lagerqvist B, Olivecrona GK, et al. Thrombus aspiration during ST-segment elevation myocardial infarction. N Engl J Med 2013;369(17): 1587–97.

11. Lagerqvist B, Frobert O, Olivecrona GK, et al. Outcomes 1 year after thrombus aspiration for myocardial infarction. N Engl J Med 2014;371(12):1111–20.

12. Jolly SS, Cairns JA, Yusuf S, et al. Randomized trial of primary PCI with or without routine manual thrombectomy. N Engl J Med 2015;372(15):1389–98.

13. Tamhane UU, Chetcuti S, Hameed I, et al. Safety and efficacy of thrombectomy in patients undergoing primary percutaneous coronary intervention for acute ST elevation MI: a meta-analysis of randomized controlled trials. BMC Cardiovasc Disord 2010;10:10.

14. Jolly SS, Cairns JA, Yusuf S, et al. Stroke in the TOTAL trial: a randomized trial of routine thrombectomy vs. percutaneous coronary intervention alone in ST elevation myocardial infarction. Eur Heart J 2015;36(35):2364–72.

15. Bhindi R, Kajander OA, Jolly SS, et al. Culprit lesion thrombus burden after manual thrombectomy or percutaneous coronary intervention-alone in ST-segment elevation myocardial infarction: the optical coherence tomography sub-study of the TOTAL (ThrOmbecTomy versus PCI ALone) trial. Eur Heart J 2015;36(29):1892–900.

16. Levine GN, Bates ER, Blankenship JC, et al. 2015 ACC/AHA/SCAI focused update on primary percutaneous coronary intervention for patients with ST-elevation myocardial infarction: an update of the 2011 ACCF/AHA/SCAI guideline for percutaneous coronary intervention and the 2013 ACCF/AHA guideline for the management of ST-elevation myocardial infarction: a report of the American College of Cardiology/American Heart Association Task Force on Clinical Practice Guidelines and the Society for Cardiovascular

Angiography and Interventions. Circulation 2015. [Epub ahead of print].

17. Jaski BE, Cohen JD, Trausch J, et al. Outcome of urgent percutaneous transluminal coronary angioplasty in acute myocardial infarction: comparison of single-vessel versus multivessel coronary artery disease. Am Heart J 1992;124(6):1427–33.

18. Muller DW, Topol EJ, Ellis SG, et al. Multivessel coronary artery disease: a key predictor of short-term prognosis after reperfusion therapy for acute myocardial infarction. Thrombolysis and Angioplasty in Myocardial Infarction (TAMI) Study Group. Am Heart J 1991;121(4 Pt 1):1042–9.

19. O'Gara PT, Kushner FG, Ascheim DD, et al. 2013 ACCF/AHA guideline for the management of ST-elevation myocardial infarction: a report of the American College of Cardiology Foundation/American Heart Association Task Force on Practice Guidelines. Circulation 2013;127(4):e362–425.

20. Hannan EL, Samadashvili Z, Walford G, et al. Culprit vessel percutaneous coronary intervention versus multivessel and staged percutaneous coronary intervention for ST-segment elevation myocardial infarction patients with multivessel disease. JACC Cardiovasc Interv 2010;3(1):22–31.

21. Toma M, Buller CE, Westerhout CM, et al. Non-culprit coronary artery percutaneous coronary intervention during acute ST-segment elevation myocardial infarction: insights from the APEX-AMI trial. Eur Heart J 2010;31(14):1701–7.

22. Vlaar PJ, Mahmoud KD, Holmes DR Jr, et al. Culprit vessel only versus multivessel and staged percutaneous coronary intervention for multivessel disease in patients presenting with ST-segment elevation myocardial infarction: a pairwise and network meta-analysis. J Am Coll Cardiol 2011;58(7): 692–703.

23. Wald DS, Morris JK, Wald NJ, et al. Randomized trial of preventive angioplasty in myocardial infarction. N Engl J Med 2013;369(12):1115–23.

24. Gershlick AH, Khan JN, Kelly DJ, et al. Randomized trial of complete versus lesion-only revascularization in patients undergoing primary percutaneous coronary intervention for STEMI and multivessel disease: the CvLPRIT trial. J Am Coll Cardiol 2015;65(10):963–72.

25. Engstrom T, Kelbaek H, Helqvist S, et al. Complete revascularisation versus treatment of the culprit lesion only in patients with ST-segment elevation myocardial infarction and multivessel disease (DANAMI-3-PRIMULTI): an open-label, randomised controlled trial. Lancet 2015;386(9994):665–71.

26. El-Hayek GE, Gershlick AH, Hong MK, et al. Meta-analysis of randomized controlled trials comparing multivessel versus culprit-only revascularization for patients with ST-segment elevation myocardial infarction and multivessel disease undergoing

primary percutaneous coronary intervention. Am J Cardiol 2015;115(11):1481–6.

27. Hochman JS, Sleeper LA, Webb JG, et al. Early revascularization in acute myocardial infarction complicated by cardiogenic shock. SHOCK Investigators. Should We Emergently Revascularize Occluded Coronaries for Cardiogenic Shock. N Engl J Med 1999;341(9):625–34.

28. Rihal CS, Naidu SS, Givertz MM, et al. 2015 SCAI/ACC/HFSA/STS clinical expert consensus statement on the use of percutaneous mechanical circulatory support devices in cardiovascular care: endorsed by the American Heart Association, the Cardiological Society of India, and Sociedad Latino Americana de Cardiologia Intervencionista; Affirmation of Value by the Canadian Association of Interventional Cardiology-Association Canadienne de Cardiologie d'intervention. J Am Coll Cardiol 2015;65(19):2140–1.

29. Reynolds HR, Hochman JS. Cardiogenic shock: current concepts and improving outcomes. Circulation 2008;117(5):686–97.

30. Hochman JS, Sleeper LA, White HD, et al. One-year survival following early revascularization for cardiogenic shock. JAMA 2001;285(2):190–2.

31. De Backer D, Biston P, Devriendt J, et al. Comparison of dopamine and norepinephrine in the treatment of shock. N Engl J Med 2010;362(9):779–89.

32. Unverzagt S, Wachsmuth L, Hirsch K, et al. Inotropic agents and vasodilator strategies for acute myocardial infarction complicated by cardiogenic shock or low cardiac output syndrome. Cochrane Database Syst Rev 2014;(1):CD009669.

33. Yoshitani H, Akasaka T, Kaji S, et al. Effects of intra-aortic balloon counterpulsation on coronary pressure in patients with stenotic coronary arteries. Am Heart J 2007;154(4):725–31.

34. Sanborn TA, Sleeper LA, Bates ER, et al. Impact of thrombolysis, intra-aortic balloon pump counterpulsation, and their combination in cardiogenic shock complicating acute myocardial infarction: a report from the SHOCK Trial Registry. SHould we emergently revascularize Occluded Coronaries for cardiogenic shocK? J Am Coll Cardiol 2000; 36(3 Suppl A):1123–9.

35. Patel MR, Smalling RW, Thiele H, et al. Intra-aortic balloon counterpulsation and infarct size in patients with acute anterior myocardial infarction without shock: the CRISP AMI randomized trial. JAMA 2011;306(12):1329–37.

36. Thiele H, Zeymer U, Neumann FJ, et al. Intraaortic balloon support for myocardial infarction with cardiogenic shock. N Engl J Med 2012;367(14):1287–96.

37. Thiele H, Zeymer U, Neumann FJ, et al. Intra-aortic balloon counterpulsation in acute myocardial infarction complicated by cardiogenic shock (IABP-SHOCK II): final 12 month results of a randomised, open-label trial. Lancet 2013;382(9905):1638–45.

38. Perera D, Stables R, Thomas M, et al. Elective intra-aortic balloon counterpulsation during high-risk percutaneous coronary intervention: a randomized controlled trial. JAMA 2010;304(8):867–74.

39. Perera D, Stables R, Clayton T, et al. Long-term mortality data from the Balloon Pump-Assisted Coronary Intervention Study (BCIS-1): a randomized, controlled trial of elective balloon counterpulsation during high-risk percutaneous coronary intervention. Circulation 2013;127(2):207–12.

40. Zeymer U, Bauer T, Hamm C, et al. Use and impact of intra-aortic balloon pump on mortality in patients with acute myocardial infarction complicated by cardiogenic shock: results of the Euro Heart Survey on PCI. EuroIntervention 2011;7(4):437–41.

41. Curtis JP, Rathore SS, Wang Y, et al. Use and effectiveness of intra-aortic balloon pumps among patients undergoing high risk percutaneous coronary intervention: insights from the National Cardiovascular Data Registry. Circulation 2012;5(1):21–30.

42. Amsterdam EA, Wenger NK, Brindis RG, et al. 2014 AHA/ACC Guideline for the Management of Patients with Non-ST-Elevation Acute Coronary Syndromes: a report of the American College of Cardiology/American Heart Association Task Force on Practice Guidelines. J Am Coll Cardiol 2014;64(24):e139–228.

43. Unverzagt S, Buerke M, de Waha A, et al. Intra-aortic balloon pump counterpulsation (IABP) for myocardial infarction complicated by cardiogenic shock. Cochrane Database Syst Rev 2015;(3):CD007398.

44. FDA Manufacturer and User Facility Device Experience (MAUDE) Impella (Abiomed, Inc) 2015. Available at: https://www.accessdata.fda.gov/scripts/cdrh/cfdocs/cfmaude/results.cfm. Accessed September 17, 2015.

45. Seyfarth M, Sibbing D, Bauer I, et al. A randomized clinical trial to evaluate the safety and efficacy of a percutaneous left ventricular assist device versus intra-aortic balloon pumping for treatment of cardiogenic shock caused by myocardial infarction. J Am Coll Cardiol 2008;52(19):1584–8.

46. O'Neill WW, Kleiman NS, Moses J, et al. A prospective, randomized clinical trial of hemodynamic support with Impella 2.5 versus intra-aortic balloon pump in patients undergoing high-risk percutaneous coronary intervention: the PROTECT II study. Circulation 2012;126(14):1717–27.

47. O'Neill W. A prospective, multicenter study to evaluate a new percutaneous ventricular assist device for right ventricular failure: the RECOVER Right Study. Paper presented at: Transcatheter Cardiovascular Therapeutics (TCT). Washington, DC, September 13–17, 2014.

48. Burkhoff D, Cohen H, Brunckhorst C, et al. A randomized multicenter clinical study to evaluate

the safety and efficacy of the TandemHeart percutaneous ventricular assist device versus conventional therapy with intraaortic balloon pumping for treatment of cardiogenic shock. Am Heart J 2006;152(3):469.e1–8.

49. Thiele H, Sick P, Boudriot E, et al. Randomized comparison of intra-aortic balloon support with a percutaneous left ventricular assist device in patients with revascularized acute myocardial infarction complicated by cardiogenic shock. Eur Heart J 2005;26(13):1276–83.

50. Thiagarajan RR, Brogan TV, Scheurer MA, et al. Extracorporeal membrane oxygenation to support cardiopulmonary resuscitation in adults. Ann Thorac Surg 2009;87(3):778–85.

51. Takayama H, Truby L, Koekort M, et al. Clinical outcome of mechanical circulatory support for refractory cardiogenic shock in the current era. J Heart Lung Transplant 2013;32(1):106–11.

52. Esper SA, Bermudez C, Dueweke EJ, et al. Extracorporeal membrane oxygenation support in acute coronary syndromes complicated by cardiogenic shock. Catheter Cardiovasc Interv 2015;86(Suppl 1):S45–50.

53. Sheu JJ, Tsai TH, Lee FY, et al. Early extracorporeal membrane oxygenator-assisted primary percutaneous coronary intervention improved 30-day clinical outcomes in patients with ST-segment elevation myocardial infarction complicated with profound cardiogenic shock. Crit Care Med 2010;38(9):1810–7.

Moving?

Make sure your subscription moves with you!

To notify us of your new address, find your **Clinics Account Number** (located on your mailing label above your name), and contact customer service at:

Email: journalscustomerservice-usa@elsevier.com

800-654-2452 (subscribers in the U.S. & Canada)
314-447-8871 (subscribers outside of the U.S. & Canada)

Fax number: 314-447-8029

Elsevier Health Sciences Division
Subscription Customer Service
3251 Riverport Lane
Maryland Heights, MO 63043

Moving?

Make sure your subscription moves with you!

To notify us of your new address, find your Clinics Account Number (located on your mailing label above your name), and contact customer service at:

Email: journalscustomerservice-usa@elsevier.com

800-654-2452 (subscribers in the U.S. & Canada)
314-447-8871 (subscribers outside of the U.S. & Canada)

Fax number: 314-447-8029

Elsevier Health Sciences Division
Subscription Customer Service
3251 Riverport Lane
Maryland Heights, MO 63043

*To ensure uninterrupted delivery of your subscription, please notify us at least 4 weeks in advance of move.

Printed and bound by CPI Group (UK) Ltd, Croydon, CR0 4YY

03/10/2024

01040298-0007